Non-Vascularised Fibular Grafts in Orthopaedic Practice

Surender Singh Yadav

Non-Vascularised Fibular Grafts in Orthopaedic Practice

Springer

Surender Singh Yadav
Department of Orthopedics
Mirpur Institute of Medical Sciences
Mirpur Rewari, Haryana, India

ISBN 978-981-95-1793-0 ISBN 978-981-95-1794-7 (eBook)
https://doi.org/10.1007/978-981-95-1794-7

This Springer imprint is published by the registered company Springer Nature Singapore Pte Ltd.
The registered company address is: 152 Beach Road, #21-01/04 Gateway East, Singapore 189721, Singapore

Preface

This is in response to the suggestions for such a work from a number of my Orthopaedic colleagues that this book has been written. They have been observing my research on non-vascularized fibular grafts (NVFG) for a long time. Our observations are related to the clinical and radiological outcomes of various orthopaedic conditions requiring bridging the defects in long bones.

While working as a lecturer in Orthopaedics at JIPMER, Pondicherry (1968), we had plenty of poor patients of Bone Tumours, and many surgeons did not treat such patients. These patients needed suitable excision and reconstruction. Such patients could not afford an endoprosthesis. Moreover, such implants were not available in those days.

I thought of the NVFG to bridge the long skeletal defects. However, due to lack of viability, such a graft did not enjoy good reputation. Left with no other choice, I picked up the NVFG from the dustbin and started thinking as how best to increase the osteogenic properties of these fibular strut grafts to successfully bridge the major bone gaps. Efforts had been made to improve the ***quality and quantity*** of the NVFG that appeared possible.

This book on improved NVFG has been a joint effort from JIPMER-Pondicherry, RML Hospital, Maulana Azad Medical College—New Delhi, PGIMS—Rohtak, and MIMS—Mirpur for over five decades. It is expected that this book carrying my personal experiences will be educational, provide the necessary resource, and will prove useful to the orthopaedic surgeons in the care of their patients.

I am not aware, if such a book has been published earlier on the NVFG with such details. All the illustrations published in this book belong to my own cases. Since I have been working on the improved NVFG in the management of different clinical conditions for a long time, it is considered desirable to publish these cases with long follow-up in the form of a book. Suggestive reading in the form of reviews and relevant original papers have been provided for those who require further information.

Rewari, India

Surender Singh Yadav

Acknowledgements

To start with, I express my gratitude to the God almighty and to my dear parents who brought me in this world and inspired me through their mentoring. My affectionate mother and two elder brothers deserve salutation for guiding me in my early life. Special thanks go to my wife, the late Dr. Shanti Yadav, for sparing me to write these chapters on NVFG. I owe my deep respects and regards to all these loving souls.

I am indebted to the late Prof. P.K. Duraiswami for playing an important role in introducing me to orthopaedics during my early career. Constructive suggestion by senior orthopaedic surgeons like Prof. S.M. Tuli from India and from abroad deserve special mention. Our dedicated team of committed residents in various institutions need a pat on their back as without their untiring efforts and co-operation all this was not possible.

My debt of gratitude goes to my affectionate patients who provided the required material for me to study the improved NVFG for over five decades. A long follow-up of such patients revealed their absolute confidence in me, as they always located me wherever I was. I owe special acknowledgement to Springer Nature for publishing this book. My thanks are also due to Mohit Kumar and Nisha Sharma for their secretarial assistance.

Surender Singh Yadav

Contents

1 General Consideration 1
1.1 General Consideration 1
1.2 Fibula 2

2 History of Bone Grafts 5
2.1 History of Bone Grafts 5
2.2 Bone Grafts Currently Used 9
Suggested Readings 10

3 Basic Science and Biology of Bone Grafts 13
3.1 Basic Science and Biology of Bone Grafts 13
3.2 Bone Graft Fixation 14
3.2.1 Mechanical Stability 14
3.2.2 Osteogenic Environment at the Host Site 14
3.3 The Biological Activity of a Successful Bone Graft 14
3.3.1 Osteoinduction 15
3.3.2 Osteoconduction 15
3.3.3 Osteogenesis 15
3.3.4 Cancellous Bone Graft 15
3.3.5 Structure of Grafts 16
3.4 Indication of Bone Grafting 16
3.4.1 Clinical Conditions Where Bone Grafts May Be Used 16
3.5 Type of Bone Grafts 17
3.5.1 Autogenous Grafts 17
3.5.2 Properties of Bone Grafts 17
3.5.3 Sources of Bone Grafts 18
3.5.4 Allografts 18
3.5.5 Cancellous Allografts 18
3.5.6 Cortical Allografts 18
3.5.7 Complications of Allograft 19
3.5.8 Demineralized Bone Matrix 20
3.5.9 Bone Morphogenetic Proteins (BMPs) 20

3.5.10 Bone Substitutes ... 20
3.5.11 Platelet-Rich Plasma ... 21
3.5.12 Hydroxyapatite ... 21
3.6 Bone Bank ... 22
Suggested Readings ... 23

4 Non-vascularized Fibular Grafts (NVFG) ... 25
4.1 Non-vascularized Fibular Grafts (NVFG) ... 25
4.1.1 Anatomy and Structure of the Fibula ... 26
4.1.2 Vascular Supply of Fibula ... 27
4.1.3 Bridging the Humeral Defects ... 27
Suggested Readings ... 28

5 Non-vascularized Fibular Grafts (NVFG) Enhanced Viability ... 31
5.1 The Existing Concept of the NVFG ... 31
5.2 Our Experience with Improved Quality and Quantity of the NVFG ... 32
5.3 Enhanced Viability of the NVFG ... 34
5.3.1 The Concept of Viable Non-vascularized Fibular Grafts (NVFG) ... 34
5.4 The Strength of the Construct ... 36
5.4.1 The Host-Graft Junction ... 36
5.5 Harvesting the Fibular Graft ... 37
5.5.1 Twin Fibular Grafts ... 37
5.5.2 Fixation of the Fibular Graft ... 37
5.6 Remodelling of the Improved NVFG ... 39
5.6.1 The Added Advantage of Twin Fibular Grafts ... 39
5.6.2 The Donor Site ... 40
5.6.3 Arthrodesis of the Neighbouring Joint ... 40
5.7 Histology of the Enhanced Quality of Non-vascularized Fibular Strut Grafts: A Project of the Indian Council of Medical Research (ICMR) ... 41
5.8 Free Vascularized Fibular Grafts (FVFG) ... 41
5.8.1 Complications of FVFG ... 42
5.8.2 Contraindications of Free Vascularized Fibular Grafts (FVFG) ... 42
Suggested Readings ... 43

6 Bone Tumours Needing Suitable Excision and Reconstruction ... 45
6.1 Bone Tumours Needing Suitable Excision and Reconstruction ... 45
6.2 Osteochondroma ... 45
6.3 Unicameral Bone Cyst ... 47
6.4 Recurrent Unicameral Bone Cyst ... 48
6.5 Aneurysmal Bone Cyst (ABC) ... 51

6.6 Giant Cell Tumour (GCT) 54
6.7 Osteosarcoma 76
6.8 Telangiectatic Osteosarcoma 83
6.9 Ewing Sarcoma 84
6.10 Malignant Fibrous Histiocytoma (MFH) 91
6.11 Adamantinoma 92
6.12 Chondrosarcoma 95
Suggested Readings 98

7 Pelvic Reconstruction with Non-vascularized Twin Fibular Grafts Stabilized with Kirschner Wires After Excision of Bone Tumour 101
7.1 Pelvic Reconstruction with Non-vascularized Twin Fibular Grafts Stabilized with Kirschner Wires After Excision of Bone Tumours 101
7.2 Chondrosarcoma 103
7.3 Giant Cell Tumour of the Pelvis 106
Suggested Reading 114

8 Post-infective Massive Bone Loss of Long Bones That Require Bridging 117
8.1 Post-infective Massive Bone Loss of Long Bones That Require Bridging 117
Suggested Readings 131

9 Post-traumatic Bone Loss of Long Bones Replaced with NVFG 133
9.1 Post-traumatic Bone Loss of Long Bones Replaced with NVFG 133
Suggested Readings 138

10 NVFG Used for Filling Bony Cavities After Curettage 139
10.1 NVFG Used for Filling Bony Cavities After Curettage 139
Suggested Readings 142

11 Twin NVFG Used for Fixation of Early Femoral Neck Fractures 143
11.1 Twin NVFG Used for Fixation of Early Femoral Neck Fractures 143
11.1.1 The Technique 143
Suggested Readings 149

12 'The Biological IM Nail': Bone-in-Bone Fixation with Osteogenic Advantage 151
12.1 Autologous Fibular Strut Used as Biological IM Nail 151
12.2 Surgical Technique 155
12.3 Advantages of the Technique 156
Suggested Reading 163

13 Biological Nail for Strengthening the Long Bones with Benign Diaphyseal Lesions ... 165
13.1 Biological Nail for Strengthening the Long Bones with Benign Diaphyseal Lesions ... 165
Suggested Readings ... 167

14 NVFG Used to Achieve Arthrodesis in Challenging Cases ... 169
14.1 NVFG Used to Achieve Arthrodesis in Challenging Cases ... 169
Suggested Reading ... 174

15 Twin NVFG Used for Achieving Stabilization of a Spinal Segment ... 175
15.1 Twin NVFG Used for Achieving Stabilization of a Spinal Segment ... 175
15.2 GCT of the Spine ... 175
Suggested Readings ... 179

16 Maternal Fibular Graft Used in Children with Congenital Pseudarthrosis of Long Bones ... 181
16.1 Congenital Pseudarthrosis of Long Bones ... 181
16.2 Congenital Pseudarthrosis of the Radius ... 181
Suggested Reading ... 184

17 Maternal Fibular Grafting in Congenital Pseudarthrosis of the Tibia ... 185
17.1 Congenital Pseudarthrosis of the Tibia (CPT) ... 185
17.2 Some of the Patients with Congenital Pseudoarthrosis of the Tibia Managed Using the Above Technique with Maternal Fibular Grafting ... 190
Suggested Readings ... 199

18 Bilateral Congenital Pseudarthroses of the Tibiae ... 203
18.1 Bilateral Congenital Pseudarthroses of the Tibiae ... 203
18.2 Conclusion ... 209
Suggested Readings ... 209

19 Tibialization of the Fibula ... 211
19.1 Tibialization of the Fibula ... 211
Suggested Readings ... 219

20 Our Experiences with Complications ... 221
20.1 Our Experiences with Complications ... 221

21 Observations Made by the Author on the Improved NVFG ... 225
21.1 Observations Made by the Author on the Improved NVFG ... 225

Chapter 1
General Consideration

1.1 General Consideration

Bone grafting has long been described and has been a subject of many experimental and clinical studies. Various types of bone grafts are being used by most orthopaedic surgeons all over the world. The biologic incorporation of bone grafts into the host bone is dependent upon the type of graft, but the aim in all the cases is to replace the graft with the host bone by bone resorption and new bone formation. It is because of the increased demand for bone graft surgery for skeletal reconstruction that the interest in this area has grown, especially in limb salvage surgery. The procedure is commonly used for reconstruction after excision of bone tumours, post-infective gaps, post-traumatic bone loss and stability of failed arthroplasties.

Bone grafting is a common procedure to achieve the regeneration of bone and results in the restoration of skeletal continuity. The reconstruction of large bone defects has been a management problem and presents a challenging subject. However, during the last few decades, significant improvement has taken place in bone graft surgery. Although the basic knowledge of bone transplant biology has advanced, further improvement is still needed to achieve an ideal bone graft in clinical practice. Bony reconstruction has been an important procedure to manage a wide variety of clinical conditions that affect the skeletal system.

Vascularized bone grafts, autografts and allografts are used to promote healing in various clinical conditions involving bone defects. An autograft is still considered the gold standard in the field of bone grafting. It is a well-described concept that some of the osteogenic cells survive on the surface of the fresh autografts and help in healing the transplant. These vital cells in allografts are dead, due to the methods that are used to diminish the immune response in such grafts.

It is over a century that non-vascularized fibular grafts have been used as means of reconstruction of skeletal defects. The fibula, a common source of cortical strut grafts, has been used to achieve bony continuity at the ends of long bone defects.

S. S. Yadav, *Non-Vascularised Fibular Grafts in Orthopaedic Practice*,
https://doi.org/10.1007/978-981-95-1794-7_1

Moreover, the mechanical properties of the fibula make it an ideal choice for the replacement of long bone defects after tumour resection and other clinical conditions that need the use of such a graft.

Since 1975, vascularized grafts have also been used. Microvascularized bone grafts include the restoration of the physiologic blood flow by surgical anastomosis of a nutrient vascular pedicle at the host site. This procedure ensures the viability of the cells within the grafted bone segment. These osteogenic cells help in the processes of bone healing and remodelling. However, the recent reconstructive procedures that have been reported to bridge such defects are extensive, require expensive equipment, are time-consuming and frequently result in complications such as infection and non-union.

The biological activity of any graft is multifactorial. The sources of bone grafts have evolved over the past decades and include autologous cortical or cancellous, freeze-dried, allogenic frozen, or processed cortical, corticocancellous and cancellous grafts and demineralized bone matrix. Recently, synthetic or engineered bone graft substitutes have been used, but they are still in the experimental stage.

1.2 Fibula

The fibula has been known and well described for vacularized and non-vacularized bone grafting procedures. The fibula is also known to bear only 15% of the axial load across the ankle, allowing it to be used as an autogenous bone graft with minimal biomechanical loss during weight-bearing of the lower limb. Since the distal end of the fibula also plays an important role during rotational stability and restraint against lateral translation, it is necessary to preserve the distal end of the fibula during graft harvest to avoid subsequent instability and deformity of the ankle joint.

It has been well described and well established that the fibula is a very good and useful donor bone. The fibula, being the strongest and a common source of strut grafts, has been commonly used for reconstruction of bony defects in long bones such as the femur, tibia and humerus. Moreover, the mechanical properties of the fibula make it suitable for replacement of long bone defects in various clinical situations which demand such a graft. Depending on the need and the site where it is required, it can be used as a single, twin or even triple strut graft. Though cortical, a strong autologous fibular graft is easily available at no cost. Moreover, this simple procedure can be performed by most orthopaedists, even at the district level. Regeneration of the fibula has been observed particularly in children.

The tricortical profile of the fibula with good bone mass is extremely well suited as an autologous graft. Its dimensions allow it to match forearm bones and can be very well used in forearm bone defects. Moreover, it can be fitted into the medullary canals of larger long bones such as the femur, tibia and humerus as a single or even a double-barrel construct where the medulla of the host bone is wide, particularly in severely osteoporotic bones. A fibular strut has been successfully used as a biological intra-medullary nail for difficult non-union of major long bones and also to strengthen weak osteoporotic long bones. Such a biological nail also strengthens a long bone affected by a benign diaphyseal lesion threatening pathological fracture.

On most occasions, an orthopaedic surgeon is in need of bone to bridge bone defects. A fibular graft may be non-vascularized or vascularized, autologous or homologous. The fibula has been established as the principal donor bone in the field of bone grafting. Though cortical, it is perhaps due to the configuration of this wonder bone that it enjoys the reputation for bridging massive bone defects in the specialty of orthopaedic surgery. Non-vascularized autologous grafts are easily available and come at no cost.

I had the opportunity/privilege to use this wonder bone in various clinical situations for over five decades. The non-vascularized fibular graft (NVFG) has been crafted non-osteogenic. The viability of NVFG has been enhanced by immediate transplantation at the host site. Immediate transfer and fixation of such a strut graft at the host site thus enhance the *quality* and *viability* of the graft for early union and consolidation at the host site. This enhanced quality along with twin grafts further adds to the *quantity* of the construct. Moreover, in twin grafts, lateral union results in a solid biological construct to provide strength to the grafts during their incorporation to the host bone. However, the construct has to be protected until repair-related changes are complete. Such an important construct has been successfully used at any age and in situations where even the host bed has poor blood supply like in post-infective gaps. The outcome has revealed that such strut grafts have revealed union of the host bone without undergoing degenerative changes, described earlier in NVFG.

There is a general perception that vascularized grafts are preferred where a long fibular graft is needed, particularly those more than 6 cm in length for long-bone reconstructions. However, this fact has not been well accepted and is debatable. Our observations reveal that the length of the autologous NVFG has no role to play in its union with the host bone. We have used 22 cm long twin NVFG with success. The literature also reveals that there is no evidence that grafts longer than 6 cm should be vascularized. Moreover, the vascularized grafts are more likely to result in surgical revision. However, the 6 cm rule requires further research. It is suggested that more observations on this topic are needed.

Moreover, due consideration should be given in selecting a technique of reconstruction which should rest upon the needs of the patient and the circumstances under which the surgeon operates. One should not thrust a technique on the patient. Such a need-based approach will enable the patient to avail the advantage of a simple, biologically oriented and cost-effective technique. Moreover, the needs and requirements of poorer patients may be a little different from those of the elite. These patients tend to prefer a single procedure even with some drawbacks rather than undergoing repeated surgeries. It is also a fact that some of the earlier reconstructive techniques described to bridge such gaps are extensive, expensive and time-consuming and may frequently result in complications.

Our observations to prove the efficacy of such an improved construct have been published in International Journals—*JBJS Am* 1990, *Orthopaedics* (International) 1995 and *JBJS Am* 2018.

Chapter 2
History of Bone Grafts

2.1 History of Bone Grafts

Medical history is as old as mankind and has had religious implications. Surgical treatment existed even in prehistoric days. Bone grafting or limb transplantation from one human being to another has been a cause of concern for many centuries. To reach the current status of bone grafting, it has been considered not only necessary but also essential to go through the history of bone grafting.

Egyptians were known for their advanced bone surgery and dental surgery. There are evidences of orthopaedic operations performed at various sites on the human body. However, there is no definite or dependable evidence to support these facts. But it is well known that the ancient Egyptians had a great knowledge of orthopaedics. Progress in this field had been made to replace body parts that had been lost during injury, illness or defects and had continued to be a cause of human concern.

The modern age starts with the research of a Dutch military surgeon Job van Meekeren (1668), who performed the first heterologous bone graft by fixing a bone fragment of dog skull into the skull of an injured soldier. Although the operation was successful, the use of an animal graft on a Christian raised religious concerns, and the soldier was then excommunicated. The success of the operation was confirmed when the patient had requested the surgeon to remove the grafted bone fragment which will enable him be readmitted into the church—by that time, the bone piece had fully united (De Boer 1988). Further research by a fellow Dutch scientist, Antonius De Heyde, had defined the process of osteogenesis. He proved, after his experimental observations on frogs, that callus forms after calcification of the blood clot around the broken bone fragments.

During the next few decades, enough research was carried on the structure of the bone which was reported for the first time by Antoni van Leeuwenhoek (1674). Duhamel (1743) published his work on experiments in animals and suggested that

S. S. Yadav, *Non-Vascularised Fibular Grafts in Orthopaedic Practice*,
https://doi.org/10.1007/978-981-95-1794-7_2

the periosteum has a vital role to play in the process of osteogenesis (De Boer 1988, Glicenstein 2000). The concepts of bony callus, implant and resorption had been described at this stage.

Some of the pioneers of bone grafting	
Jobi Van Meekeren	1668
Philips von Walter	1820
Leopord Ollier	1861
Sir William Macewen	1880
Albee FH	1911
Phemister DB	1914
Abbott	1947
Ray RD	1972
Taylor GI	1975

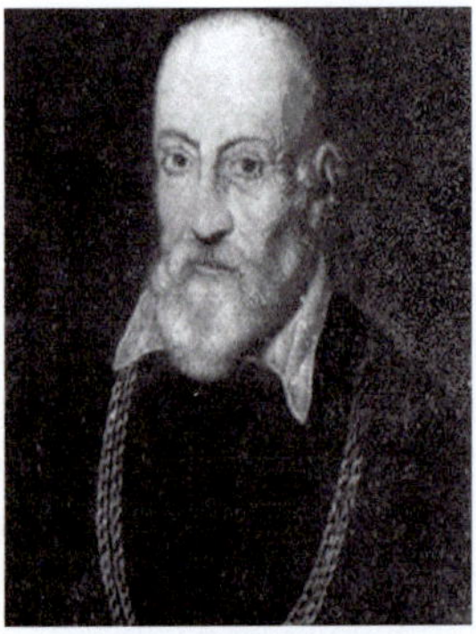

Jobi Van Meekeren
(1565-1676)

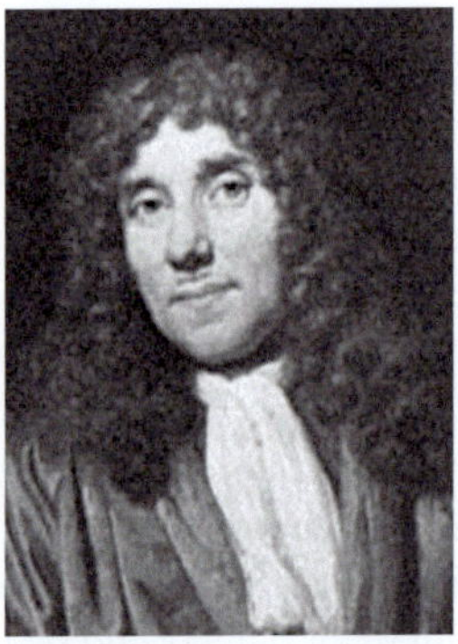

Antony Van Leeuwenhoek
(1632-1723)

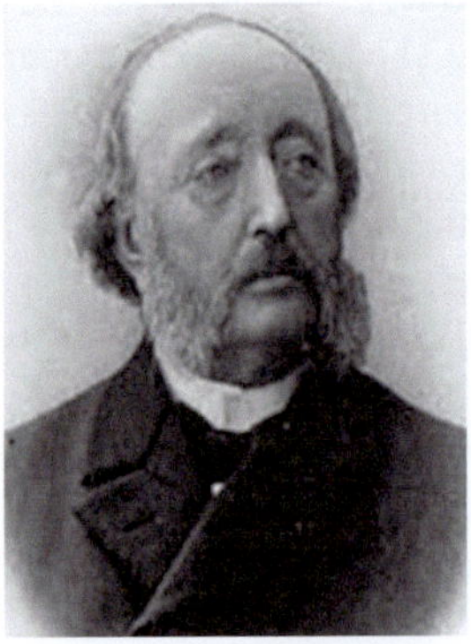

Leopold Ollier
(1830-1900)

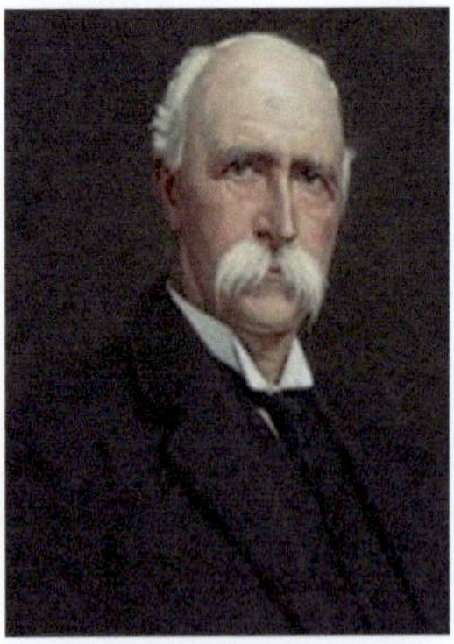

Sir William Macewen
(1848-1924)

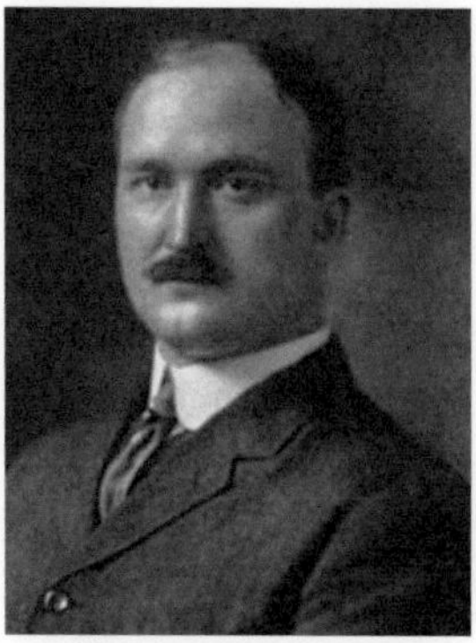

Frederick Houdlette Albee
(1876-1945)

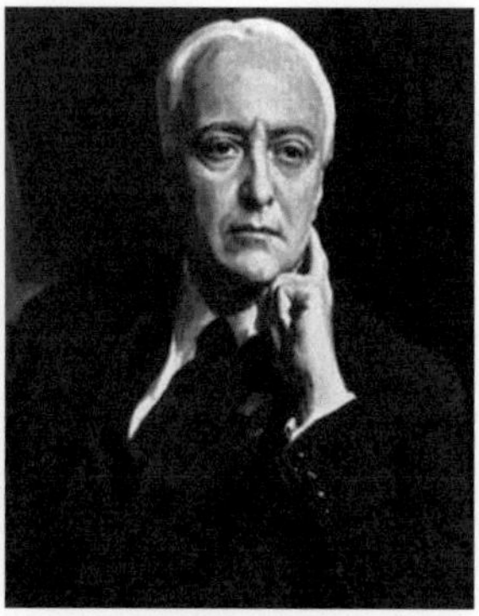

Vittorio Putti
(1880-1940)

Frenchman Leopold Ollier (1861) from Lyon published his work and coined the term 'bone graft' for the first time. He reported that 'implanted bone is viable, if it includes the periosteum, which is the most vital viability factor of the graft' (Putti 1912, De Boer 1988). Putti also reported Ollier's work as 'an immortal work on bone generation'. However, at that time, Barth reported different results and stated that the bone, periosteum and the bone marrow in the graft die and are replaced by newly formed bone. The osteogenic cells of the implanted bone would die within a few days, and the dead bone starts getting absorbed and replaced by newly formed bone produced by the cells of the surrounding living bone. The difference of opinion between Ollier and Barth encouraged their fellow colleagues to study this phenomenon for further research.

Philips Von Walter (1820) performed the first clinical autologous graft in Germany Putti (2007). Ollier described that autografts can be viable. Barth later reported absorption of the dead tissues of the bone graft. This was followed by formation of new bone, which grew into the graft from the surrounding cells of the living bone. Curtis first reported his observation on the presence of Haversian canals. Phemeister supported the opinion and added that there is simultaneous removal of necrotic tissues of the non-vascularized bone and subsequent formation of new bone.

Bone grafts used by Ollier (1860) and others at the same time were of autologous origin. Grafts other than autologous origin were not taken into consideration for many years. The reason for this is not known, may be because of the memory of Van Meekeren's operation performed two centuries ago. It was Scottish surgeon William Macewen (1880) who performed the first allograft surgery. He inserted a graft of the tibia from a child suffering from rickets into the infected humerus of another child (De Boer 1988). However, Phelps (1891) followed Curtis' hypothesis that 'an ideal implant is formed by living bone that fits the gap perfectly and continues to live without getting reabsorbed' (Urist et al. 1994).

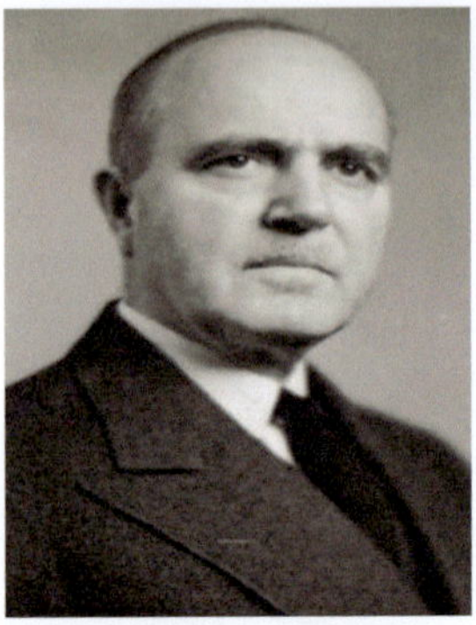

Dallas B. Phemister
(1882-1951)

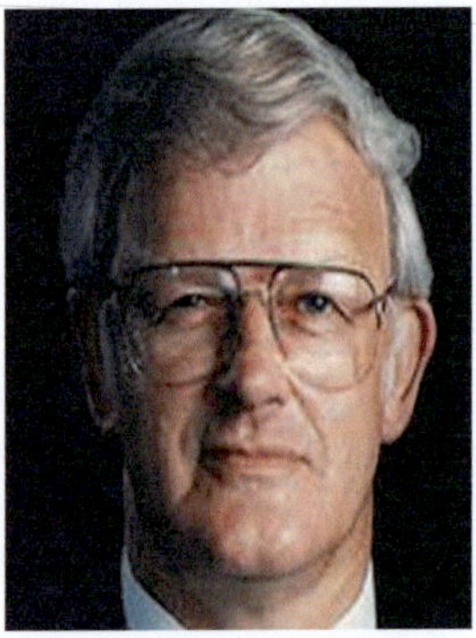

Prof. Geoffrey Ian Taylor
1957-2008

Putti (1912) reviewed the work of earlier researchers and described the clinical and experimental observations made on animals by several workers, especially the work of Ollier, Barth, Axhausen and Macewan including his own personal experiences. He reported the contrasting research of Ollier and Barth. However, he supported Ollier's theory regarding the osteogenic capacity of the periosteum in both autologous and homologous grafts. Later, it was accepted that it is only in autologous grafts that some osteogenic cells are able to survive and take part in the process of osteogenesis. This advantage is not possible in homoplastic grafts.

Phemister (1914) took a step forward and introduced the modern concept of bone reabsorption, which he described as a phenomenon called 'creeping substitution' of old bone by the new bone and further stated that, 'the living cells on the graft surface proliferate and get deposited around the graft lamellae of new bone. This gradually replace the dead part inside the graft. The time period needed to accomplish this process may range from many months or even longer depending on the size and thickness of the graft' (Phemister 1914). Phemister's description of the time to replace the graft revealed that the histological interpretation of bone viability had not been very clear.

Contradictory opinions about the biological activity of graft survival still existed. Ollier stated that the autogenous graft survives and is renewed by cells of the periosteum and the bone marrow. Barth reported that the whole graft dies and the connective cells of the host regenerate it. Axhausen described that the graft substance undergoes necrosis except for some thin layers under the periosteum and Haversian canals. Instead, he reported that the periosteum and medullary regions survive and are responsible for the formation of new bone. Macewen further stated that the osteocytes of the graft are not damaged during surgery and help in the healing process. He reported this regardless of the cellular elements of the periosteum and bone marrow which are not indispensable for bone formation.

It was only after the publication of Albee's book (1915) *Bone Graft Surgery* that bone grafting was well understood and became a commonly performed surgical procedure. It is only after this that the metallurgic age of the speciality had started. Tylor (1975) suggested the concept of vascularized fibular grafts with advantage over non-vascularized fibular grafts.

2.2 Bone Grafts Currently Used

Majority of bone autografts are now used to enhance fracture healing or to reconstruct skeletal defects. The allografts, consisting of a part of or a whole bone, from bone banks have renewed interest in reconstruction of large skeletal defects. Several reports have discussed the clinical advantage of allograft reconstruction. However, further analyses of the results indicate that numerous problems still remain unsolved. Fresh allografts are associated with immune response that is primarily cellular but has some humoral component. Many studies have reported the techniques to diminish this immune response. Because of the process to reduce the immunogenicity of the allografts, the cellular complex undergoes necrosis. Hence, the allograft serves only as a non-viable construct to which the soft tissues can get attached.

While waiting for an ideal bone graft of the future, like the insertion of living bone which will fit the gap and will continue to live without absorption' (Fig. 2.1a, b). It was not until the concept of microsurgery was advanced in 1960 with the development of the operating microscope and improvements of microsurgical instruments that vascularized bone grafts became possible. The work of Ostrup stimulated the new type of bone transplantation. Taylor (1975), from Australia, performed the first free vascularized fibular graft. However, the procedure is extensive, expensive and has its own complications.

Recently, a combination of an allograft and a vascularized bone graft has been introduced. This technique provides both viability and strength for reconstruction of large skeletal defects. However, the definitive management of large skeletal defect continues to be a subject of further research.

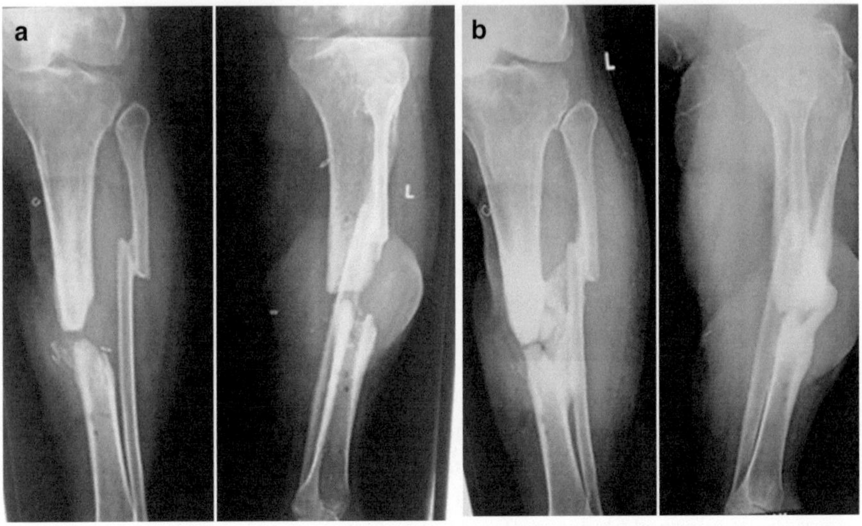

Fig. 2.1 (**a**) AP and lateral radiograph of a 40-year-old man with frank non-union of the tibia and union of the fibular fracture. Because of extensive scar at the fracture site, a full-thickness skin graft was carried out at the previous centre. (**b**) AP and lateral radiograph after cancellous bone grafting at the site of tibial non-union between the tibial and fibular shaft. The stability at the site was provided by the united fibula. A further support to this construct by provided by an above-knee POP cast. The operation was carried out based on the original principle of the Huntington procedure. The radiograph after 6 months revealed union between tibial and fibular shafts, even at the non-union site of the tibia. This case testifies that simple and biological procedures have a place in the management of challenging non-union of the long bones

Suggested Readings

1. Donati DM, Zolezzi C, Tomba P, Vigano A. Bone grafting: historical and conceptual review, strating with an old manuscript by Vittorio Putti. Acta Orthop. 2007;78(1):19–25.
2. De Boer HH. The history of bone grafts. Clin Orthop Relat Res. 1988:292–8.
3. Donati D, Zolezzi C, Tomba P, Vigano A. Bone grafting: historical conceptual revie, starting with an olds manuscript by Vittorio Putti. Acta Orthop. 2007;78(1):19–25.
4. Gross TP, Cox Q, Jinnah RH. History and current application of bone transplantation. Orthopaedics. 1993;16:895–900.
5. Albee FH. Bone graft surgery. Philadelphia: WB Saunders; 1915.
6. Barth A. Ueber histologische Befunde nach Knochenimplantationen. Arch Klin Chir. 1893;46:409.
7. Carrel A, Guthrie CC. Results of replantation of the thigh. Science. 1906;23:393–7.
8. Curtis BF. Cases of bone implantation and transplantation for cyst of tibia, osteomyelitic cavities and ununited fractures. Am J Med Sci. 1893;106:30.
9. Finemeier CG. Bone grafting and bone graft substitutes. J Bone Joint Surg Am. 2002;84A(3):454–64.
10. Hamada G, Rida A. Orthopaedics in acient and modern Egypt. Clin Orthop. 1972;89:253–68.
11. Van Leeuwenhoek A. Microscopical observations about blood, milk, bone, the brain, spittle, cuticula, sweat, fat and tears. Philos Trans R Soc Lond. 1674;9:125.
12. Macewen W. Observations concerning transplantation on bone. Proc R Soc Lond. 1881;32:232.

13. Van Meekeren J. Heel en geneeskonstige aanmerkingen. Amsterdam: Commelijin; 1668.
14. Older J. Introduction: history and research on bone transplantation. In: Older J, editor. Bone implant grafting. Springer-Verlag; London, 1992. p. XV–XVIII.
15. Ollier L. Traite de la regeneration des os. Paris: Victor Mason et Fils; 1867.
16. Phemister DB. The fate of transplanted bone and regenerative power of its various consituents. Surg Gynecol Obstet. 1914;19:303.
17. Putti V. I trapianti ossei. Arch Orthop. 1912;29:294–334.
18. Taylor GI. Microvascular free bone transfer. Orthop Clin North Am. 1977;8:425.
19. Taylor GI, Miller GDH, Ham FJ. The free vascularized bone graft: a clinical extension of microvascular techniques. Plast Reconstr Surg. 1975;55:533–44.
20. Walter P. von: Wiedereinheilung der bei der Trapanation ausgebohrten Knochenscheibe. Journal der Chirurgie und Augen-Heilkunde. 1821;2:571.
21. Walter M. Resection de I'extremite inferieur de radius pour osteosarcoma. Bull Et Mem Soc de Chir de Par. 1911;37:954.

Chapter 3
Basic Science and Biology of Bone Grafts

3.1 Basic Science and Biology of Bone Grafts

Bone grafting is a surgical procedure used to promote osteogenesis in various clinical situations which lack biological potential. It facilitates biologic augmentation/osteogenesis. The choice of bone graft depends on the needs of a particular patient. The described bone grafts have the capacity to provide active bone formation, to augment bone formation by the cells of surrounding soft tissues and to serve as a substrate for bone formation. This biological property of any graft is multifactorial. Its function represents the sum of its inherent biological property, its ability to activate the surrounding host tissues and its osteoinductive capacity, which is mediated by bioactive activity within the matrix. Ultimately, its ability to support the ingrowth of osteogenic tissues through its osteoconductive property also plays a role in its behaviour. Autogenous bone grafting is considered the best material for grafting as it has all the three vital elements needed for bone regeneration, namely osteoinduction, osteoconduction and osteogenic cells. However, the healing of the bone graft is mainly influenced by the host environment in which it is transplanted.

There are two basic and important principles involved for the success of a bone graft:

1. Mechanical stability of the graft fixation.
2. Osteogenic environment at the host site.

S. S. Yadav, *Non-Vascularised Fibular Grafts in Orthopaedic Practice*,
https://doi.org/10.1007/978-981-95-1794-7_3

3.2 Bone Graft Fixation

3.2.1 Mechanical Stability

Bone healing is a continuous and active process, and the stability of a graft plays one of the key roles in this process. For healing to occur, both adequate mechanical stability and good blood supply are required. In case a structural support is necessary, a cortical autograft can be used. Because the mechanical stabilization is under the control of the surgeon, it can affect signalling pathways that are important for bone healing. Depending on the site, there are many techniques to stabilize a graft. A stable graft fixation results in minimum failure rates. A graft that has mechanical stability needs a good biological environment at the host site for healing.

3.2.2 Osteogenic Environment at the Host Site

What happens to a bone graft when transplanted? It has been observed that some of the transplanted osteogenic cells survive at the endosteal or periosteal surface of a fresh autograft. Also, over time, the old bone is replaced by newly formed bone. The remodelling takes place by osteoclastic resorption and formation of new vascular channels with new bone formation.

The bone graft serves as a surface on which the cells are attached and differentiate. The surrounding cells are converted into undifferentiated perivascular mesenchymal cells. This cascade results in formation of osteoprogenitor cells with the capacity to form new bone. Earlier researchers demonstrated that, in addition, some cells survive and participate in new bone formation. However, the percentage of such cells that survive transplantation is not known. The survival of these vital cells appears to be improved by minimizing the interval between graft harvest and implantation and by keeping the graft moist with blood-soaked mops at physiologic temperatures. These living periosteal and endosteal cells and other osteoblasts transplanted with such grafts are osteogenic. These vital cells in an immediately transplanted graft can survive to produce new bone.

3.3 The Biological Activity of a Successful Bone Graft

Based on their biological actions, ideal bone graft properties can be divided into three groups:

3.3.1 *Osteoinduction*

Osteoinduction is an active process through which a signal is sent to influence new bone formation. At this stage, a cascade to produce healing starts. The graft is surrounded by inflammatory cells, encouraging the undifferentiated perivascular mesenchymal stem cells to become active osteoblasts. The osteoinductive property of living bone graft cells is related to its production of osteoinductive factors, including bone morphogenic proteins (BMPs) and other growth factors. These factors are known to influence the differentiation of the mesenchymal cells into bone-forming cells. BMPs are also capable of signalling the differentiation of mesenchymal cells and finally result in cartilage and bone formation.

3.3.2 *Osteoconduction*

Osteoconduction acts as the scaffolding over which new bone grows for healing to take place. It is also a continuous but passive process of bone resorption and bone formation where reparative growth is carried out by the natural bone itself. The osteoclasts create a tunnel, and the newly formed osteoblasts fill in the tunnel. The newly created Haversian systems provide a pathway for the blood vessels. This process is called ‘creeping substitution’. The process provides strength and stiffness to the construct and increases the capacity to form new bone.

3.3.3 *Osteogenesis*

Osteogenesis is the synthesis of new bone formation by donor cells derived either from the graft or from the cells at the host site. Osteogenesis depends on the ability of the graft to form bone by its vital cellular elements, through either differentiation of mesenchymal cells or recruitment of osteoblasts and osteocytes. Because an autologous bone graft contains all the three characteristics, namely osteoinduction, osteoconduction and osteogenesis, it remains the gold standard.

3.3.4 *Cancellous Bone Graft*

Cancellous bone graft is the commonly used form of autologous bone graft. It contains a high concentration of osteoblasts and osteocytes that provide a much better healing through its superior osteogenic potential. Additionally, its large trabecular surface area encourages the process of revascularization and graft incorporation at the host site.

The success of cancellous bone graft is a well-established phenomenon, characterized by formation of new bone over a necrotic graft bed through the twin processes of resorption and substitution. Following transplantation of a cancellous autograft, a local hematoma is formed that is rich in inflammatory cells and chemotactic mitogens and low in oxygen tension. This results further in the recruitment of mesenchymal cells.

3.3.5 *Structure of Grafts*

Cortical bone is primarily used for structural support and cancellous bone grafts for osteogenesis. Cortical and cancellous bone grafts may be combined. This is one of the prime advantages of using bone graft. In cortical bone, the process of replacement is considerably slower than in spongy or cancellous bone. Although cancellous bone is more osteogenic, it is not strong enough to provide efficient structural support. Once a graft has united with the host and is strong enough to permit unprotected use of the part, remodelling of the construct takes place which depends on the functional demands.

3.4 Indication of Bone Grafting

Bone grafting is performed due to the iatrogenic reduction of the biologic potential that has occurred at the host site. If the alignment and fixation can be achieved biologically, then bone grafting could be optional and rests on the judgment of the treating surgeon.

Hypertrophic and oligotrophic non-unions have their biologic potential, with a blood supply sufficient to allow for healing. Atrophic non-union lacks biologic potential and thus requires bone grafting, with autografts still considered the gold standard. In cases that also require structural support, a cortical autograft may be used.

Bone grafts are used in a wide variety of surgical methods augmenting or stimulating the formation of new bone where it is needed.

3.4.1 *Clinical Conditions Where Bone Grafts May Be Used*

1. Cortical bone grafts are used to bridge major bone defects and establish continuity of long-bone ends.
2. Cancellous bone grafts are used to promote union and fill defects in delayed union, fresh fractures or osteotomies.

3. To pack cavities or defects resulting from cysts, tumours and other causes.
4. To bridge joints requiring arthrodesis.
5. To establish union in pseudarthrosis.
6. To augment the acetabular surface in congenital dislocation of the hip.
7. To provide bone needed for revision total hip and knee arthroplasty.

3.5 Type of Bone Grafts

3.5.1 Autogenous Grafts

An autograft (autogenous autologous) is from the same individual. Autologous bone graft continues to be the gold standard because it contains all three characteristics, namely osteoinduction, osteoconduction and osteogenesis.

3.5.2 Properties of Bone Grafts

Type of graft	Osteoconduction	Osteoinduction	Osteogenesis	Mechanical strength	Vascularity
Bone marrow	+/−	+	++	−	−
Cancellous autograft	++	+	++	+	−
Cortical autograft	+	+/−	+	++	−
Vascularized	++	+	++	++	++

When a major bone graft is required, autogenous bone is most preferred because there is no risk of graft rejection because the graft originated from the patient's own body. As indicated in the chart above, such a graft would be osteoinductive and osteogenic, as well as osteoconductive. The only negative aspect of autologous grafts is that an additional surgical site is required.

A cancellous autograft from the anterior superior iliac spine may also be performed without a solid bony structure. In this case, there is an osteoinductive and osteogenic action; however, there is no osteoconductive action, as there is no solid bony structure.

Pedicle grafts: Local muscle-pedicle bone grafts.

Shift of one bone for the other: Leg (Huntington's procedures and single bone forearm)

Turn-Grafts: Mainly at the knee (not used these days)

3.5.3 Sources of Bone Grafts

Cancellous bone	Iliac crest—anterior or posterior and others
Cortical bone	Fibula—cascularized and non-vascularized
Cortico-cancellous	Combination of the two-cortical and cancellous graft
Allograft	Homogenous (homologous)—from the same species
Composite	Autograft + Allografts

Heterogeneous graft-Bone from the other species (not recommended).

Hydroxyapatite and tricalcium phosphates (for cancellous bone). Porous materials are invaded by blood vessels and osteogenic cells. Ceramics are also used.

3.5.4 Allografts

An allograft bone, like autogenous bone, is derived from humans; the difference is that an allograft is harvested from a different individual than the one receiving the graft. Allograft bone is taken from cadavers, and after processing, it can be used for living people who are in need. An allograft is typically sourced from a bone bank. Cortical allografts provide structural support, are readily available and can be used in conjunction with other multiple bone repair techniques. Allografts come in a variety of forms, including osteochondral, cortical, cancellous and highly processed bone derivatives such as demineralized bone matrix (DBX). In most instances, allografts do not include viable cells and are therefore not osteogenic.

3.5.5 Cancellous Allografts

Cancellous allografts are produced in the form of small cuboid chips. They are used to pack osseous defects, such as those seen in retroacetabular osteolysis associated with total hip arthroplasty. Like autogenous cancellous grafts, cancellous allografts confer little mechanical strength. They are osteoconductive grafts.

3.5.6 Cortical Allografts

Cortical allografts provide structural support, are readily available in bone banks and can be used in combination with multiple other bone repair techniques. Like cortical autografts, allografts can also be used to fill large bone defects and depend on the stability of their fixation. They are also frequently used to provide stablilzation to the femoral shaft in the setting of periprosthetic hip fracture.

The types of allograft available include:

1. Fresh frozen bone.
2. Freeze-dried bone allograft.
3. Demineralized freeze-dried bone allograft.

There is no donor site morbidity, and minimal surgical time makes the allograft a good alternative to autologous bone graft. However, due to the high costs and risks such as viral transmission, allograft is not considered an ideal choice.

3.5.7 Complications of Allograft

1. **Non-union at the host-graft junction**

   Non-union at the host-graft junction may take place within a year. The reasons reported could be fractures, infection and the type and size of the graft. The number of revision surgeries and chemotherapy may also add to the complications.

2. **Fractures**

   Fractures in allografts are not rare and usually occur during the stage of revascularization which generally occurs after 6 months. Most fractures (75%) are known to occur during the first 3 years after implantation.

3. **Infection**

   Infection is one of the most devastating causes of allograft failure. It is associated with other complications and a worse outcome. The reported incidence has been up to 30%. About 75% are diagnosed within 3 months after implantation. The principal organism is usually *Staphylococcus aureus* or *Staphylococcus epidermidis*. Polymicrobial infection may be present in 50% of cases.

4. **Graft disease transmission**

   A detailed check-up of the donor is essential. Screening is the first step in preventing the use of contaminated grafts. The detailed guidelines regarding the medical history as well as clinical tests are essential. Screening is currently done for HIV, hepatitis B virus, hepatitis C virus, human transmissible spongiform encephalopathy, syphilis, human T-lymphotropic virus and cytomegalovirus. However, after a thorough check-up, allograft contamination is not common.

3.5.8 Demineralized Bone Matrix

Demineralized bone matrix (DBM) is an easily available and well-known type of bone graft, comprising nearly 50% of all allografts. DBM is derived from human bone. In order to remove the mineral matrix, demineralized bone matrix is acid-treated. It is considered necessary to retain the organic matrix and growth factors such as bone morphogenetic protein (BMP), insulin growth factor (IGF), transforming growth factor (TGF) or fibroblast growth factor (FGF). The use of DBM also avoids donor-site morbidity including possible complications at the host site. However, during the preparation, most of the osteogenic capacity is lost and studies showed a comparable pain intensity after the surgical procedure compared to autograft procedures. Nevertheless, a large rate of the osteogenic capacity of the bone is lost during its processing. Most of the DBM preparations are admixed with cortical and/or cancellous bone chips to confer additional osteoconductive properties. Hence, DBM is used only for filling purposes and generally not as an independent bone substitute.

3.5.9 Bone Morphogenetic Proteins (BMPs)

Since their discovery almost 50 years ago, BMPs have become the subject of orthopaedic research. Over the past few decades, their evolving orthopaedic indications and promising clinical outcomes have attracted considerable interest. Out of more than 20 identified BMPs, all but one are members of the TGF-beta superfamily, a class of closely related biologic molecules thought to function in complex signalling pathways of osteoblastic differentiation and osteogenesis.

Bone morphogenetic proteins (BMPs) are well-known osteoinductive growth factors included in transforming growth factor B (TGF-B). They are produced by osteoblasts and are mainly involved in the osteogenic process that enables ectopic bone formation. BMPs are reported to play a role in the recruitment of osteoprogenitor cells in bone formation. Genetic engineering allows to synthetize recombinant human BMP (rhBMP-2 and rhBMP-7). The history of the safety of BMPs has been eventful. There are reports of complications up to 50%. The use of BMPs is still not fully established. Moreover, their high cost makes their use prohibitive in most settings.

3.5.10 Bone Substitutes

Bone transplantation has been practised for many decades with various materials of natural origin, but it had rarely met success until the late nineteenth century. Recently, many different types of bone substitutes are in use. They can be derived from biological products such as demineralized bone matrix, platelet-rich plasma, hydroxyapatite, adjunction of growth factors (like bone morphogenetic protein) or synthetic materials such as calcium sulfate, tricalcium phosphate ceramics, bioactive glasses or polymer-based substitutes. All these substitutes are not suitable for every clinical use, and they have to be selected carefully which depends on the indication where it is used. Bone substitutes are thus classified into two main categories: bone substitutes derived from biological products and synthetic bone substitutes.

Synthetic calcium bone substitutes are an osteoconductive alternative to both autologous and allogenic grafts. Since they are strictly osteoconductive, their biologic role in bone healing is limited. Bone substitutes come in a variety forms, including powders, putty, pellets or as coatings on implants, such as hydroxyapatite-coated joint prostheses. Additionally, they can be mixed with additives such as antibiotics, making them significant in the setting of infection-associated osseous defects. Research on synthetic bone substitutes is underway to test their efficacy.

3.5.11 Platelet-Rich Plasma

Platelet-rich plasma (PRP) is easily obtained with the patient's blood and is used as a gel. Blood is centrifuged through gradient density, and the resulting blood platelets are mixed with thrombin and calcium chloride. PRP includes a useful concentration of platelets and fibrinogen as well as growth factors such as platelet-derived growth factor (PDGF), vascular endothelial growth factor (VEGF), IGF and TGF. PRP is expected to show pro-coagulant effects due to platelets. However, there is no evidence that the addition of PRP accelerates bone healing. PRP may also show limited infectious risks and adverse effects as it is derived from the patient's own blood. It does not possess any mechanical resistance and is not justified as an important stand-alone bone substitute. PRP may be used as a supplement with other materials.

3.5.12 Hydroxyapatite

Hydroxyapatite (HA) is a crystalline compound and extremely biocompatible, has osteoconductive properties and does not add to an inflammatory response. Hydroxyapatite alone may not be very effective. HA comes in both natural and synthetic forms. Ceramics are usually preferred over HA alone. A few composite materials containing HA and collagen are available, and their combination enhances osteoblast differentiation and accelerates osteogenesis. HA-collagen composites have little mechanical advantages over HA alone. The ductile properties of collagen allow an increase in poor fracture toughness of the hydroxyapatite. Its advantage and prolonged osteogenic properties are still the subject of laboratory and clinical research.

No doubt autogenous bone graft continues to be the gold standard for reconstruction of various types of bone defects. Autogenous cancellous bone grafting has been recommended for achieving union in cases of non-union and delayed union. Unless considerable strength is needed, cancellous graft is useful to manage any clinical requirement. Since the osteogenic cells in the graft remain viable, clinical results suggest that cancellous grafts unite with the host bone much earlier than do cortical grafts.

3.6 Bone Bank

Many decades ago, there were articles published on various type of bone grafts. Inclan (1942) published an article in the *Journal of Bone and Joint Surgery* and presented a large number of operations performed with autologous and homologous implants and also described the problems that he encountered in finding grafts suitable for clinical use. The problems related to the immune response were reported. It was observed that when the autologous graft is not possible, a homologous graft between living patients of the same blood group can be performed, whereas grafts from cadavers cannot be used. Inclan and many other researchers had already begun to hint at the modern concept of storing bone material for different clinical uses. The preservation techniques reported consisted of putting the graft, immersed in the donor's blood or that of the host, in a sterile glass container. The graft was then kept in a refrigerator at a temperature of 2–5 °C until it was used. During the period of preservation, necessary bacteriological tests were performed every 3–14 days (Inclane 1942).

The modern bone bank to store blood for use was only possible after cooling techniques were developed. Bush and Wilson (1947) reported the need to preserve bone grafts at a temperature of 20 °C, and they managed to build a bone bank for small fragments of bone. Mouly and Sicard (1951) and Herbert founded the first bone bank in France. The first large bank for frozen osteoarticular grafts was already functioning in 1970.

For necessary preservation of the allograft material, a bone bank is required after a thorough screening of the donor, rapid procurement and safe, sterile processing. The screening must be carried out for bacterial and viral (HIV and hepatitis) infections, malignancies, metabolic bone disease and the presence of toxins, all of which are contraindications to donation. It has been accepted that the guidelines set by the American Association of Tissue Banks (A.A.T.B.) should be followed as the standard for the use of preserved allogenic bone. However, opinions differed. Allografts have osteoconductive properties and may serve as a substitute for autografts. Though rare, they do carry the risk of disease transmission.

Suggested Readings

1. Abbott LC, Schottstaedt ER, Saunders JB, De CM, Bost FC. The evaluation of cortical and cancellous bone grafting material: a clinical and experimental study. J Bone Joint Surg. 1947;29A:381.
2. Blick SS, Brumback RJ, Lakatos R, et al. Early prophylactic bone grafting of high-energy tibial fractures. Clin Orthop Relat Res. 1989;240:21–41.
3. Bush LF. The use of homogenous bone grafts. J Bone Joint Surg. 1947;29:620–8.
4. Bassett CAL. Current concepts of bone formation. J Bone Joint Surg. 1962;44A:1217.
5. Bassett CAL. Clinical implications of cell function in bone grafting. Clin Orthop. 1972;87:49.
6. Bieber EJ, Wood MB. Bone reconstruction. Clin Plast Surg. 1986;12:645.
7. Allsopp BJ, Hunter-Smith DJ, Rozen WM. Vascularized versus non-vascularized bone grafts: what is the evidence? Clin Orthop Relat Res. 2016;474(5):1319–27.
8. Burchardt H. The biology of bone graft repair. Clin Orthop. 1983;174:28.
9. Chalmers J. The transplantation immunity in bone homografting. J Bone Joint Surg. 1959;41B:160.
10. Chase SW, Herndon CH. The fate of autogenous and homogenous bonegrafts. Bone Joint Surg. 1955;37A:809.
11. Cutting CB, McCarthy JG. Comparison of residual osseous mass between vascularized and non-vascularized onlay bone transfers. Plast Reconstr Surg. 1983;72:672.
12. Connolly JF. Clinical use of marrow osteoprogenitor cells to stimulate osteogenesis. Clin Orthop Relat Res. 1998;355:S257–66.
13. Delloye C, Cornu O, Druez V, Barbier O, Bone allografts. What they can offer and what they cannot. J Bone Jont Surg. 2007;89B:574–9.
14. Doppelt SH, Tomford WW, Lucas AD, Mankin HJ. Operational and financial aspects of a hospital bone bank. J Bone Joint Surg. 1981;63A:244.
15. Enneking WF, Burchardt H, Puhl JJ, Piotrowski G. Physical and biologic aspects of repair in dog cortical bone transplants. J Bone Joint Surg. 1975;55A:232.
16. Enneking WF, Eady JL, Burchardt H. Autogenous cortical boen grafts in the reconstruction of segmental skeletal defects. J Bone Joint Surg. 1980;62A:1039.
17. Finkermeier CG. Bone grafting and bone-graft substitutes. J Bone Joint Surg. 2002;84(3):454–64.
18. Friedlaender GE, Mankin HJ. Bone banking: current methods and suggested guidelines. In: Murray D, editor. AAOS instructional course lectures, vol. 30. St. Louis: CV Mosby; 1981.
19. Geideman W, Early JS, Brodsky J. Clinical results of harvesting autogenous graft from the ipsilateral proximal tibiafor use in foot and ankle surgery. Foot Ankle Int. 2004;25(7):451–5.
20. Groves EWH. Methods and results of transplantation of bone repair of defects caused by injury of disease. Br J Surg. 1917;5:185.
21. Heiple KG, Chase SW, Herndon CH. A comparative study of the healing process following different types of bone transplantation. J Bone Joint Surg. 1963;45A:1593.
22. Inclan A. The use of preserved bone graft in orthopaedic surgery. J Bone Joint Surg. 1942;24A:81.
23. Ilizarov GA. Basic principles of transosseous compression and distraction osteosynthesis. Ortop Travmatol Protez. 1971;32(11):7–15.
24. James TM, Mruce HZ. Use of solid and cancellous autologous bone graft for fractures and non-unions. Orthop Clin N Am. 2010;41:15–26.
25. Kurz LT, Garfin SR, Booth RE Jr. Harvesting autogenous iliac bone grafts: a review of complications and techniques. Spine. 1989;14(12):1324–31.
26. Lacroix P. Organizers and the growth of bone. J Bone Joint Surg. 1947;29A:292.
27. Langer F, Czitrom AA, Pritzker KP, Gross AE. The immunogenicity of fresh frozen allogenic bone. J Bone Joint Surg. 1975;57A:216.
28. Levander G. On the formation of new bone in bone transplantation. Acta Chir Scand. 1934;74:425.

29. Mankin HJ, Doppelt SH, Tomford WW. Clinical experience with allograft implanation. The first ten years. Clin Orthop. 1983;174:69.
30. Mankin HJ, Hornicek FJ, Raskin KA. Infection in massive bone allografts. Clin Orthop Relat Res. 2005;432:210–6.
31. Muschler GF, Boehm C, Easley K. Aspiration to obtain osteoblast progenitor cells from human bone marrow: the influence of aspiration volume. J Bone Joint Surg. 1997;79(11):1699–709.
32. Ostrup LT, Frederickson JM. Distant transfer of a free living bone graft by microvascular anastomoses: an experimental study. Plast Reconstr Surg. 1974;54:274.
33. Phemister DB. Treatment of ununited fractures by onlay bone grafts without screw or tie fixation and without breaking down of the fibrous union. J Bone Joint Surg. 1947;29(4):946–60.
34. Ray RD. Vascularization of bone grafts and implants. Clin Orthop. 1972;87:43.
35. Ring D, Allende C, Jafarnia K, et al. Ununited diaphyseal forearm fractures with segmental defects: plate fixation and autogenous cancellous bone-grafting. J Bone Joint Surg. 2004;86(11):2440–5.
36. Roberts TT, Rosebbaum AJ. Bone grafts, bone substitutes and orthobiologics. The bridge between basic science and clinical advancements in fracture healing. Organogenesis. 2012;8(4):114–24.
37. Rodringo J, Chapman MW. Bone grafting, bone graft substitutes and growth factors. In: Chapman MW, Szabo RM, Marder RA, et al., editors. Chapman's orthopaedic surgery. 3rd ed. Philadelphia: Lippincott Williams & Wilkins; 2001. p. 81–211.
38. Siffert RS, Barash ES. Delayed bone transplantation: an experimental study of early host-transplant replationship. J Bone Joint Surg. 1961;43A:407.
39. Shaffer JW, Field GA, Goldberg VM, Davy DT. Fate of vascularized and non-vascularized autografts. Clin Orthop Relat Res. 1985;197:32–43.
40. Tomford WW, Doppelt SH, Mankin HJ, Friedlander GE. 1983 bone bank procedures. Clin Orthop. 1983;174:15.
41. Turner J, Bassett CAL, Pate JW, Sawyer PN. An experimental comparison of freeze-dried and frozen cortical bone graft healing. J Bone Joint Surg. 1955;37A:1197.
42. Urist MR. The physiologic basis of bone graft surgery, with special reference to the theory of induction. Clin Orthop. 1953;1:207.
43. Urist MR, Delange RJ, Finerman GA. Bone cell differentiation and growth factors. Science. 1983;220:680.
44. Urist MR, O'Connor BT, Burwell RG. Bone graft, derivatives and substitutes. Cambridge: Butterworth-Heinemann; 1994. p. 3–102.
45. Weiland AJ, Moore JR, Daniel RK. Vascularized bone autograft: experience with 41 cases. Clin Orthop. 1983;174:87.
46. Westrich GH, Geller DS, O'Malley MJ, et al. Anterior iliac crest bone graft system. J Orthop Trauma. 2001;15(7):500–6.
47. Wilkins RM, Chimenti BT, Rifkin RM. Perutaneous treatment of long bone nonunions: the use of autologous bone marrow and allograft bone matrix. Orthopaedics. 2003;26(5):S549–54.
48. Wilson PD. Experiences with a bone bank. Ann Surg. 1947;126:932–46.
49. Wood MB, Cooney WP. Vascularized bone segment transfer for management of chronic osteomyelitis. Orthop Clin North Am. 1984;15:461.
50. Wood MC, Cooney WP, Irons GB. Post traumatic lower extremity reconstruction by vascularized bone graft transfer. Orthopedics. 1984;7:255.
51. Ziran BH, Smith WR, Morgan SJ. Use of calcium based demineralized bone matrix/ allograft for nonunions and post-traumatic reconstruction of the appendicular skeleton: preliminary results and complications. J Trauma. 2007;63(6):1324–8.

Chapter 4
Non-vascularized Fibular Grafts (NVFG)

4.1 Non-vascularized Fibular Grafts (NVFG)

The fibula is well recognized as a cortical graft and is reported to be a long bone flap. It is long and straight, has good bone strength, has a tricortical structure and can be used as a graft up to 22 cm in size (Fig. 4.1a, b). Its dimensions permit it to anatomically match forearm bones and can also be used as a single graft to repair forearm bone defects. It can also be fixed into the medullary canals of major long bones like the femur, tibia and humerus (Fig. 4.2). The fibula derived its direct arterial supply from the peroneal artery. The outer third of the bone has profuse periosteal circulation.

Major bone gaps resulting from excision of osseous tumours, more so in the lower extremity, still continue to be a challenge to the treating surgeon. The existing reconstructive procedures described to bridge such bone defects are extensive and time-consuming. They require expensive equipment and frequently result in complications such as non-union, which is usually accompanied by infection. It is also a fact that the host bone is often osteoporotic, and hence, metallic implants may not be suitable for all patients. It is, therefore, necessary to suggest alternative reconstructive procedures that are biologically sound especially in active and young patients, who need them more often. Although non-vascularized fibular grafts had been used sporadically to bridge bone defects earlier, they also have their limitations and the results reported were poor. Hence, such grafts could not be popularized.

S. S. Yadav, *Non-Vascularised Fibular Grafts in Orthopaedic Practice*,
https://doi.org/10.1007/978-981-95-1794-7_4

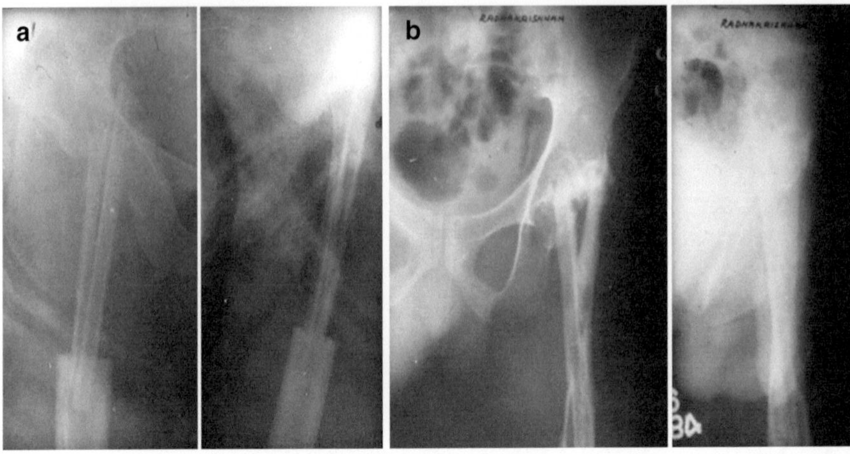

Fig. 4.1 (**a**) Radiograph reveals twin fibular grafts put together and wedged into the parent bone on either side and were supported by spica cast (this was one of the earlier cases when the grafts were not stabilized with internal fixation). (**b**) Radiograph revealing union and healing with lateral union in between the struts. It took 18 months to achieve healing

4.1.1 Anatomy and Structure of the Fibula

Structurally, the fibula is extremely well suited as a cortical graft and is considered to be a long-bone flap. The size, straight configuration and good bone mass of the fibular graft makes it suitable to be fitted into the medullary canal of long bones. Its shape and size also match the forearm bones, and it has been commonly used to reconstruct major bone defects of the radius and ulna.

For so long, the fibula has been recognized as a favourable choice for non-vascularized bone grafting procedures. The fibula is known to bear only 15% of the axial load across the ankle. It also permits its use as an autogenous bone graft with minimal biomechanical consequences on weight-bearing. The distal fibula also plays an important role in maintaining rotational stability and restraint against lateral translation of the talus. It is considered essential to preserve the distal third of the fibula during graft retrieval to avoid subsequent ankle instability and deformity.

The shape and size of the proximal articular surface of the fibula simulate those of the lower end of the radius. After excision of tumours at the lower end of the radius, transplantation of the upper end of the fibula permits a satisfactory range of pain-free motion at the wrist joint. Although the hyaline cartilage degenerates and results in fibrocartilage, it provides functional activities at the wrist.

4.1.2 *Vascular Supply of Fibula*

The vascular supply to the fibula is derived from the nutrient artery which enters the posterior fibular cortex at the junction of the proximal one-third and distal two-thirds. This nutrient artery is a branch of the peroneal artery, which is a branch of the posterior tibial artery and runs along the posterior aspect of the fibular diaphysis. The peroneal artery is located at the posterior aspect of the intermuscular septum of the lateral compartment, between the tibialis posterior and flexor halluces longus muscles in the posterior compartment. In addition to the nutrient artery, the fibula gets additional vascularity through a number of segmental musculo-periosteal vessels which also arise from the peroneal artery.

4.1.3 *Bridging the Humeral Defects*

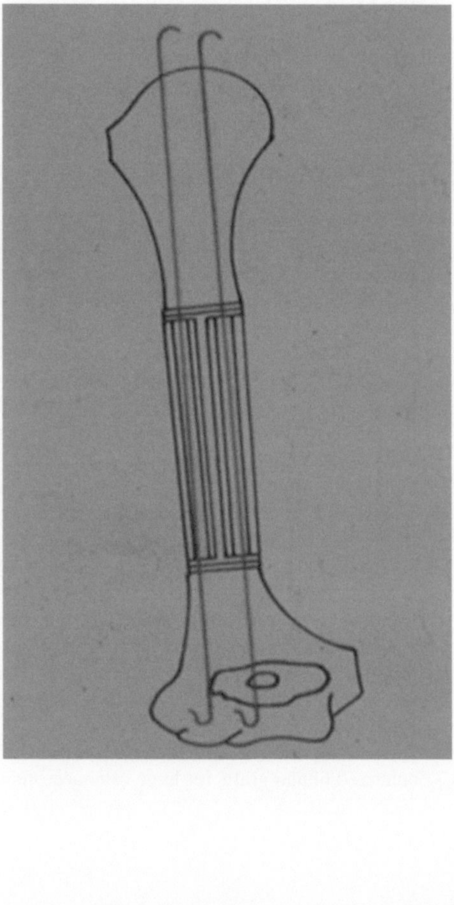

Fig. 4.2 Diagrammatic representation of a case with loss of diaphysis of the humerus bridged by twin fibular grafts stabilized with long Kirschner wires bent on either side to lock the construct. The twin fibular struts simulate the diameter of the parent bone

Suggested Readings

1. Arai K, Toh S, Tsubo K, Nishikawa S, Narita S, Miura H. Complications of vascularized fibula graft for reconstruction of long bones. Plast Reconstr Surg. 2002;109(7):2301–6.
2. Akiyama T, Clark JC, Miki Y, Choong PF. The non-vascularised fibular graft: a simple and successful method of reconstruction of the pelvic ring after internal hemipelvectomy. J Bone Joint Surg. 2010;92(7):999–1005.
3. Benlidayi ME, Gaggl A, Buerger H, Kürkcü M, Ünlügenç H, Önal D, Polat S, Sencar L. Comparison of vascularized osteoperiosteal femur flaps and nonvascularized femur grafts for reconstruction of mandibular defects: an experimental study. J Oral Maxillofac Surg. 2009;67:1174–83.
4. Benlidayi ME, Gaggl A, Bürger H, Brandner C, Kurkcu M, Unlugenç H. Comparative study of the osseointegration of dental implants after different bone augmentation techniques: vascularized femur flap, non-vascularized femur graft and mandibular bone graft. Clin Oral Implants Res. 2010;22:594–9.
5. Berggren A, Weiland AJ, Ostrup LT. Bone scintigraphy in evaluating the viability of composite bone grafts revascularized by micro vascular anastomoses, conventional autogenous bone grafts, and free non-revascularized periosteal grafts. J Bone Joint Surg. 1982;64:799–809.
6. Bus M, Bramer J, Schaap G, Schreuder H, Jutte P, Van der Geest I, Van de Sande M, Dijkstra P. Hemicortical resection and inlay allograft reconstruction for primary bone tumours. J Bone Joint Surg. 2015;97(9):738–50.
7. De Boer HH, Wood MB. Bone changes in the vascularised fbular graft. J Bone Joint Surg. 1989;71(3):374–8.
8. Dell PC, Burchardt H, Glowczewskie FP. A roentgenographic, biomechanical, and histological evaluation of vascularized and non-vascularized segmental fibular canine autografts. J Bone Joint Surg. 1985;67:105–12.
9. El-Sayed M, El-Hadidi M, El-Adl W. Free non-vascularised fibular graft for treatment of post-traumatic bone defects. Acta Orthop Belg. 2007;73(1):70–6.
10. Enneking WF, Eady JL, Burchardt H. Autogenous cortical bone grafts in the reconstruction of segmental skeletal defects. J Bone Joint Surg. 1980;62(7):1039–58.
11. Funovics PT, Bucher F, Toma CD, Kotz RI, Dominkus M. Treatment and outcome of parosteal osteosarcoma: biological versus endoprosthetic reconstruction. J Surg Oncol. 2011;103(8):782–9.
12. George B, Abudu A, Grimer RJ, Carter SR, Tillman RM. The treatment of benign lesions of the proximal femur with non-vascularized autologous fibular strut grafts. J Bone Joint Surg. 2008;90(5):648–51.
13. Gilbert A. A free transfer of the fibula shaft. Int J Microsurg. 1979;2:100.
14. Gross AE, McKee N, Farine I, Czitrom A, Langer F. Reconstruction of skeletal defects following en bloc excision of bone tumours: current concepts of diagnosis and treatment of bone and soft tissue tumours. Berlin: Springer-Verlag; 1984. p. 163.
15. Grzegorzewski A, Pogonowicz E, Sibinski M, Marciniak M, Synder M. Treatment of benign lesions of humerus with resection and non-vascularized, autologous fibular graft. Int Orthop. 2010;34(8):1267–72.
16. Hariri A, Mascard E, Atlan F, Germain MA, Heming N, Dubousset JF, Wicart P. Free vascularized fibular graft for reconstruction of defects of the lower limb after resection of tumour. J Bone Joint Surg. 2010;92(11):1574–9.
17. Kim SY, Kim YG, Kim PT, Ihn JC, Cho BC, Koo KH. Vascularized compared with nonvascularized fibular grafts for large osteonecrotic lesions of the femoral head. J Bone Joint Surg. 2005;87:2012–8.

18. Krieg AH, Davidson AW, Stalley PD. Intercalary femoral reconstruction with extra corporeal irradiated autogenous bone graft in limb-salvage surgery. J Bone Joint Surg. 2007;89(3):366–71.
19. Krieg AH, Lenze U, Gaston MS, Hefti F. The outcome of pelvic reconstruction with non-vascularized fibular grafts after resection of bone tumours. J Bone Joint Surg. 2010;92(11):1568–73.
20. Lawal YZ, Garba ES, Ogirima IL, Maitama K, et al. Use of non-vascularized autologous fibula strut graft in the treatment of segmental bone loss. Ann Afr Med. 2011;10:25–8.
21. Lenze U, Kasal S, Hefti F, Krieg AH. Non-vascularized fibular grafst for reconstruction of segmental and hemicortical bone defects following meta/diaphyseal tumour resection at the extremities. BMC Musculoskelet Disord. 2017;18:289.
22. Liu T, Liu Z, Zhang Q, Guo X, Zhang X. Hemicortical resection and reconstruction using pasteurized autograft for parosteal osteosarcoma of the distal femur. Bone Joint J. 2013;95(9):1275–9.
23. Liu T, Zhang Q, Guo X, Zhang X, Li Z, Li X. Treatment and outcome malignant bone tumours of the proximal humerus: biological versus endoprosthetic reconstruction. BMC Musculoskelet Disord. 2014;15:69.
24. Bumbasirevic M, Stevanovic M, Bumbasirevic V, Lesic A, Atkinson HDE. Free vascularised fibular grafts in orthopaedics. Int Orthop. 2014;38(6):1277–82.
25. Nather A, Goh JC, Lee JJ. Biomechanical strength of non-vascularised and vascularised diaphyseal bone transplants: an experimental study. J Bone Joint Surg. 1990;72:1031–5.
26. Omololu B, Ogunlade SO, Alonge TO. Limb conservation using non vascularised fibular graft. West Afr J Med. 2002;21:347–9.
27. Parrish FF. Allograft replacement of all or part of the end of a long bone following excision of a tumour: report of twenty-one cases. J Bone Joint Surg. 1973;55A:1.
28. Plakseychuk AY, Kim SY, Park BC, Varitimidis SE, Rubash HE, Sotereanos DG. Vascularized compared with nonvascularized fibular grafting for the treatment of osteonecrosis of the femoral head. J Bone Joint Surg. 2003;85:589–96.
29. Rabitsch K, Maurer-Ertl W, Pirker-Fruhauf U, Wibmer C, Leithner A. Intercalary reconstructions with vascularized fibula and allograft after tumour resection in the lower limb. Sarcoma. 2013;
30. Soucacos PN, Korompilias AV, Vekris MD, Zoubos A, Beris AE. The free vascularized fibular graft for bridging large skeletal defects of the upper extremity. Microsurgery. 2011;31(3):190–7.
31. Taylor GI. Microvascular free bone transfer. Orthop Clin North Am. 1977;8:425.
32. Taylor GI, Miller GDH, Ham FJ. The free vascularized bone graft: a clinical extension of microvascular techniques. Plast Reconstr Surg. 1975;55:533–44.
33. Tsuchiya H, Tomita K, Minematsu K, Mori Y, Asada N, Kitano S. Limb salvage using distraction osteogenesis. A classification of the technique. J Bone Joint Surg. 1997;79(3):403–11.
34. Villemagne T, Bonnard C, Accadbled F, et al. Intercalary segmental reconstruction of long bones after malignant bone tumour resection using primary methyl methacrylate cement spacer inter position and secondary bone grafting: the induced membrane technique. J Pediatr Orthop. 2011;31(5):570–6.
35. Wang JW, Weng LH. Treatment of distal femoral nonunion with internal fixation, cortical allograft struts and autogenous bone-grafting. J Bone Joint Surg. 2003;85(3):436–40.
36. Weiland AJ, Kleinert HE, Kutz JE, Daniel RK. Free vascularized bone grafts in surgery of the upper extremity. J Hand Surg. 1979;4:129.
37. Weiland AJ, Moore JR, Daniel RK. Vascularized bone autografts: experience with 41 cases. Clin Orthop Relat Res. 1983;174:87–95.
38. Wood MB, Cooney WP, Irons GB. Skeletal reconstruction by vascularized bone transfer: indications and results. Mayo Clin Proc. 1985;60:729.

39. Wood MB. Free vascularized fibula grafting- 25 years experience: tips, techniques and pearls. Orthop Clin North Am. 2007;38(1):1–12.
40. Yadav SS. Enhanced viability status of non-vascularised free fibular strut grafts. A report of 600 cases and experiences over five decades. Indian J Orthop:1–10.
41. Yadav SS. Dual fibular grafting for massive bone gaps in the lower extremity. J Bone Joint Surg. 1990;72(4):486–94.
42. Yadav SS. Bridging of large skeletal defects by twin fibular grafts supported by L-plate fixation. Orthopaed Int Edition. 1995;3:213–21.
43. Bi Z, HAN X, Fu C, Cao Y, Yang C. Reconstruction of large limb bone defects with a double-barrel free vascularized fibular graft. Chin Med J. 2008;121(23):2424–8.

Chapter 5
Non-vascularized Fibular Grafts (NVFG) Enhanced Viability

5.1 The Existing Concept of the NVFG

Non-vascularized fibular grafts have been well known to bridge major bone defects of the extremities. However, we still lack knowledge about their incorporation to the host bone. The existing concept has been that majority of the transplanted cells in such grafts undergo necrosis and that almost all the new bone formation is generated from the host site. These grafts are known for their delayed rate of revascularization and remodelling. Vascular penetration of the graft by the host tissue only happens after resorption of the cortical surface by the osteoclasts (Lieberman and Friedlander 2005). These grafts are known to become radiolucent and significantly weaker than normal bone. This is known to last for months and depends on the graft size and implantation site of these grafts. However, the union of such grafts depends on the establishment of their blood supply. Non-union may also develop because of relative ischemia or lack of adequate immobilization.

It has been reported that a significant number of osteoblasts exist on the graft of a mature bone (Ray 1972). If these osteogenic and functional cells are kept viable, they are capable of new bone formation by inducing surrounding unspecialized cells by either diffusion or cell-to-cell contact (Urist 1968). However, it had been debatable (Bessett 1972). Prolonged exposure of these cells outside

S. S. Yadav, *Non-Vascularised Fibular Grafts in Orthopaedic Practice*,
https://doi.org/10.1007/978-981-95-1794-7_5

the body and delays in the fixation process can destroy these vital osteogenic cells, as well as the diffusible bone morphogenetic protein (BMP), which is known to promote osteogenesis by stimulating the surrounding host mesenchymal cells. It has been debatable to obtain a definite evidence of vascularization of such grafts. Many controversial points were yet to be solved about the viability process of these transplants.

5.2 Our Experience with Improved Quality and Quantity of the NVFG

Massive bone defects of the long bones have been a challenging clinical situation. Reconstruction after resection of malignant bone tumour continues to be a major challenge. In 1968 while working at JIPMER, Pondicherry, many poor patients came with bone tumours needing salvage procedures. A suitable prosthesis was not available in those days. Bone gaps were also observed in infected cases after premature diaphyseal sequestration. Under the circumstances, an attempt was made to improve the osteogenic property of the non-vascularized fibular grafts for successfully bridging the major bone defects.

During the last five decades, we have been using improved non-vascularized fibular grafts in different clinical situations needing single and twin fibular struts. Twin fibular grafting with adequate fixation has been reported to bridge large bone defects, particularly in the femur, tibia and humerus for the first time (Yadav 1990). It has been our regular practice to use twin fibular struts to replace a full intercalary segment of the major bone. The technique described has considerably increased the viability of these grafts. The rate of union and remodelling of the twin grafts have been as good as reported in any other bone grafting method (Figs. 5.1a–c and 5.2a, b).

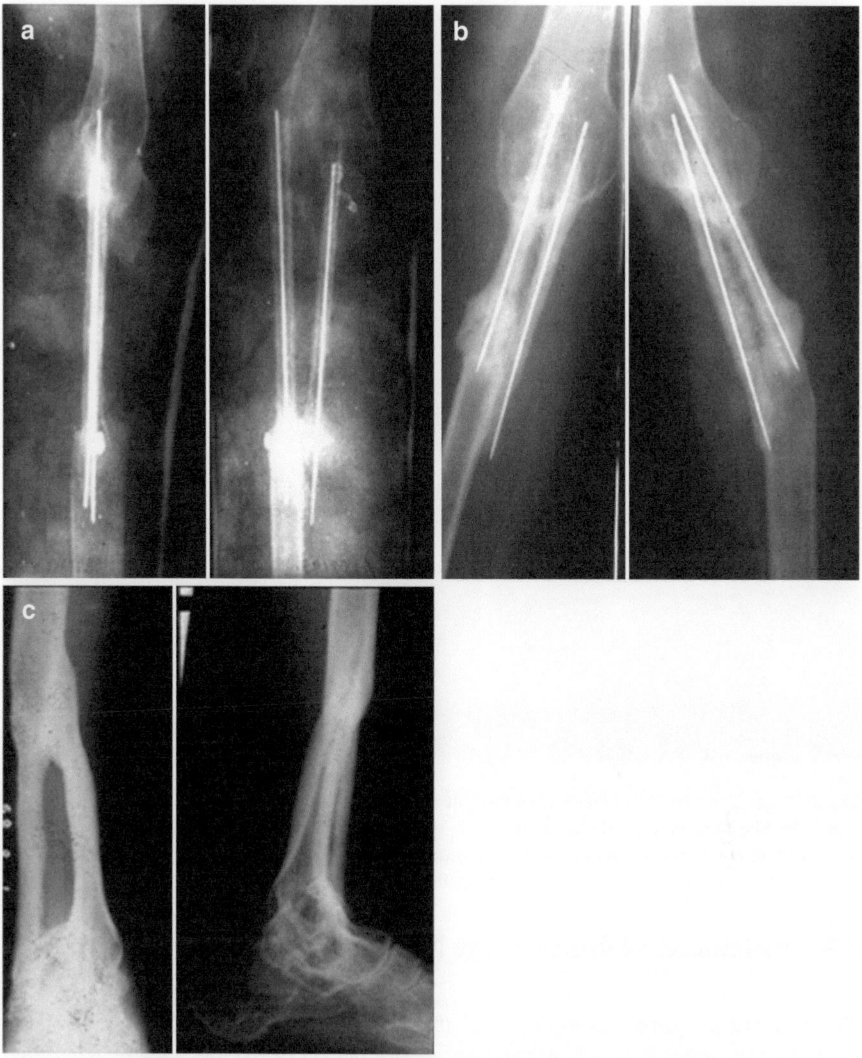

Fig. 5.1 (**a**) Twin fibular grafts stabilized with Kirschner wires and a screw supported with POP cast revealing early healing. (**b**) Twin fibular grafts stabilized with Kirschner wires show healing. These grafts have not undergone degenerative changes. (**c**) Twin fibular grafts attempted to bridge a gap after excision of large giant cell tumour at the lower end of the tibia. The fibular struts revealed sound union after 6 months. The shape of the ankle is maintained

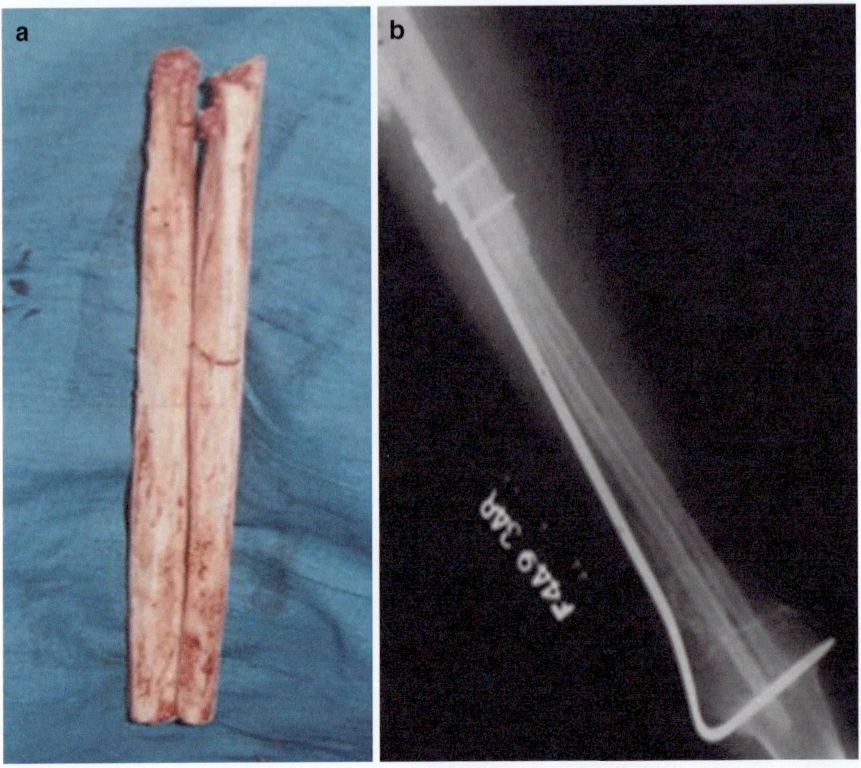

Fig. 5.2 (**a**) Long twin fibular strut grafts put together simulate the diameter of the major long bone. (**b**) The twin grafts stabilized with an L-plate reveal lateral union throughout the length of the graft that simulates the diameter of the femoral shaft. It was after en-bloc excision of an osteosarcoma of the lower end of the femur that resulted in such a gap

5.3 Enhanced Viability of the NVFG

The concept of enhanced viability of the NVFG described and the observations made by the author in nearly 1000 cases over a period of five decades revealed that these grafts can also be qualitatively more osteogenic. The improved concept and the advantages of the suggested technique are as follows:

5.3.1 The Concept of Viable Non-vascularized Fibular Grafts (NVFG)

5.3.1.1 Improved Quality

It is well known that osteogenic cells exist on the surface of fresh autologous grafts (Ray 1972). Through 'immediate transplantation' of these grafts at the host site, these vital osteocytes can become oxygenated and derive their nutrition from the

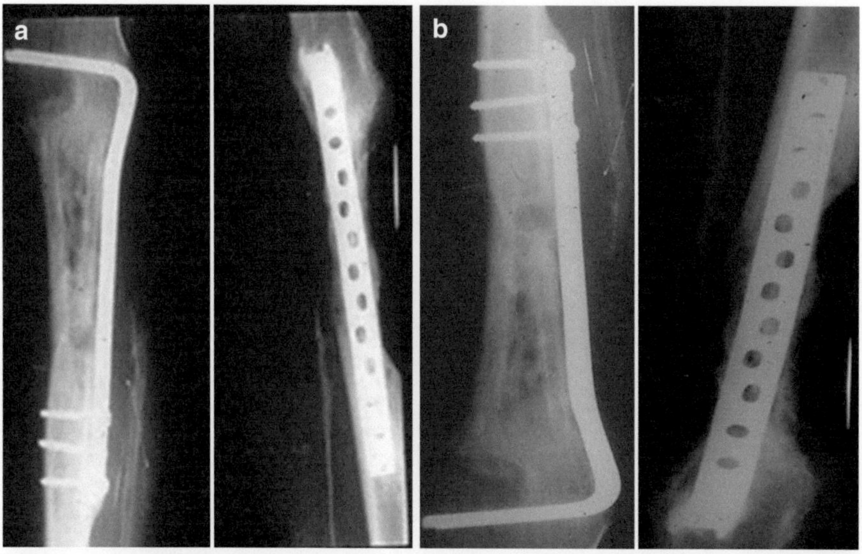

Fig. 5.3 (**a**, **b**) Twin fibular struts put together simulate the diameter of the parent bone like the femur, tibia and the humerus wherever they are required. Lateral union takes place between the struts. Twin fibular grafts stabilized with an L-plate attempted to bridge a gap at the lower end of the femur. Note the lateral union in between the fibular struts

blood of the host site, and they can be preserved before these cells undergo necrosis. In this way, the graft experiences only a 'transient ischemia'. With the preservation of these osteogenic cells, the graft remains viable and its quality is enhanced. The survival of these cells results in viable interaction with the mesenchymal cells of the host bone ends and permits simultaneous new bone formation. It is, therefore, essential that the graft be retrieved only after the host site is ready to receive the graft.

5.3.1.2 Added Quantity

Twin fibular struts also add to the 'quantity' of the construct in bridging bone defects. Moreover, the additional strut makes the construct similar to the diameter of the parent host bone like the femur, tibia and humerus (Fig. 5.3a, b).

5.3.1.3 The 'Lateral Union' Between the Twin Grafts

Since twin fibular struts are put together, a new concept of 'lateral union' has been coined which occurs between the strut grafts. This breakthrough in this significant process of lateral union takes place throughout the length of the grafts including the host-graft junctions. If necessary, additional cancellous graft can be attempted between the twin struts. It further enhances the 'lateral union', which results in a solid sheet of bone with a diameter similar to that of a major long bone (Fig. 5.4).

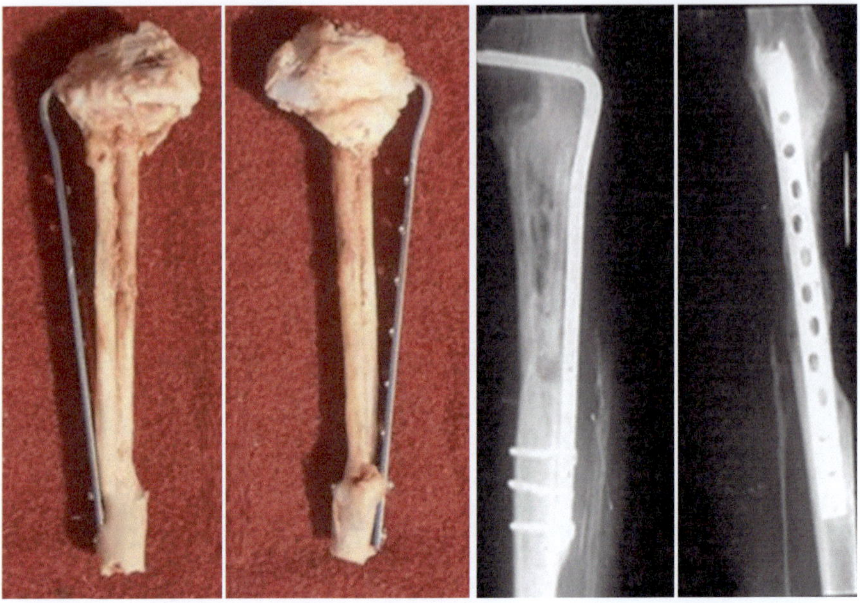

Fig. 5.4 A post-mortem specimen of a girl with osteosarcoma of the proximal end of the tibia. The twin fibular grafts were stabilized with an ordinary L-plate. Note the lateral union in between the struts, simulating the diameter of the tibia

5.4 The Strength of the Construct

The additional fibular strut graft not only provides *added quantity* to the bone but also strengthens the construct to prevent fractures that are known to commonly occur in the centre of such grafts. The lateral union also sustains the rotational forces acting on the construct during the process of their incorporation with the host bone. The twin fibular graft fixation also provides additional and the much needed *double contact* at the ends of the host bone. This also enhances the strength and stability at the host-graft junction, improves the rate of osteogenesis and also minimizes the undesirable forces acting on the construct.

5.4.1 The Host-Graft Junction

Fashioning the twin fibular graft to fit the viable host bone provides double contact with the host bone ends and plays a definite role in the incorporation of the graft construct. Moreover, the twin fibular struts put together are equivalent in diameter to the host bone. In most patients, the graft has been quite stable after about 16–24 weeks and is consolidated in about 36 weeks. The rate of union was not influenced by the size or polarity of the graft. It is suggested that stable internal fixation of these grafts with an L-plate or any other suitable device results in early incorporation of the graft at both ends. Union occurred in all patients in whom the ends of the graft were wedged inside the medullary canal of the host bone. In such cases, guarded stress also stimulates repair and further strengthens the grafts. Union also occurs at the host-graft junction, irrespective of the length of the graft. However, these grafts need to be protected until radiological union occurs.

5.5 Harvesting the Fibular Graft

A postero-lateral incision is made over the leg. The cleavage between the peroneus longus anteriorly and soleus posteriorly is identified. The fibular diaphysis is exposed globally preserving the periosteum. Extending the dissection proximally, care is exercised to retract and preserve the peroneal nerve. Distally, the fibula is exposed, leaving behind nearly 8 cm of the distal end for stability of the ankle. The intramuscular septum is now divided according to the length of the graft required. The graft is now ready to be removed for immediate transplantation at the host site.

5.5.1 Twin Fibular Grafts

In situations where the length of the bony defect is up to 10–12 cm, the entire length of the ipsilateral fibula (including the head) can be harvested, leaving behind the distal end, as stated. The 25-cm graft can now be divided into two struts of 10–12 cm each and is ready to be used. In case the bony defect is more than 13 cm, the contralateral fibular strut graft can also be obtained. Once the recipient site is prepared, the fibular graft is transferred immediately to the desired site and fixed to the host bone.

However, during the removal of the fibular graft, three points should be observed: (1) The peroneal nerve must be preserved. (2) The distal fourth of the fibula must be retained. (3) The peroneal muscles should not be damaged.

5.5.2 Fixation of the Fibular Graft

Fixation of the fibular grafts to the host bone depends on the site and the requirement of an individual patient. Depending on the clinical condition at the host site, where the available bone ends are small, a plate could not be used. The fibular strut grafts are stabilized with long Kirschner wires. The wires are passed through the host bone end, fibular strut and to the other end of the bone. This has been based on the principle of three-point fixation. At other sites such as the ankle and wrist, the fibular strut is stabilized with the help of multiple screws and cross Kirschner wires.

For fixation of large bone gaps around the knee and hip, the fibular struts are fixed with an L-plate. The adequacy of stable fixation created a better physiological condition at the host-graft junction, resulting in early union and minimizing the period of immobilization of the extremity. The L-plate fixation used in this series provided contour-based fixation at the knee and hip regions and provided the much-needed protection to the twin grafts. Although the L-plate stabilizes the host-graft junction adequately, it does not come into direct contact with the grafts, thereby allowing circumferential osteogenic activity on all surfaces of the graft (Fig. 5.5a–d). It also protects the construct from rotational movement at the distal extremity and helps prevent fracture of the graft.

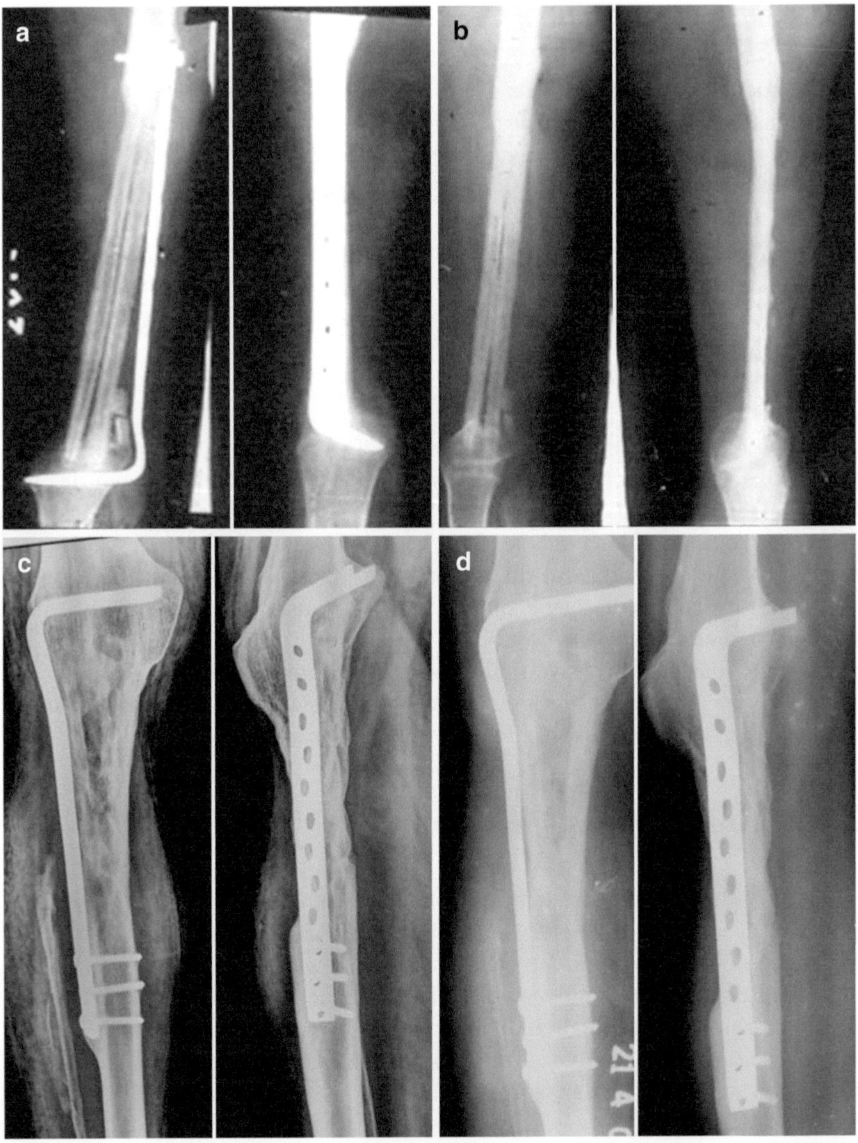

Fig. 5.5 (**a**) Twin fibular strut grafts stabilized with an L-plate at the lower end of the femur showing early healing. (**b**) Complete healing of the struts with lateral union which provided strength to the construct. However, the long struts were still protected in a brace after removal of the plate. (**c**) The radiograph reveals twin fibular graft used at the proximal end of the tibia stabilized with an L-plate. (**d**) Note the advanced stage of lateral union between the strut grafts. It has resulted in a sheet of bone and got remodelled simulating the proximal tibia

The construct can be stabilized with any of the following methods:

1. Wedging (press-fit fixation) supported with a POP cast.
2. Intramedullary insertion of Kirschner wires.
3. L-plate fixation and arthrodesis of the neighbouring joint.
4. Fibular strut graft as 'biological nail'.

5.6 Remodelling of the Improved NVFG

Twin fibular struts of enhanced quality, when put together, result in early and sound union. This process of lateral union takes place throughout the length of the struts and finally results in a sheet of bone which is equal to the diameter of the parent bone like the femur, tibia and humerus. Remodelling of such a construct had taken place in twin grafts that simulated the diaphysis of the parent bone.

5.6.1 The Added Advantage of Twin Fibular Grafts

Twin free fibular grafts, when placed together and fixed adequately to the host bone ends, have double contact with the host bone and unite comparatively earlier than a single graft. Lateral union takes place throughout the length of the graft, and this becomes a solid biological construct. Such a construct also offers a better mechanical advantage for early and reliable union, and it has the advantage in terms of remodelling in response to stress forces. Gradual and protected weight-bearing also results in early healing, as well as hypertrophy and remodelling of the twin grafts.

The concept of immediate fixation of the twin grafts and lateral union appears to have addressed the age-old drawbacks associated with non-vascularized fibular grafts. The incorporation of the graft with the host bone in a relatively short time also reveals the viability of these grafts. Because of lateral union between the two struts throughout the length of the graft, the construct becomes a solid sheet of bone, and it also offers a better mechanical advantage for early and dependable union and remodelling.

Initially, the grafts were stabilized by wedging them into the major bone ends on either side, supported by a suitable cast. Soon, it was realized that a suitably sized inlay Kirschner wire could better hold the graft by fixing the ends of the host bone. We procured 18-in.-long Kirschner wires with 1.5 to 2.5 diameters which could be passed through the fibular strut based on the principle of three-point fixation. The construct proved useful in stabilizing the graft. In the later years, we had used an L-plate to stabilize the twin grafts with the host bone ends. This, no doubt, had afforded a better fixation. In such cases, application of a cast was not required. The time for union with such a construct had also improved to 16–24 weeks. Moreover, the complications have been minimal.

However, like any other graft, these grafts also need to be protected until radiological union is complete. The insertion of Kirschner wires inside the single fibular struts prevented/minimized stress fractures. Union occurred in all patients whose graft ends were wedged inside the medullary canal of the host bone and stabilized with a POP cast. Union has also taken place at the host-graft junction, irrespective of the length of the graft. In the lower extremity, guarded stress further stimulates repair and strengthens the construct.

5.6.2 The Donor Site

Fibular grafts of various sizes have been harvested by a postero-lateral approach. Fibular grafts up to 22 cm can be removed including the head of the fibula after preservation of the lateral popliteal nerve. However, 6–8 cm of the distal end must be preserved to avoid ankle instability and subsequent valgus deformity at the ankle. Regeneration of the fibula has been observed in younger patients. A regenerated fibular graft can be used if a graft is needed for some other condition needing such a graft.

It has been reported that vascularized fibular grafting is an extensive and expensive procedure that may result in more complications at the donor site.

5.6.3 Arthrodesis of the Neighbouring Joint

Considering the seriousness of the disease, the long-term stability provided by arthrodesis of the adjacent joint has been accepted by the patients. Arthrodesis of the neighbouring joint is a small price to pay for resolution of the original pathology, when the result is a stable joint, with no risk of failure of the implant or repeated surgeries. The aim of the operation is replacement of the affected bone and restoration of the skeletal continuity and function of the extremity. It is simple, reliable, less time-consuming and economic one-time procedure. No bone bank is needed. Arthrodesis of the neighbouring joint has proved stable and painless, more so in the lower extremity. It is of great advantage to the manual labourers who need a stable, painless and dependable joint. Moreover, arthrodesis is a one-time and lifelong treatment.

The advantages of improved NVFG:

1. An easier operative technique.
2. Short operative time.
3. Capacity of early healing and remodelling.

In conclusion, the improved NVFG seems to have changed the existing concept that the NVFG are non-osteogenic. The enhanced quality and added quantity of the twin free vascularized fibular grafts (FVFG) have been used for over five decades with successful clinical and radiological outcomes. With 'lateral union', the improved twin NVFG may prove as a considerable alternative to the single vascularized fibular graft.

Moreover, it may not be justified to subject the patient to a challenging and riskier surgical procedure.

5.7 Histology of the Enhanced Quality of Non-vascularized Fibular Strut Grafts: A Project of the Indian Council of Medical Research (ICMR)

After the encouraging clinical and radiological success of these grafts, it was decided to carry out the histological assessment of the struts in vivo. It was considered essential to further prove the viability of these grafts.

After excision of the tumour around the knee, reconstruction was carried out with twin fibular struts stabilized using an L-condylar plate immediately after they were retrieved from the donor site. Three weeks after the surgery, biopsy was obtained with a core biopsy needle. The biopsy material proved the presence of viable osteoblasts and osteocytes. Histopathology had been carried out in 50 patients. In 44 of the 50 patients, osteogenic cells have been observed on the surface of the graft. Histological assessment proved that these grafts had not been undergoing degenerative changes as observed in a conventional non-vascularized fibular graft. The observations made coincided with the radiological assessment during the process of healing. None of our twin fibular strut grafts had undergone the changes described earlier in the NVFG.

The histology of such fibular struts has been carried out in a research project of the Indian Council of Medical Research for a period of 3 years. The study revealed that after observing the suggested steps, viability of these grafts have improved. The enhanced quality of these fibular strut grafts seems to have revised the concept about NVFG. In our experience for over five decades, these improved fibular grafts have made their presence felt.

5.8 Free Vascularized Fibular Grafts (FVFG)

Vascularized fibular grafts, by definition, retain their blood supply and thus remain viable. First described by Taylor (1975) from Australia, the vascularized fibular graft has become an important tool in the treatment of skeletal defects resulting from tumour resection, trauma and post-septic loss of bone. These grafts are said to have higher potential for hypertrophy and for remodelling. This kind of graft is known as a vital bone graft.

The harvesting of vascularized bone graft requires preservation of its vascular supply. It is essential to preserve the nutrient, artery and additional perforating vessels for anastomosis of both arteries and veins. In vascularized grafts, the graft osteocytes and other osteoprogenitor cells are preserved. These viable grafts are incorporated through primary or secondary bone healing and not through creeping substitution. This may increase the graft osteogenic potential and prevent the initial loss of graft strength typically seen with non-vascularized cortical grafts. Commonly utilized vascularized grafts include free fibular strut grafts, free iliac crest grafts and distal radius grafts.

Despite its many theoretical applications and advantages, free vascularized fibular grafting is technically challenging and has its own inherent risks and potential complications. Sound microsurgical technique is essential in performing the required arterial and venous anastamoses and ensuring long-term graft viability. The middle one-third of the fibula also can be used as a vascularized free autograft based on the peroneal artery and vein pedicle using the microvascular technique. Portions of the iliac crest also can be used as free vascularized autografts. Furthermore, donor site morbidity has been well documented in these patients. If fibular harvest is not performed with proper care and technique, patients may subsequently develop ankle pain, instability and progressive valgus deformity. Given these considerations, free vascularized fibular grafting should only be employed in specific clinical situations. The use of free vascularized autografts has limited indications, requires expert microvascular technique and is not without donor site morbidity. However, should the anastomosis/graft fail for technical reasons, the outcome may be no different from that observed with non-vascularized grafts.

5.8.1 *Complications of FVFG*

Complications can occur at acute, subacute and delayed stages at both the donor and recipient sites. Early complications include uncontrolled bleeding at the site of microvascular anastomosis or following failure of adequate haemostasis, thrombosis of the anastomosis and torsion of the vascular pedicle. Subacute vessel thrombosis and compartment syndrome occur if the deep fascia is closed too tightly.

Late complications include non-union and inadequate graft hypertrophy, which often reflect insufficient vascularization. Infection can also occur. Some studies have reported even tibial stress fractures in some cases. There are many reports of donor-site morbidity, muscle weakness, pain and valgus deformity of the ankle.

5.8.2 *Contraindications of Free Vascularized Fibular Grafts (FVFG)*

During preoperative planning for FVFG, patients with peripheral vascular disease, deep venous thrombosis or previous damage to their blood vessels should be excluded.

FVFG is also contraindicated if there is absence of vessels at the donor or recipient site.

5.8.2.1 Future of Bone Grafts

The future holds tremendous promise because of current research, especially in 3D printing and bone tissue engineering, which aim to provide grafts that have all the ideal characteristics and are available in unlimited amounts. Bone tissue engineering aims to act as a source for unlimited autogenous bone tissue. Human mesenchymal stem cells have been the subject of several studies and experiments aimed at bone tissue engineering with promising outcomes being yielded. The patient's bone marrow is used as the source for human mesenchymal stem cells, which are multipotent undifferentiated cells which are capable of undergoing chondrogenesis and osteogenesis. The idea is to use a polymer scaffold onto which these cells grow while in the presence of bone-stimulating factors.

Suggested Readings

1. Adani R, Delbroix L, Innocenti M, et al. Reconstruction of large post-traumatic skeletal defects of the forearm by vascularized free fibular graft. Microsuergy. 2004;24(6):423–9.
2. Aldlyami E, Abudu A, Grimer RJ, Carter SR, Tillman RM. Endoprosthetic replacement of diaphyseal bone defects. Long term results. Int Orthop. 2005;29(1):25–9.
3. Arai K, Toh S, Yasumura M, Okamoto Y, Harata S. One bone forearm formation using vascularized fibula graft for massive bone defect of the forearm with infection: case report. J Reconstr Microsurg. 2001;17:151–3.
4. Agarwal A, Kumar A. Fibula regeneration following non-vascularized graft harvest in children. Int Orthop. 2016:1–7.
5. Bradley JA, David JHS, Warren MR. Vascularized versus non-vascularized bone grafts: what is the evidence? Clin Orthop Relat Res. 2016;474(5):1319–27.
6. Chew WY, Low CK, Tan SK. Long-term results of free vascularized fibular graft: a clinical and radiographic evaluation. Clin Orthop Relat Res. 1995;311:258–61.
7. Davis PK, Mazur JM, Coleman GN. A torsion strength comparison of vascularized and non-vascularized bone grafts. J Biomech. 1982;15:875–80.
8. Krieg AH, Hefti F. Reconstruction with non-vascularised fibular grafts after resection of bone tumours. J Bone Joint Surg. 2007;89:215–21.
9. Minami A, Kasashima T, Iwasaki N, Kato H, Kaneda K. Vascularized fibular grafts. An experience of 102patients. J Bone Joint Surg. 2000;82(7):1022–5.
10. Houdek MT, Bayne CO, Bishop AT, Shin AY. The outcome and compliations of vascularised fibular grafts; 2017.
11. Schuh R, Panotopoulos J, Puchner SE, Willegger M, Hobusch GM, Windhagar R, Funovics PT. Vascularized or non-vascularized autologous fibular grafting for the reconstruction of a diaphyseal bone defect after resection of a musculoskeletal tumour. Bone Joint J. 2014;96(B):1258–63.
12. Steinlechner CW, Mkandawire NC. Non-vascularised fibular transfer in the management of defects of long bones after sequestrectomy in children. J Bone Joint Surg. 2005;87:1259–63.

13. Vail TP, Urbaniak JR. Donor site morbidity with use of vascularized autogenous fibular grafts. J Bone Joint Surg. 1996;78(2):204–11.
14. Wood MB. Free vascularized fibula grafting- 25 years experience: tips, techniques and pearls. Orthop Clin North Am. 2007;38(1):1–12.
15. Yadav SS. Enhanced viability and clinical outcomes of non-vascularized fibular strut grafts: a 50-year experience of 621 cases. Indian J Orthop. 2025:1–10.
16. Yadav SS. Dual fibular grafting for massive bone gaps in the lower extremity. J Bone Joint Surg. 1990;72(4):486–94.
17. Yadav SS. Bridging of large skeletal defects by twin fibular grafts supported by L-plate fixation. Orthop Int Edition. 1995;3:213–21.

Chapter 6
Bone Tumours Needing Suitable Excision and Reconstruction

6.1 Bone Tumours Needing Suitable Excision and Reconstruction

In the past, malignant bone tumours of the extremities were managed by performing an amputation. Currently, limb salvage procedure has become popular with a definite advantage of preserving the limb. When possible, limb salvage is preferred to an amputation. However, an amputation is still the treatment of choice in large and inoperable malignant bone tumours.

Limb salvage procedure includes two steps: (1) en bloc excision of the lesion after achieving safe margins and (2) a suitable reconstruction of the large bone gap created after excision. In case the desired excision is not possible, an attempt to save the extremity should not be made because the chances of recurrence are almost certain which will result in an amputation, adding to the morbidity and even mortality.

Many techniques of reconstruction have been described. Different types of endoprosthesis, the Ilizarov technique, vascularized fibular grafts (VSG) and non-vascularized fibular grafts (NVFG) are some of the well-known procedures used to bridge such gaps.

Over the past five decades, the author has used NVFG for reconstruction of such gaps after excision of aggressive bone tumours of the extremities.

6.2 Osteochondroma

A patient with solitary exostosis usually is brought in by a parent who has just noticed a mass adjacent to a joint. Occasionally, a patient has loss of motion in the adjacent joint due to the size of the mass. The patient often has been aware of the mass for months to years and reports that it has been slowly enlarging. It may result in repeated trauma, pressure on adjacent neurovascular bundle or inflammation in an overlying bursa.

S. S. Yadav, *Non-Vascularised Fibular Grafts in Orthopaedic Practice*,
https://doi.org/10.1007/978-981-95-1794-7_6

Ordinarily, an osteochondroma is managed by excision. However, a massive osteochondroma may require excision and reconstruction (Fig. 6.1a–e).

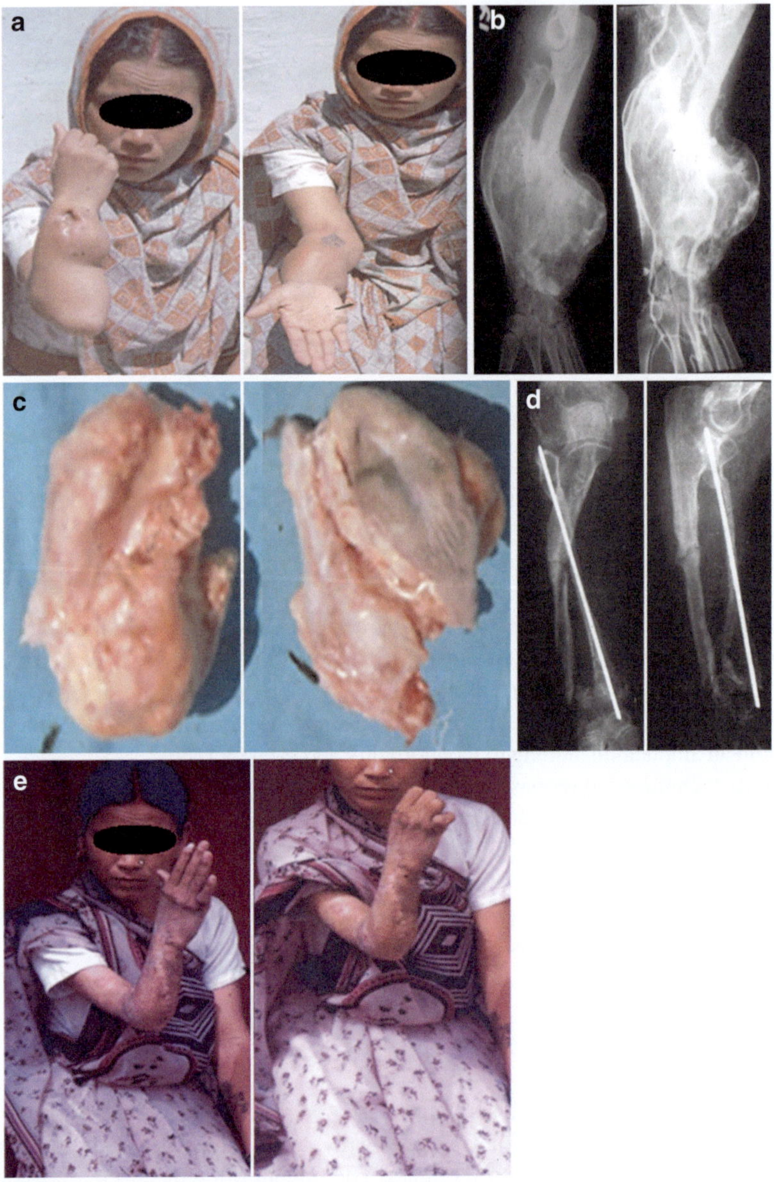

Fig. 6.1 (**a**) Huge swelling of the right distal forearm, gradually increasing for 8 years and had become painful. Biopsy proved osteochondroma. (**b**) Radiograph reveals massive osteochondromas of the distal half of the radius and ulna. An excision of the tumour was attempted, and the gap was bridged by fibular grafts stabilized with long Kirschner wires. (**c**) The front and back of the excised specimen. (**d**) Radiograph taken 5 months after bridging the gap with fibular graft stabilized with Kirschner wires, arthrodesing the wrist joint. The Kirschner wire from ulna has been removed. (**e**) The final function of the hand with fist closed and open. She had been able to perform her house hold duties

6.3 Unicameral Bone Cyst

Unicameral bone cysts may be noted incidentally in the first two decades of life. It is usually diagnosed after a pathologic fracture. These lesions typically occur in metaphyses of the proximal humerus or proximal femur. Radiographs of these benign lesions reveal a sharp marrow zone of transition between the cyst and surrounding bone.

Unicameral bone cysts are not always unicameral and are also called simple bone cysts. After a pathological fracture, these lesions may show signs of healing. However, in advance cases, a pathological fracture should be avoided with an intramedullary support (Fig. 6.2a, b).

Numerous methods have been used for management, but none has been universally successful. Operative treatment with curettage and autogenous bone graft is reserved for lesions that do not respond to repeated injections of corticosteroids (Fig. 6.3a–c). The injection of autogenous bone marrow is a new technique that has not been completely evaluated.

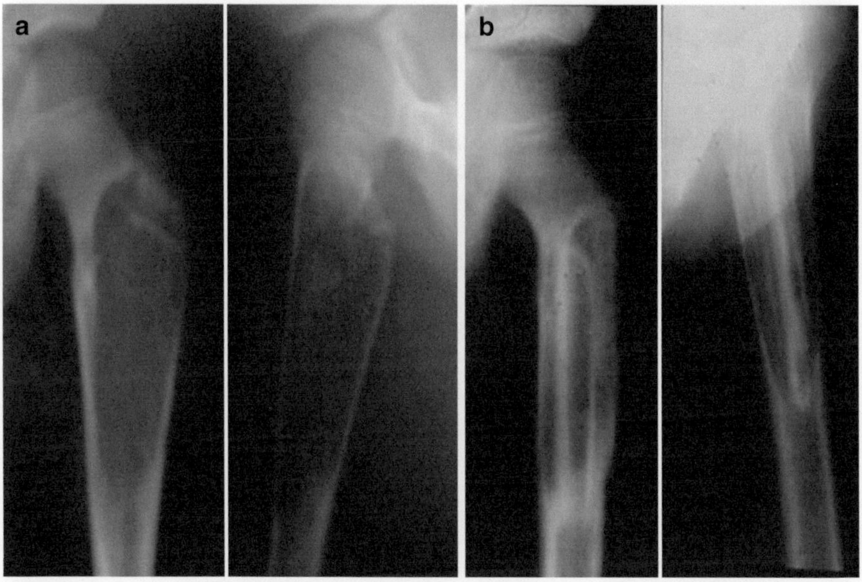

Fig. 6.2 (**a**) A case of simple bone cyst of the proximal femur threatening a pathological fracture. (**b**) Curettage and placement of a single fibular strut of appropriate size lead to healing. Note the graft has merged with the host bone that shows remodelling

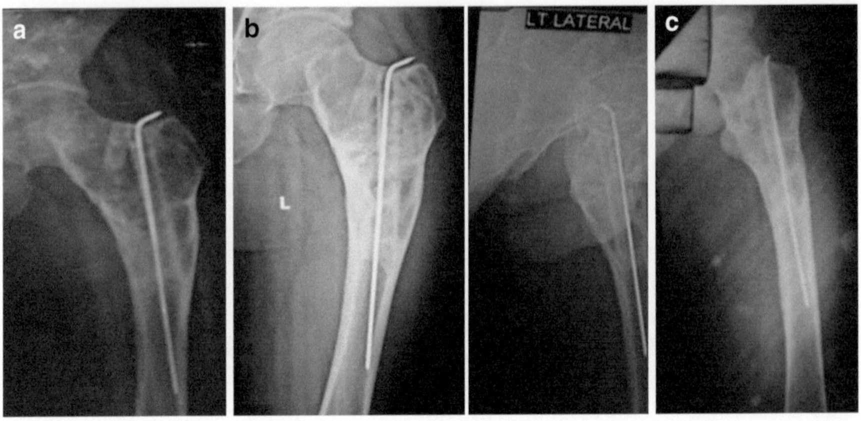

Fig. 6.3 (**a**) A case of simple bone cyst of the proximal end of the femur. A fibular strut has been a stabilized in the cavity with a Kirschner wire in the strut. (**b**) Note the healing of the cyst after 2 months. (**c**) The bone reveals complete healing and remodeling

6.4 Recurrent Unicameral Bone Cyst

We had a very unusual but known case of bone cyst of the right humerus in a boy of 14 years which was curetted five times (in other centres) and had recurred (Fig. 6.4a–e). This large and aggressive cyst had expanded the bone to the extent that the cortex of the bone was very thin (pencil line) and had also revealed a pathological fracture (Fig. 6.5a, b).

No other procedure could be indicated/possible except excision of the cyst and reconstruction of the diaphysis. This was achieved by twin NVFG fixed to the host bone ends with a pair of suitable long Kirschner wires. The final result demonstrated healing, with the help of lateral union between the struts, which together simulated the humeral shaft (Fig. 6.5c–h).

The reason for recurrences in such case could be because of an associated aggressive lesion (like an aneurysmal bone cyst) with this bone cyst.

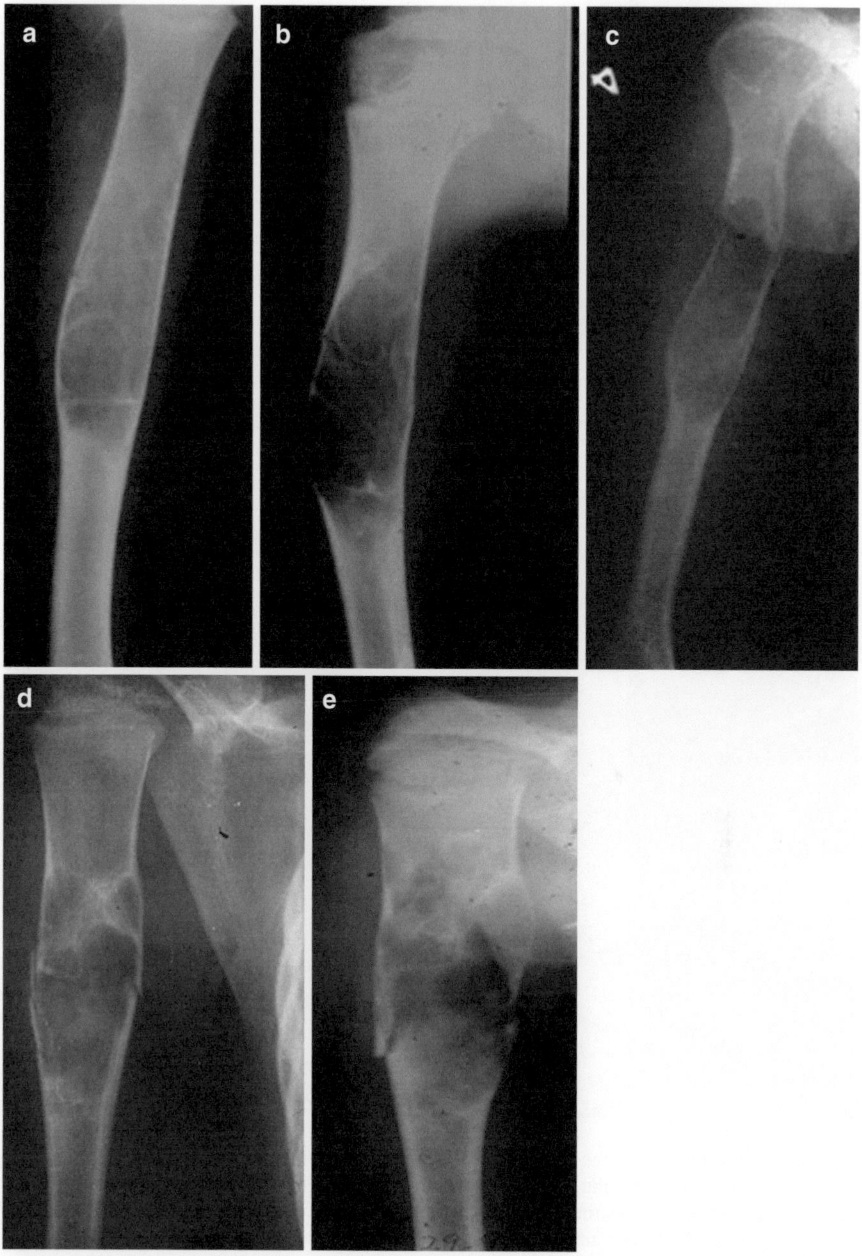

Fig. 6.4 (**a**–**e**) Radiograph reveals a unicameral bone cyst of the right humerus which had migrated distally. This cyst was curetted five times in different centres and had recurred. Patient with bone cyst at the proximal humerus with complete destruction of diaphysis with pathological fracture

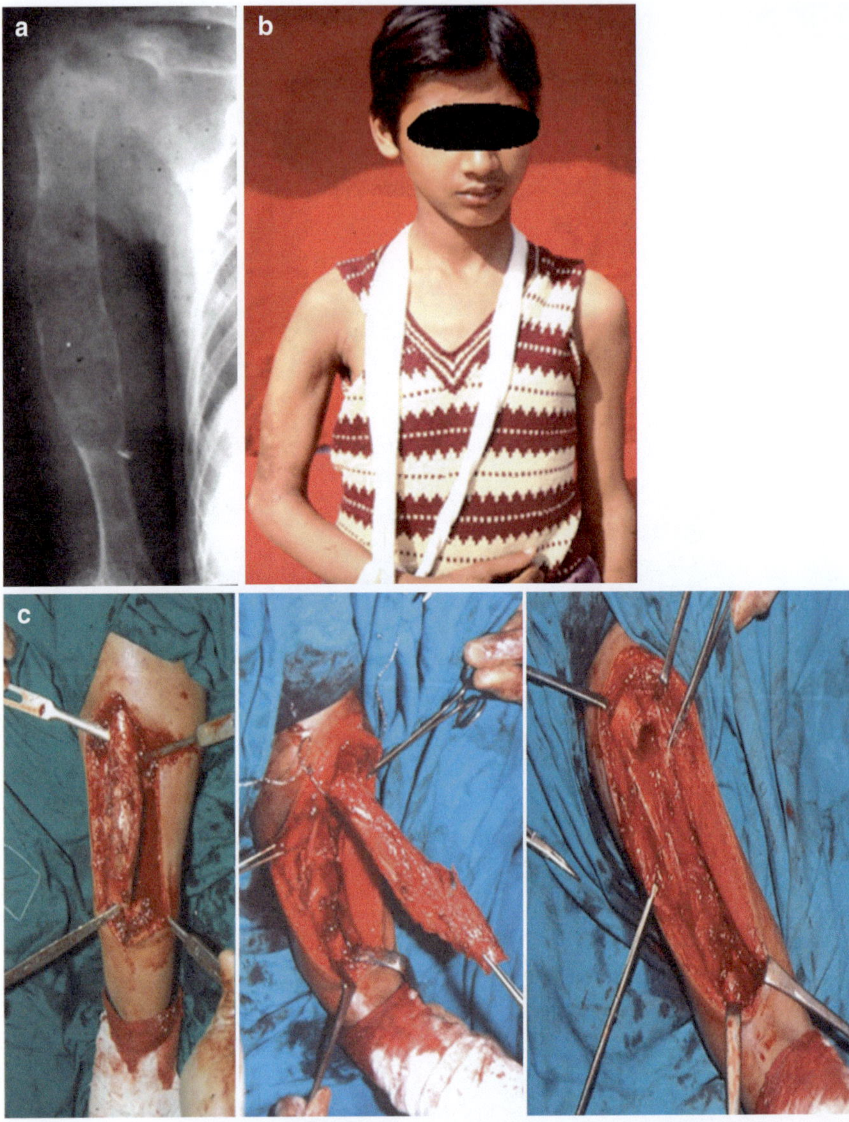

Fig. 6.5 (**a**) Radiograph of the patient when he attended our outpatient department. (**b**) Clinical picture of the patient. Since the last radiograph revealed extensive involvement, it was decided to excise the lesion and reconstruct with twin fibular grafts. (**c**). Intraoperative pictures during the excision of the cyst. (**d**) The anterior and posterior views of the excised specimen.The bone was extensively involved with complete destruction of the cortex. (**e**) Twin fibular grafts in situ bridging the gap, stabilized with long twin Kirschner wires. Note the bent wires at the tip of the shoulder. (**f**) Radiograph showing lateral union between the two struts. (**g**) Radiograph revealed complete healing which simulated the shaft of the humerus. (**h**) Clinical picture of the patient showing abduction at the shoulder and flexion at the elbow. This proves that even long NVFG, when used with the suggested technique of improved quality and quantity, do not result in degenerative changes previously described in NVFGs

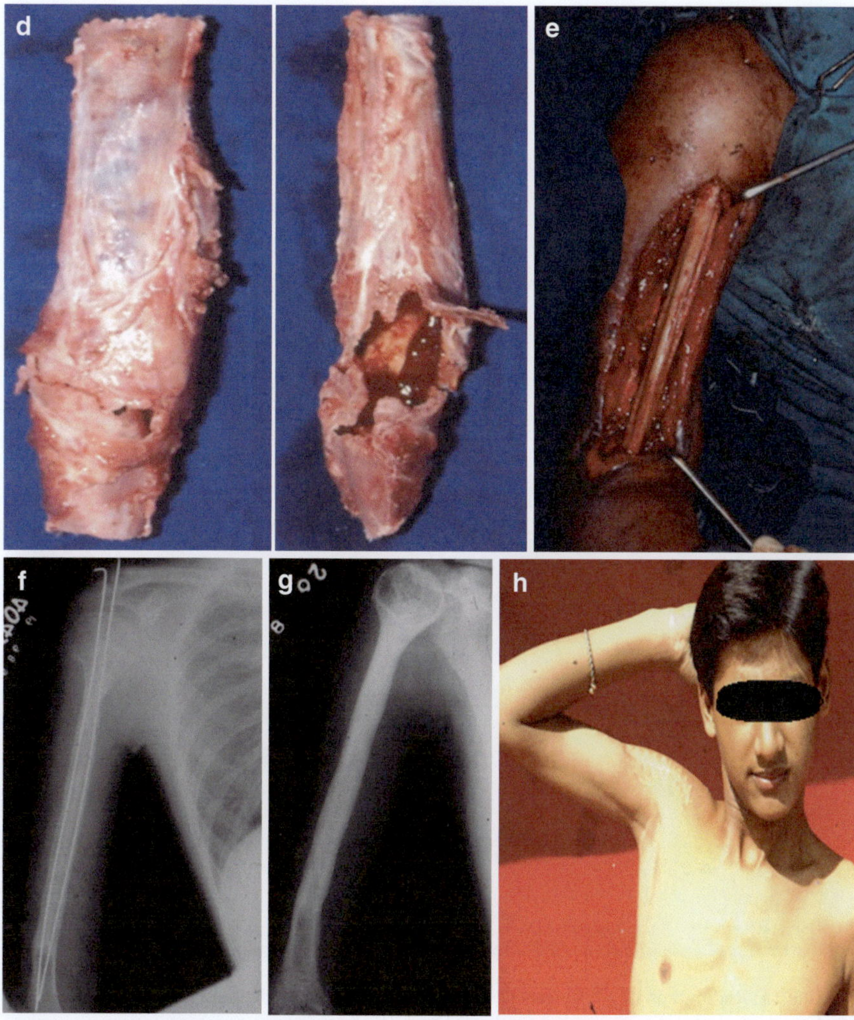

Fig. 6.5 (continued)

6.5 Aneurysmal Bone Cyst (ABC)

Aggressive aneurysmal bone cysts should be biopsied to establish diagnosis and then curetted and packed with bone graft. However, in aggressive large lesions, a curettage may not be enough. In such cases, a suitable resection of the cyst is required followed by suitable reconstruction (Figs. 6.6a–d, 6.7a–d, and 6.8a–e).

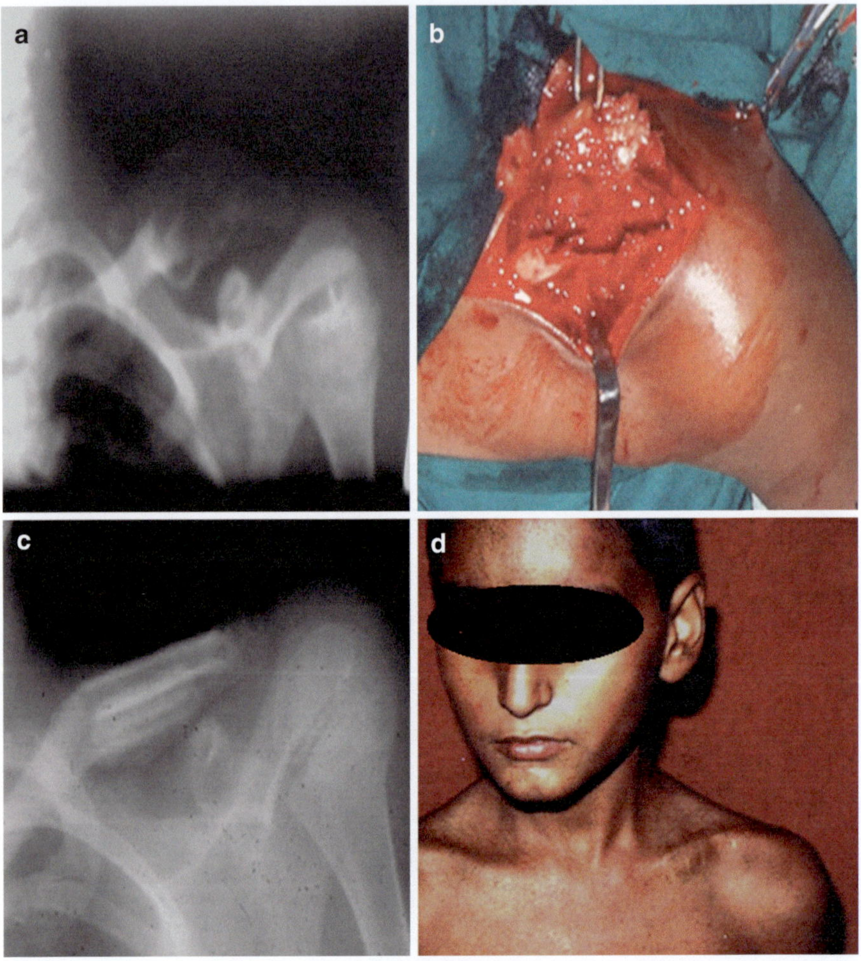

Fig. 6.6 (**a**) Radiograph of a 13-year-old boy with huge aneurysmal bone cyst of the left clavical. The bone had almost disappeared at the lateral end. (**b**) Intraoperative picture during excision of the lesion. (**c**) Roentgenogram shows twin fibular grafts stabilized with Kirschner wires (wires removed). The construct had healed completely. (**d**) Postoperative picture of the patient 2 year after surgery

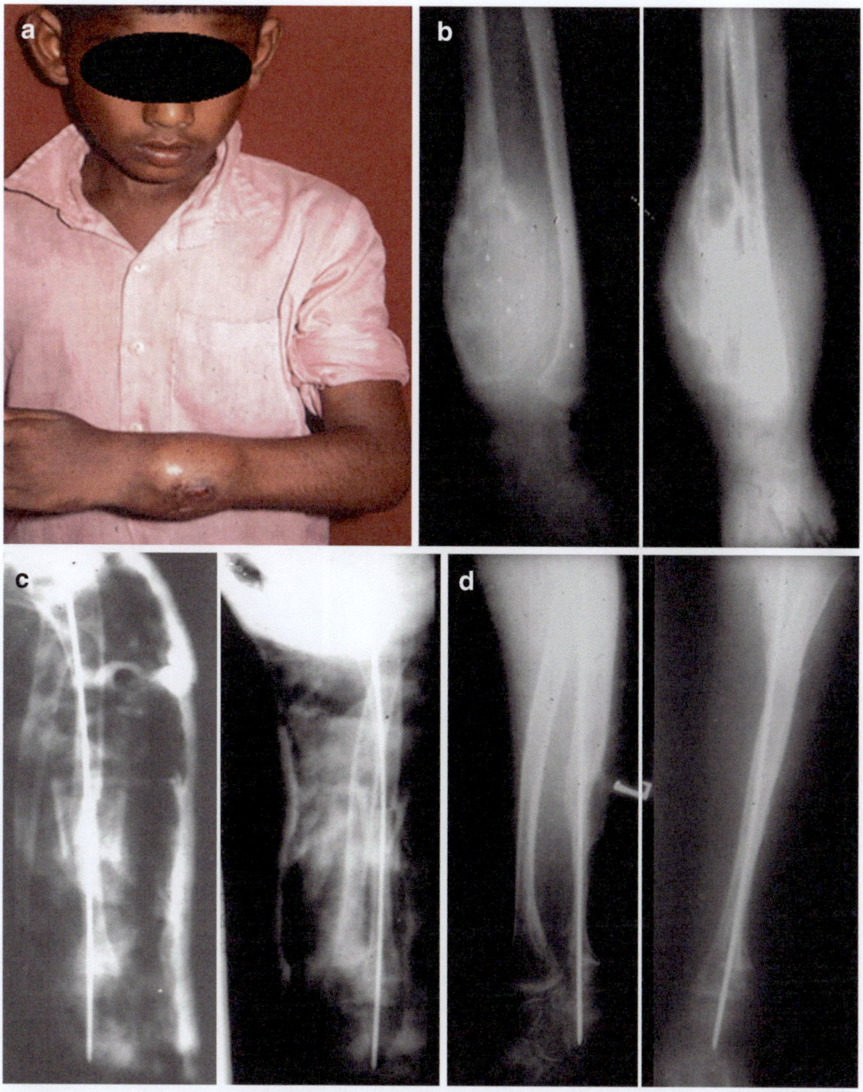

Fig. 6.7 (**a**) A 10-year-old boy with swelling at the lower end of the left distal forearm on the left side. (**b**) Roentgenogram reveals evidence of a huge aneurysmal bone cyst at the distal end of the ulna. (**c**) The lesion was excised, and a single graft from the proximal fibula (turned upside down) stabilized with a Kirschner wire was attempted. (**d**) Radiograph reveals complete healing of the graft at both its ends

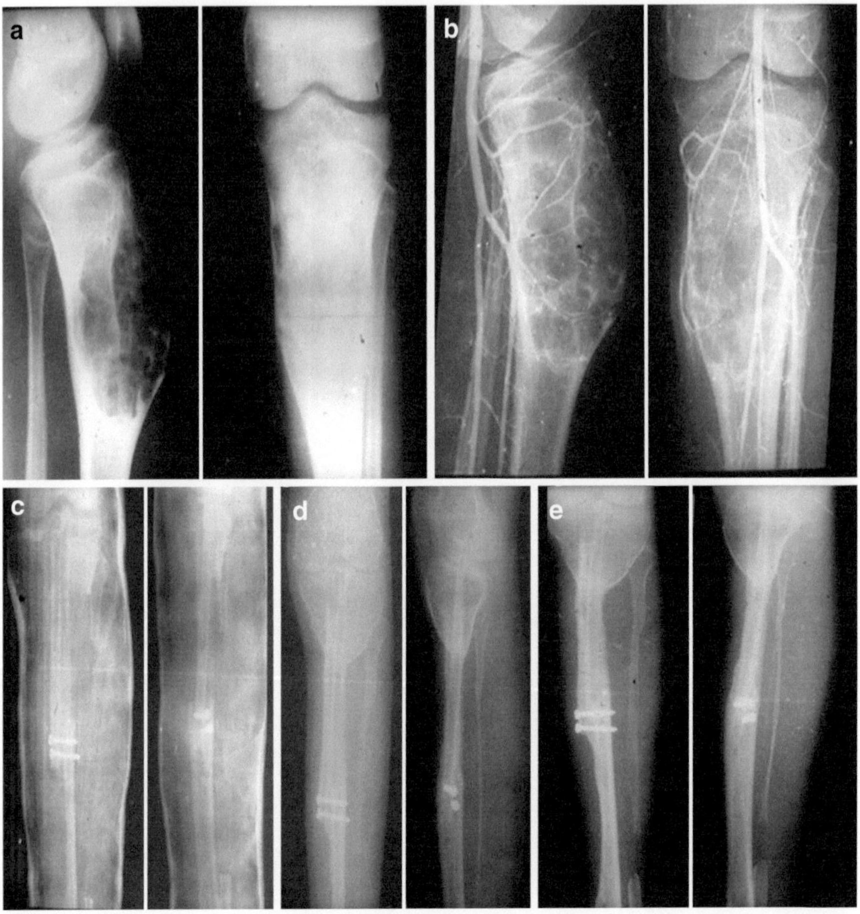

Fig. 6.8 (**a**) Radiograph revealing huge ABC of the proximal end of the right tibia involving the major part of the bone. (**b**) Angiogram revealing the blood supply of the lesion. Note the major involvement of the bone by the lesion. (**c**) The lesion was excised, and the gap was bridged by bisecting the diaphysis of the tibia which was then slid upwards, along with one fibular strut graft. The graft was wedged into the proximal tibia, with screw fixation at its distal end. The construct was further stabilized with a POP cast. (**d**) The grafts reveal healing after 6 months. (**e**) Complete healing and hypertrophy of the construct after a year. Note the regeneration of the fibula. This is one of our earlier cases—a technique not practiced these days

6.6 Giant Cell Tumour (GCT)

A giant cell tumour of bone occurs predominantly in the late teenage years or during the third or fourth decade and is rare in patients with an open epiphysis. The patient complains of a mild, dull pain and often has symptoms suggestive of an internal derangement of the adjacent joint. It is not uncommon to see a patient with a pathologic fracture through the lesion. The patient is more likely to be a girl with

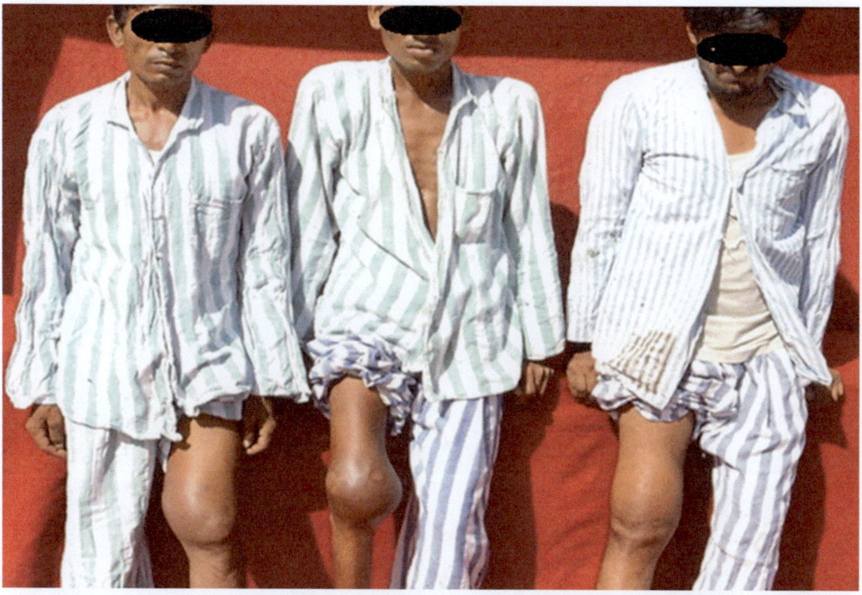

Fig. 6.9 Three cases of giant cell tumours at the lower end of the femur, admitted on a single day

symptoms in the knee. More than 50% of cases arise in the distal femur and proximal tibia (Fig. 6.9). The distal radius, proximal humerus, proximal fibula and sacrum are other common sites. But a giant cell tumour of bone may occur in any bone (Figs. 6.10, 6.11, 6.12, 6.13, 6.14a–e, and 6.15a–c). Radiolucent lesions in the vertebral body of a young patient are usually giant cell tumours.

On physical examination, atrophy of the muscles that control the joint adjacent to the tumour may be observed. Frequently, especially in those lesions arising from the distal radius, an extraosseous mass can be palpated. This mass is warm, firm and slightly tender. The entire skeleton should be examined because a giant cell tumour of bone may present with multiple lesions. The patient's parathyroid glands should be examined because hyperparathyroidism may produce brown tumour that are radiographically and histologically similar to a giant cell tumour of bone.

The plain radiograph of a giant cell tumour is almost diagnostic (Fig. 6.10a–f). The tumour is a radiolucent lesion that involves the epiphysis and metaphysis of a long bone. It invariably extends to and sometimes through the subchondral bone. An angiogram demonstrates the hypervascularity of the lesion but does not significantly contribute to the evaluation. The CT and MRI scans show the extent of the tumour better than the plain films and demonstrate cortical destruction more accurately. A giant cell tumour of bone has an increased uptake on the technetium bone scan. Histopathology demonstrates multiple tumour giant cells (Figs. 6.12a, b and 6.13a, b).

Earlier in the past, the majority of giant cell tumours of bone were treated by simple curettage and bone grafting. Because of the frequency of local recurrence

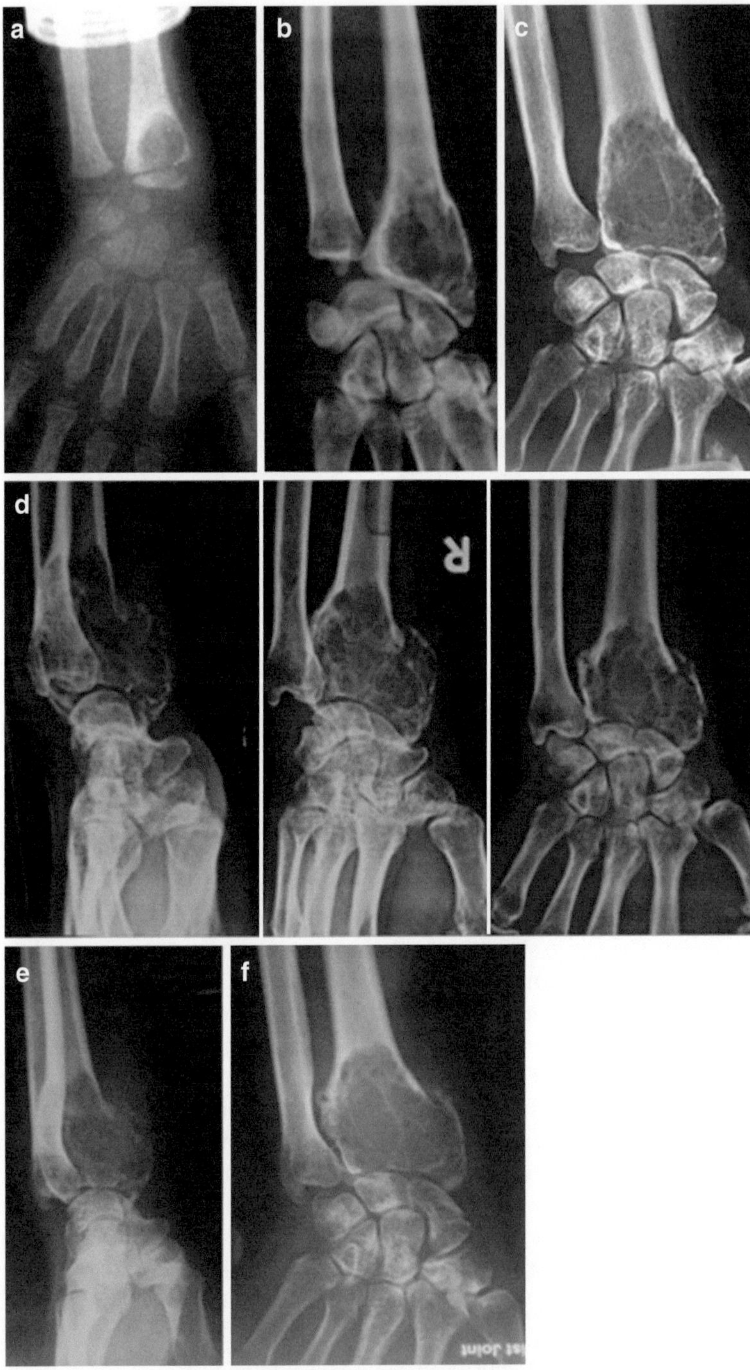

Fig. 6.10 (**a–f**) These radiographs serially reveal lytic lesions at the distal end of the radius which clearly suggest the possibility of a giant cell tumour. (**d–f**) Radiographs reveal a large growth of the lesion which has resulted in pathological fracture. The lower end of the radius is the third common site for the GCT

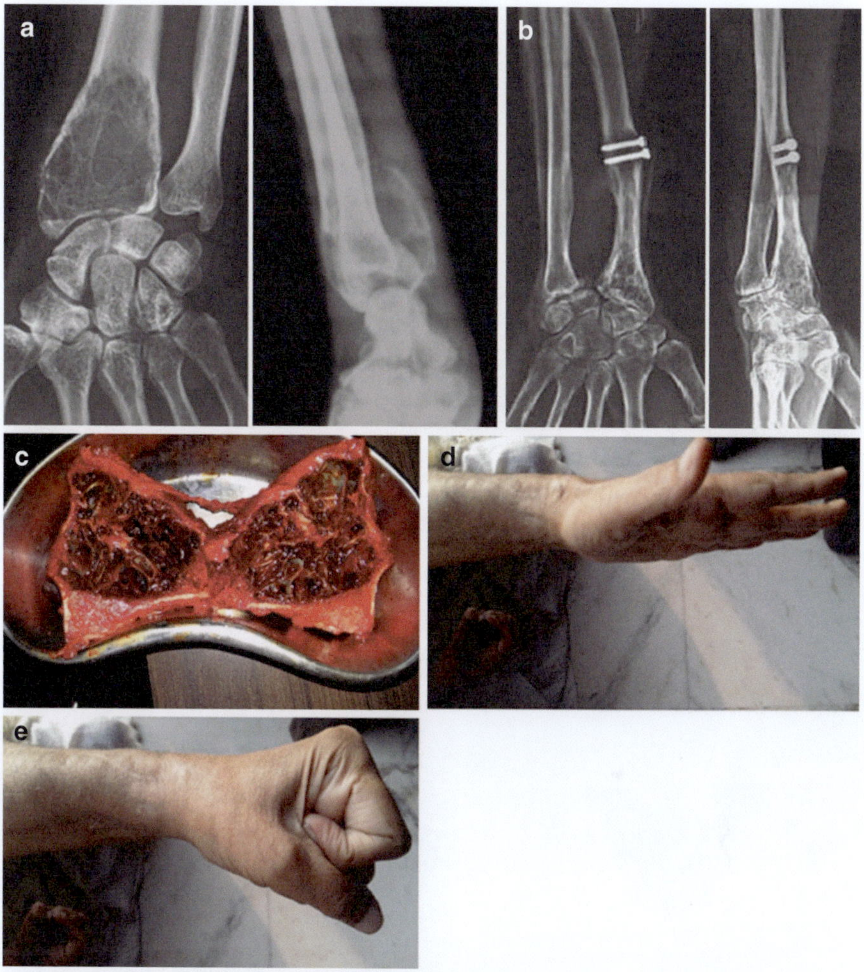

Fig. 6.11 (**a–e**) AP and lateral radiographs reveal a large GCT (still within the bone). The lesion was excised, and reconstruction was performed with the proximal end of the fibula stabilized with screws proximally and Kirschner wires distally (removed) 27 years ago. This 'Sadhu-Guru' has a very good function of the hand with full flexion and extension of the wrist and the fingers

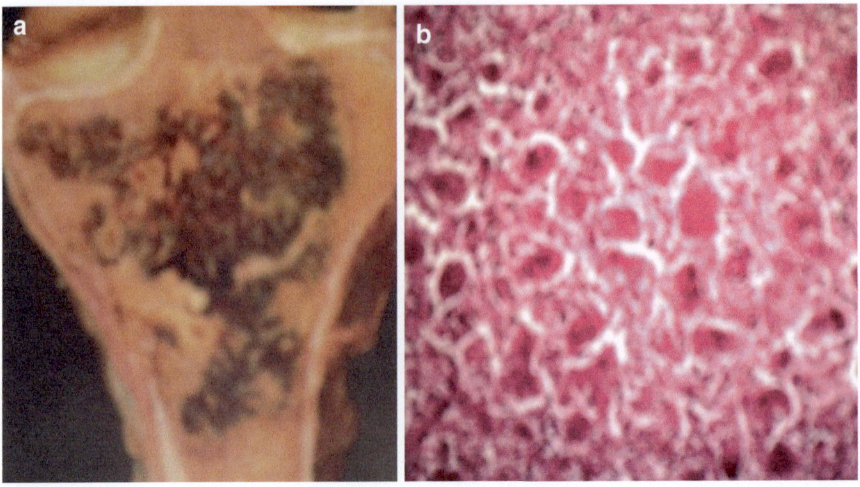

Fig. 6.12 (**a**) The gross appearance of the GCT. The tumour varies from yellow to brown in colour. (**b**) GCT (low magnification) consists of numerous mononuclear cells along with multinucleated giant cells

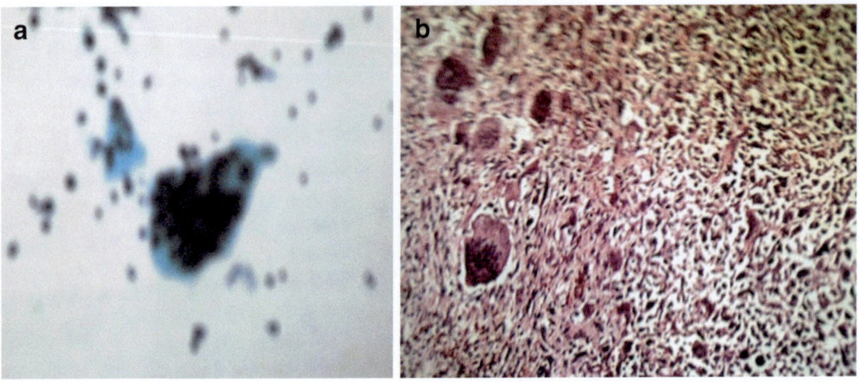

Fig. 6.13 (**a**) An aspiration biopsy of the GCT reveals many multinucleated giant cells. (**b**) The lesion reveals a typical benign GCT along with a clear picture of a sarcomatous component

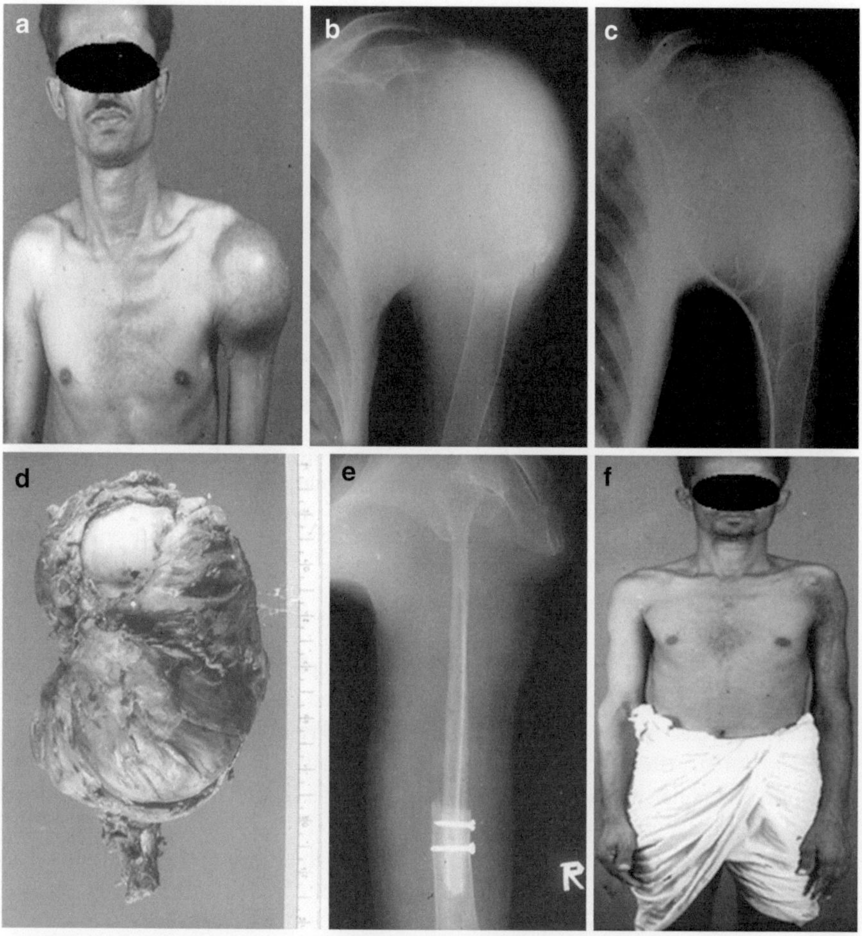

Fig. 6.14 (**a**) A huge GCT of the proximal end of the left humerus. (**b**) Roentgenogram revealing the lesion. (**c**) An angiogram revealing displacement of the left axillary artery. (**d**) The excised specimen of the proximal end of the humerus. (**e**) The gap was bridged by a long, single fibular strut, stabilized proximally in the glenoid and distally inlaid into the proximal end of the remaining humerus, fixed with a pair of screws (this was one of our earlier cases). Now, we use twin fibular grafts with shoulder arthrodesis. (**f**) Clinical picture of the patient

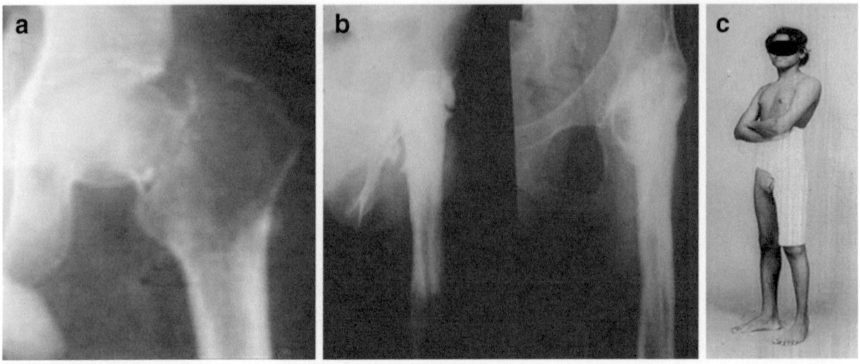

Fig. 6.15 (**a**) Radiographs reveal a GCT of the trochanteric region of the left femur. (**b**) Excision was done, and reconstruction was attempted with a twin fibular graft after wedging the graft at both ends supported by a POP hip spica cast (one of our earlier cases). The radiograph shows complete healing of the of the construct with lateral union after 18 months of arthrodesis of the hip joint. (**c**) The patient could stand and walk a little in this short hip spica. Note the sound union with improved quality and added quantity of the twin NVFG with no complication (nowadays, fixation of the graft was achieved using an L-plate)

and the inability to predict the behaviour of giant cell tumours, surgical resection became popular. Although these resections controlled giant cell tumours better than curettage, it occasionally results in functional loss (Figs. 6.11a–e, 6.16a–c, 6.17a, b, 6.18, and 6.19). After excision, the gap was bridged with fibular grafts stabilized with long Kirschner wires (Figs. 6.20a–f, 6.21, 6.26a–g, and 6.27a–c). At the knee and hip, the fibular struts were fixed with an L-plate (Figs. 6.18a–d, 6.19a, b, 6.22a–f, 6.23a–d, 6.24a–d, 6.25, 6.26, and 6.27). GCTs at the lower end of the radius and at the distal tibia were stabilized with cross Kirschner wires and screws (Figs. 6.28a, b, 6.29a–e, 6.30a–e, and 6.31a–d).

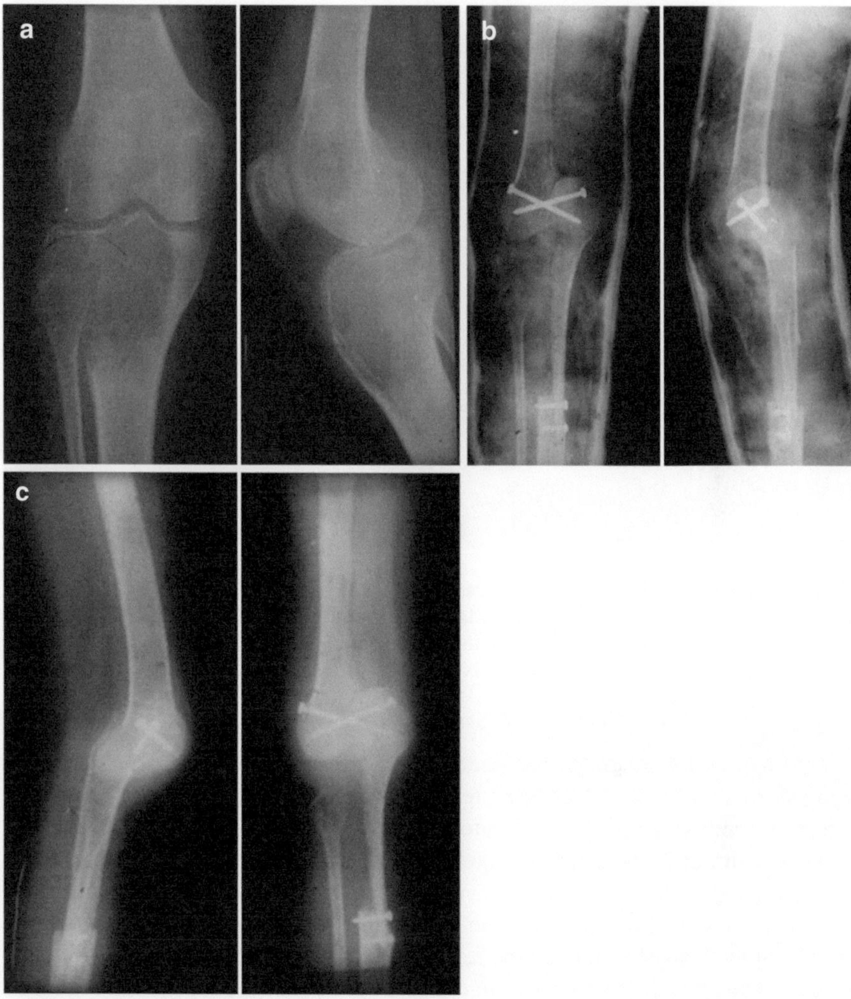

Fig. 6.16 (**a**) AP and lateral radiograph showing a GCT of the proximal end of the right tibia. (**b**, **c**) Radiograph reveals an old method of bridging a bone defect after bisection of the distal femur and turning it down, stabilized with screws. This procedure is not practised these days

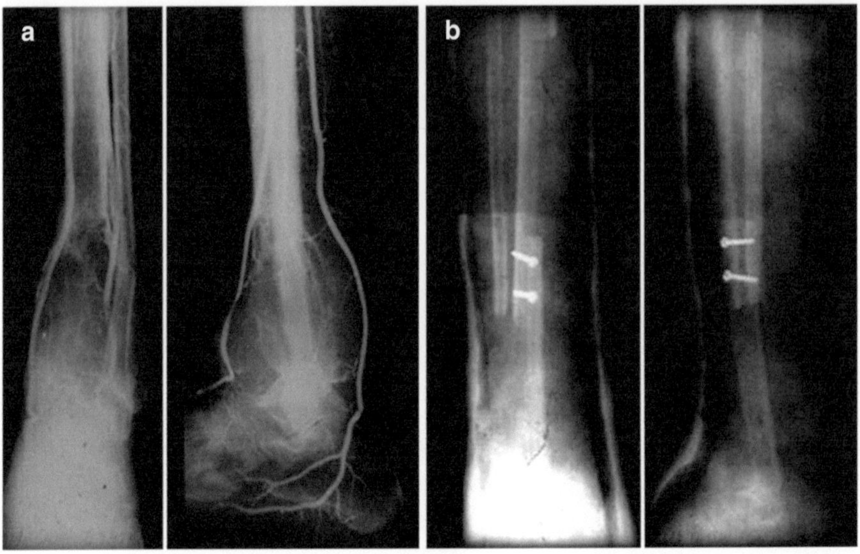

Fig. 6.17 (**a**) Angiogram reveals the vascularity of a GCT involving the distal end of the left tibia and reveals near-normal vascularity of the lesion. (**b**) After excision of the lesion, the tibia was bisected and slid down to bridge the gap, then stabilized distally by arthrodesis and proximally fixed with a pair of screws. This procedure is also not practiced nowadays

Less aggressive treatment has been used as an initial management. Numerous adjuvant treatments to reduce local recurrence have been tried. The most popular treatment method is an extended curettage with the use of a high-speed burr and packing with polymethylmethacrylate (PMMA) or bone. The most important part of the curettage is to see the entire cavity at the time of the operation. A wide opening in the bone must be made, and the curettage must be complete beyond the reactive rim of the bone surrounding the lesion. Cryosurgery (freezing of the lesion) has been used and has been successful in eradicating the tumour, but it has a high incidence of complications.

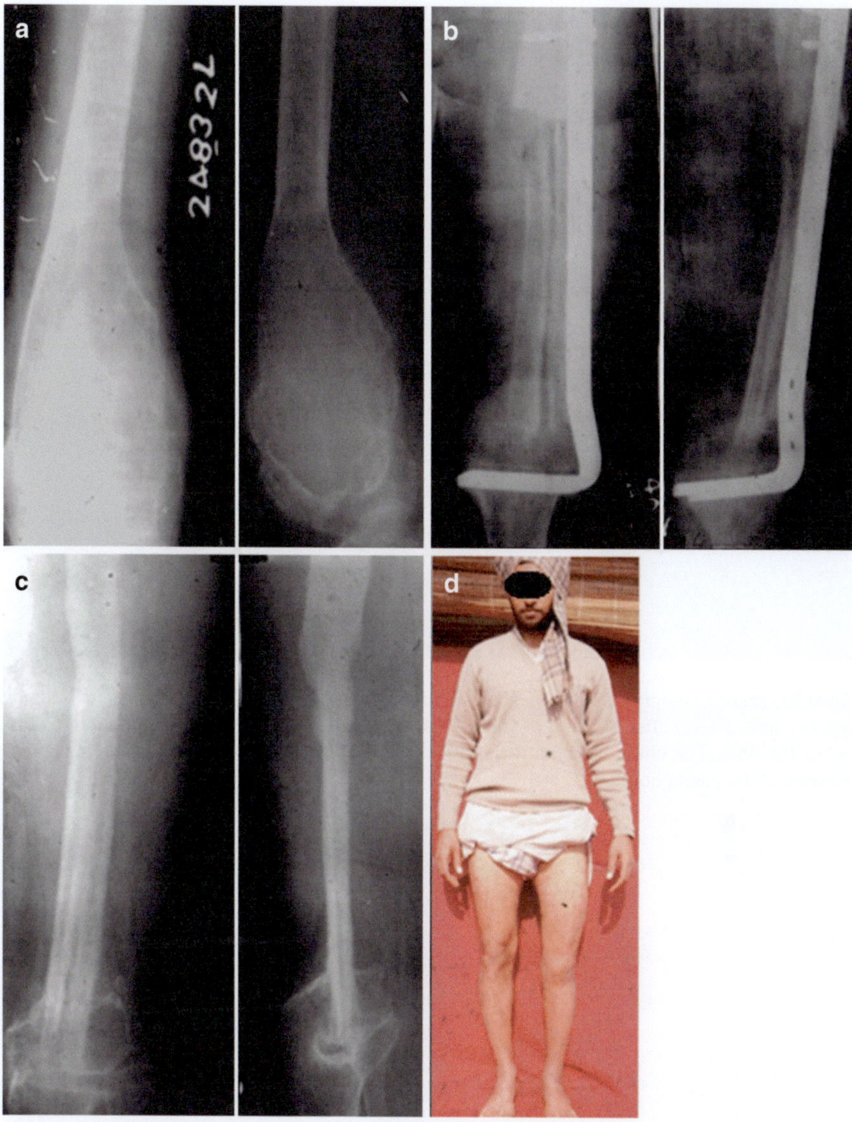

Fig. 6.18 (**a**) AP and lateral radiograph illustrates a large giant cell tumour involving the lower end of the femur. (**b**) A 34-year-old male with a GCT (grade III) of the lower end of the femur. En bloc excision was performed, followed by reconstruction using a dual fibular graft stabilized with an L-plate. (**c**) Roentgenogram with 'lateral union' between two struts with hypertrophy of the construct. The plate has been removed after 10 months. (**d**) Clinical picture of the patient

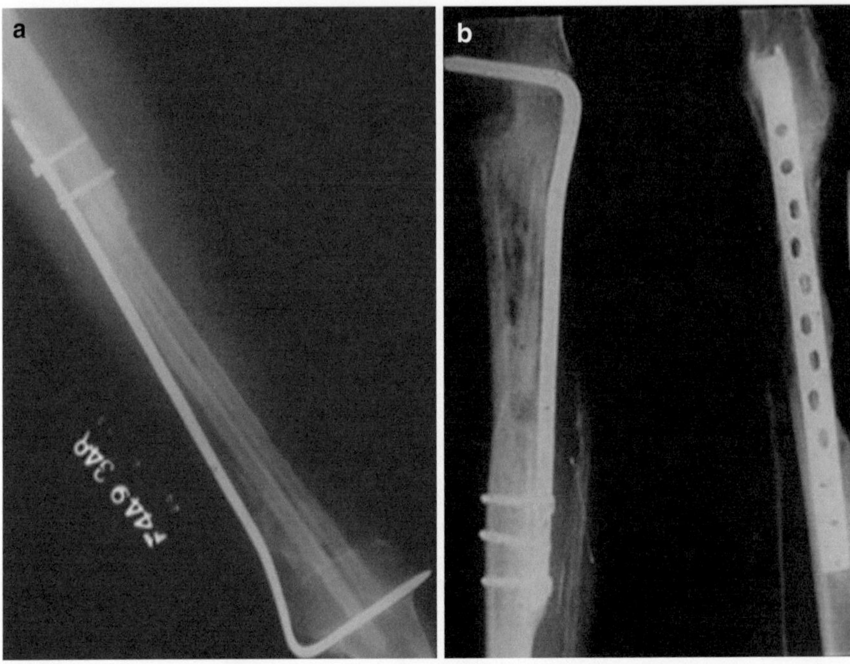

Fig. 6.19 (**a**, **b**) Radiographs illustrate the twin fibular struts stabilized with an L-plate in bridging massive bone defects after excision of various lesions at the lower end of the femur and proximal end of the tibia. The union between the struts takes place by lateral union which simulates the diameter of the parent bone

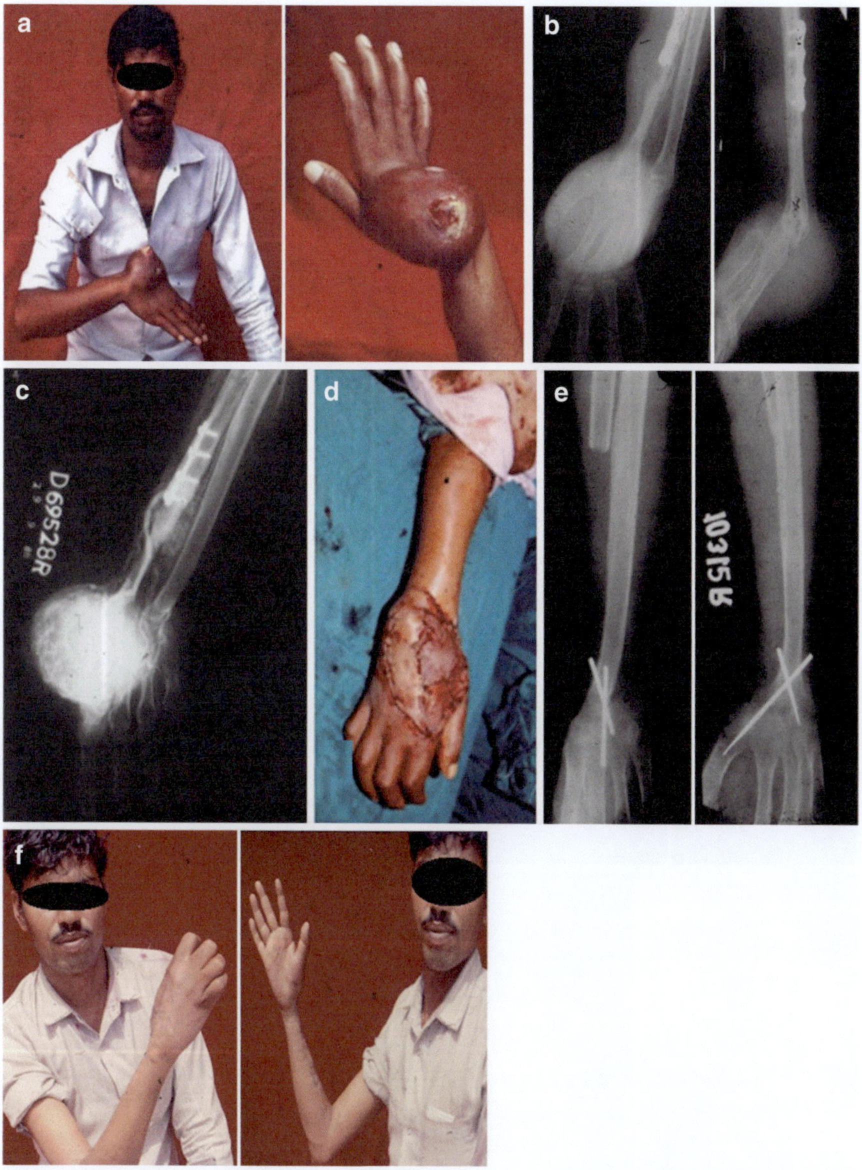

Fig. 6.20 (**a**) Clinical picture of a huge, recurrent and infected GCT of the distal radius on the right side. (**b**, **c**) Radiograph and angiogram of the recurrent and infected lesion, which was previously excised and reconstructed with a fibular graft fixed with a plate (in other centre), reveals huge recurrence. (**d**) The lesion was excised, and split skin graft was done on the dorsal aspect of the hand. (**e**) The radiograph illustrates a single bone forearm between the distal ulna and carpal bones arthrodesing the wrist joint. (**f**) The forearm and the function of the hand 8 months after surgery. The hand had been functional

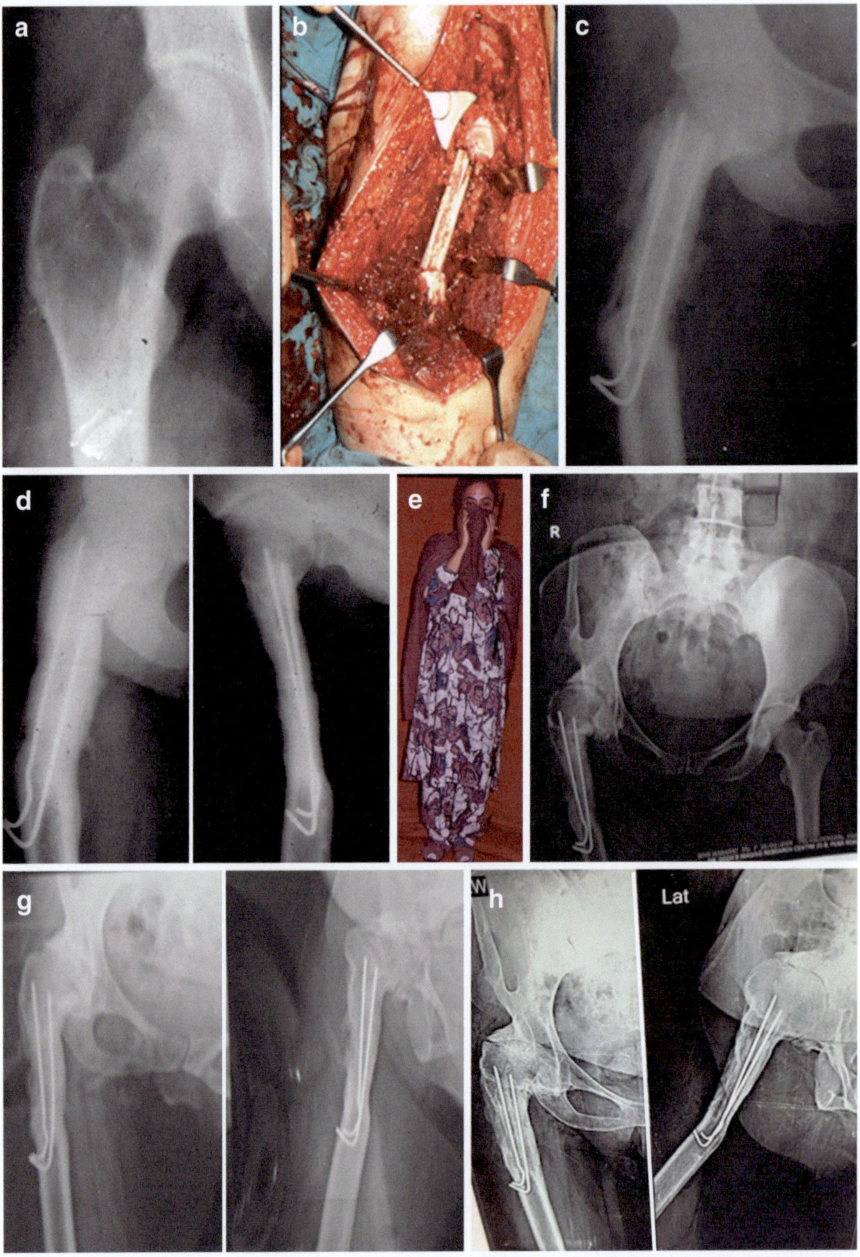

Fig. 6.21 (**a–e**) A 22-year-old girl had a giant cell tumour of the trochanteric region of the right femur. The lesion was resected, and dual fibular grafts were placed proximally between the head and the remaining neck and distally with the proximal end of the femur, stabilized by twin Kirschner wires (a three-point fixation). The construct was further supported by POP spica for 5 weeks. Complete healing, hypertrophy and lateral union took place in 10 months, and the patient had been active. (**f–h**) A 30-year follow-up of the same patient reveals signs of AVN (avascular necrosis) with osteoarthrosis. However, she could still manage her household duties with 2.5 cm shoe raise

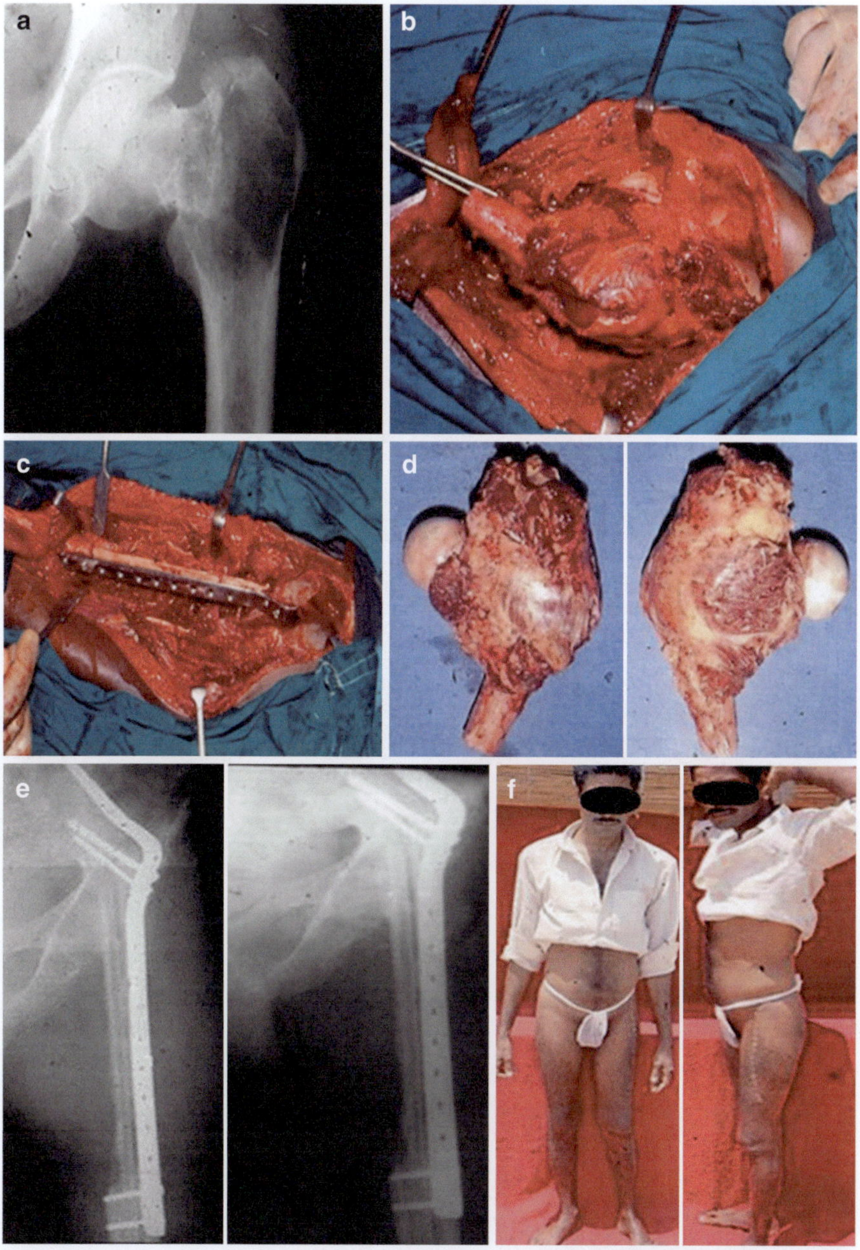

Fig. 6.22 (**a**) Radiograph reveals a large GCT of the trochanteric area with pathological fracture. (**b**) Intraoperative picture during excision. (**c**) Intraoperative picture showing twin fibular grafting with L-plate fixation. (**d**) The front and back of the excised specimen. (**e**) Radiograph illustrating the twin fibular graft stabilized with an L-plate and screws arthrodesing the hip joint. The construct has healed with lateral union between the struts. (**f**) The front and side view of the patient 8 months after the surgery. A long operative scar is visible on the thigh

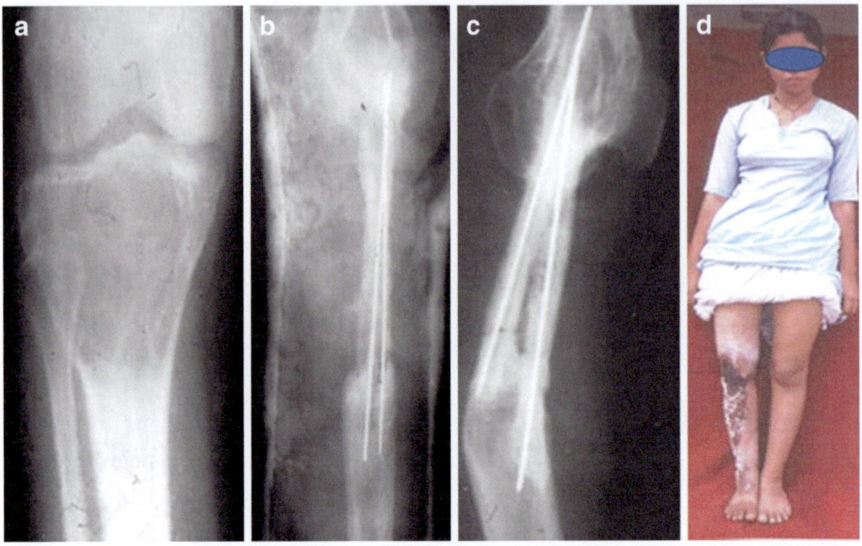

Fig. 6.23 (**a**) A 19-year-old girl had a GCT of the upper end of the right tibia. (**b**) Excision of the lesion was followed by twin fibular grafts, with Kirschner wires fixed to the remaining host bone on either side, and further stabilized by a POP cast. (**c**) Although the fixation was not very sound, healing took place in 12 months. The result reveals the enhanced osteogenic capacity of the NVFG we have been using. (**d**) Clinical picture of the patient (one of our earlier cases; now, we use an L-plate for fixation as shown earlier)

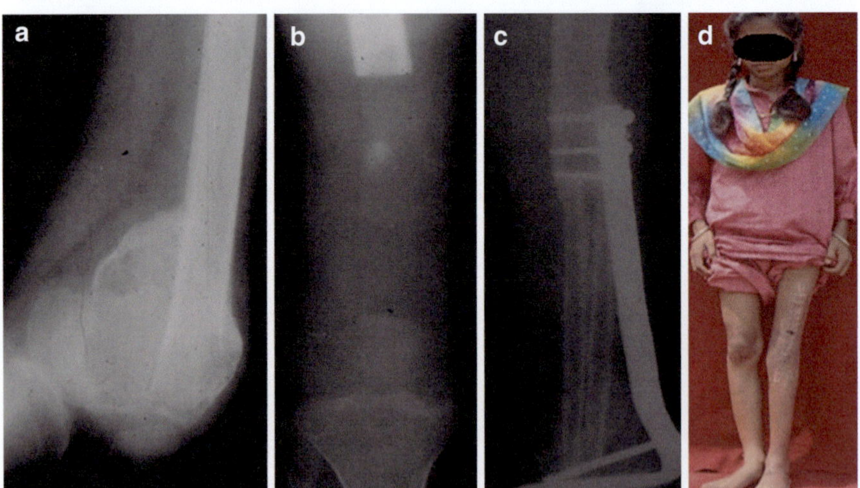

Fig. 6.24 (**a–d**) A 26-year-old girl had a GCT of the lower end of the left femur with neglected pathological fracture with mal-union. The lesion was excised as it is, and skeletal traction was applied as the first stage. After gaining the required length, dual fibular grafting was stabilized by an L-plate. The construct revealed union in 10 months. Clinical picture of the patient

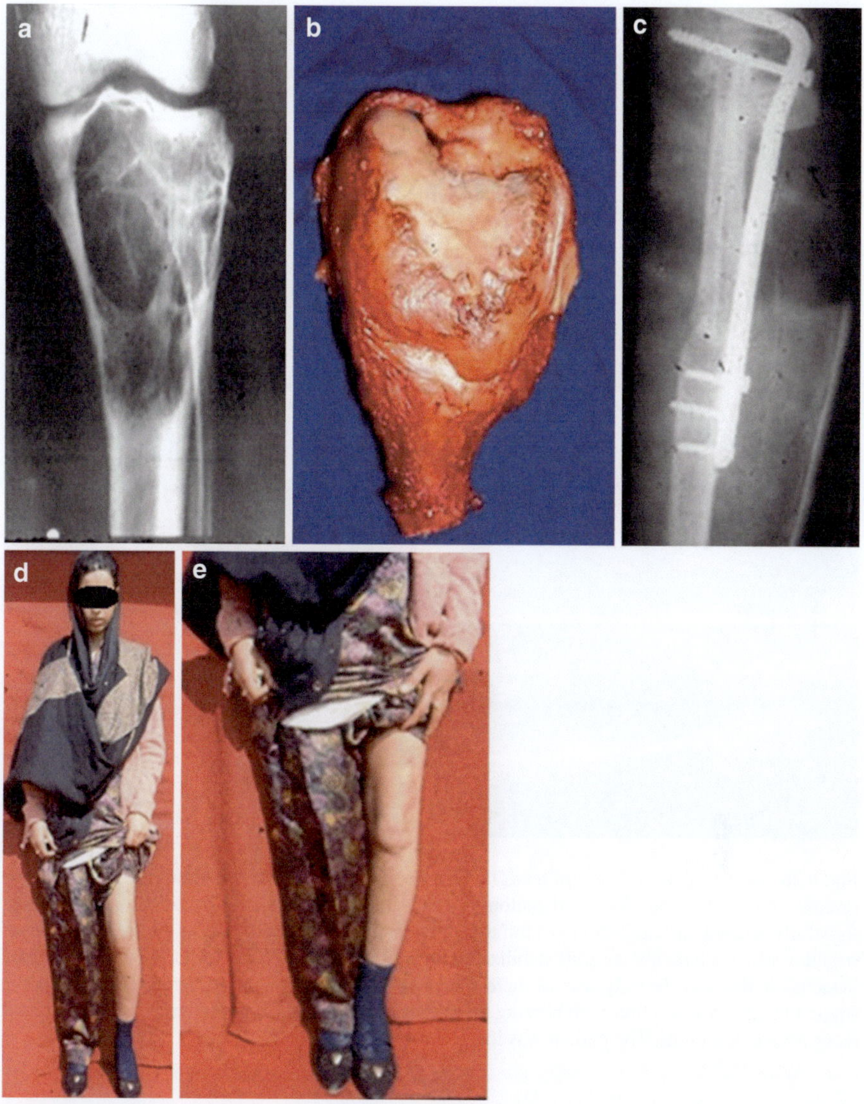

Fig. 6.25 (**a**) The radiograph reveals a GCT involving the epiphysio-metaphyseal area of the left proximal tibia. (**b**) The excised specimen. (**c**) Reconstruction was attempted with twin fibular grafts stabilized with an L-plate. The radiograph shows complete healing with lateral union. (**d**, **e**) Clinical picture of the patient 1 year after surgery

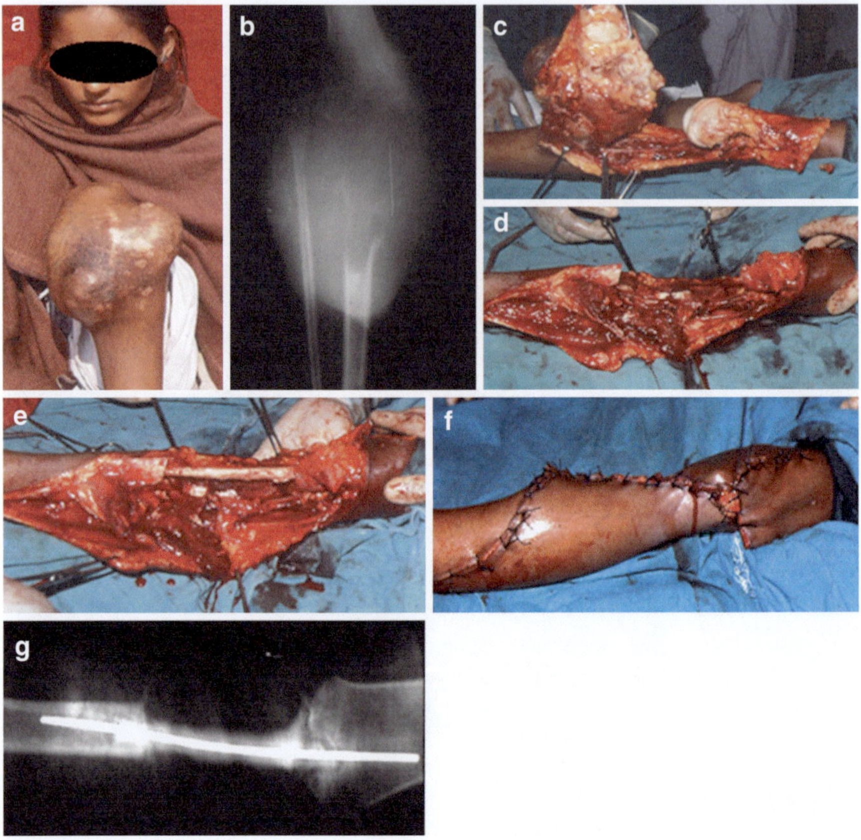

Fig. 6.26 (**a**) An advanced case of a GCT of the proximal end of the left tibia. (**b**) AP radiograph reveals a huge GCT with disturbed anatomy. This was a fit case for an amputation, but the patient forcefully refused the suggestion. (**c**) Intraoperative pictures of the excision of the mass and reconstruction with a single fibular graft stabilized with a long Kirschner wire. (**d–f**) Though it appeared inadequate, this was the only way as there was gross loss of skin. (**g**) Radiograph reveals that the single fibular reconstruction is stabilizing the graft at both its ends, showing early healing without recurrence at 8 months. The patient was lost to follow-up

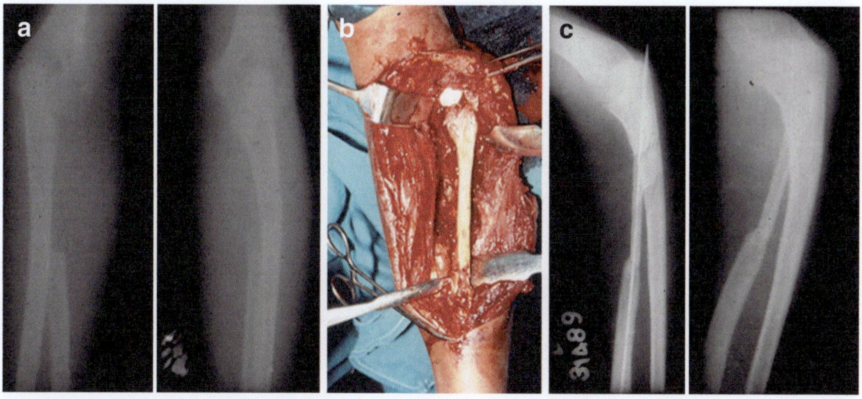

Fig. 6.27 (**a**) Radiograph reveals a huge GCT of the proximal radius. (**b**) Intraoperative picture after excision of the lesion and reconstruction with the proximal end of the fibula (simulating the radial head) stabilized with a long Kirschner wire. (**c**) The wire was removed after healing took place in 10 months

Nearly 5% of patients with a giant cell tumour of bone develop pulmonary metastasis. Although irradiation also has been used, resections are reserved for the neglected large lesions, lesions with pathologic fracture, or recurrent giant cell tumours. Patients with a metastatic giant cell tumour of bone usually are cured by surgical resection.

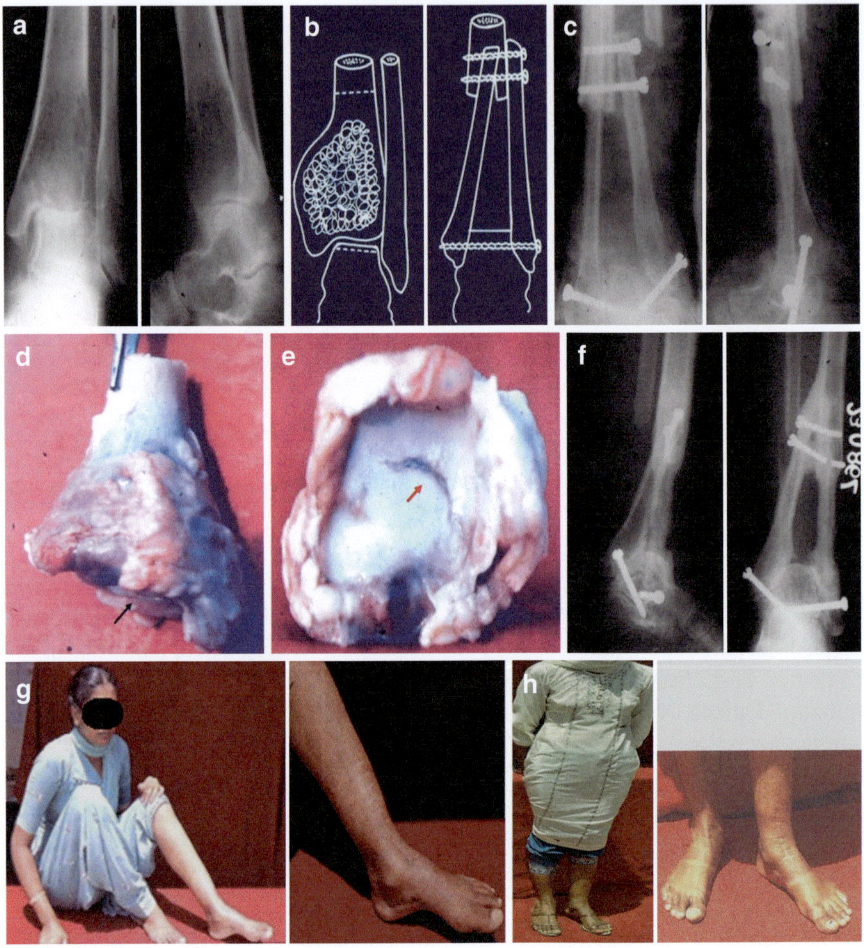

Fig. 6.28 (**a**) Roentgenogram of a 25-year-old lady revealed a GCT at the distal end of the left tibia involving the ankle joint. (**b**) A diagrammatic presentation of the excision and reconstruction plan with twin fibular grafts. The distal fibula has been medialized, and the proximal third of the fibula has been stabilized turning its head down. (**c**) Postoperative roentgenogram reveals the proposed excision and reconstruction. (**d**) The excised specimen reveals extension into the ankle joint (black arrow). (**e**) The specimen reveals a crack in the articular surface (red arrow which is usually not appreciated even on an MRI). (**f**) Roentgenogram taken after 8 months reveals complete healing and hypertrophy of the fibular struts. (**g**, **h**) Clinical pictures of the patient and the ankle reveal a near-normal appearance. The turned-down placement of the head of the fibula simulates the medial malleolus of the tibia

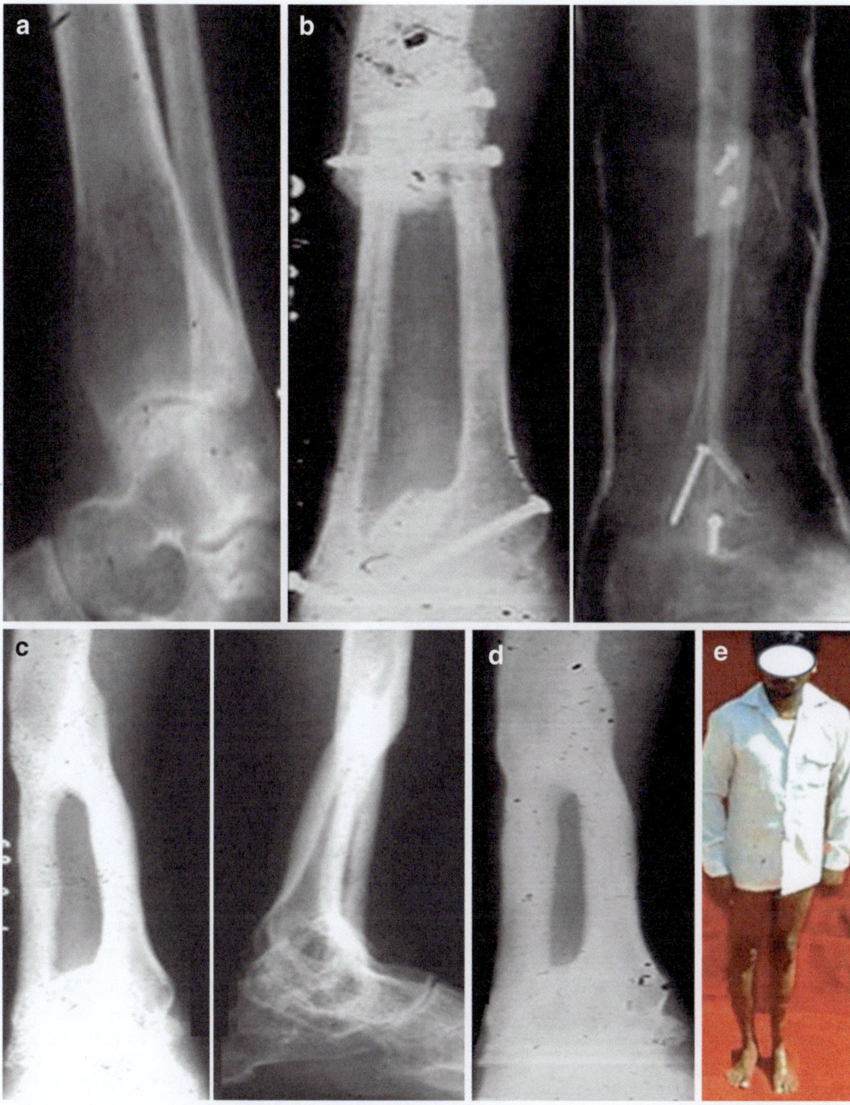

Fig. 6.29 (**a**) Roentgenogram of a 29-year-old man reveals a GCT of the distal end of the left tibia. (**b**) En bloc excision followed by twin fibular grafts fixed to the distal end of the tibia and body of the talus with screws. (**c**) En bloc excision followed by twin fibular grafts fixed to the distal end of the tibia and body with screws (screws have been removed). Note the hypertrophy of the fibular struts after 1 year. (**d**) AP and lateral roentgenogram after 2 years showing good union with hypertrophy of the fibular struts. (**e**) The clinical picture of the patient after surgery. Cosmetically, the left ankle simulates the right ankle

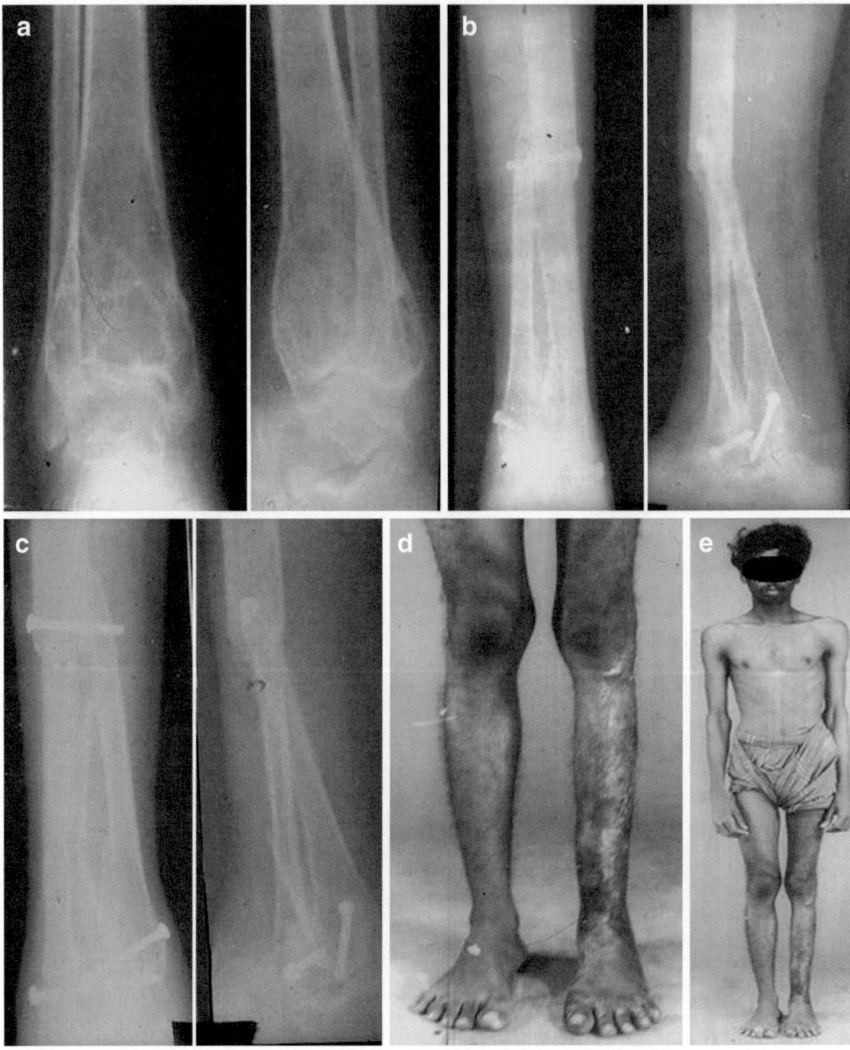

Fig. 6.30 (**a**) Roentgenogram reveals a GCT of the lower end of the left tibia. (**b**) Excision of the lesion and twin fibular grafting as suggested in the earlier case. (**c**) Follow-up roentgenogram taken 10 months after surgery reveals complete healing. (**d**, **e**) Clinical picture of the patient. The inverted head of the fibula now simulates the medial malleous

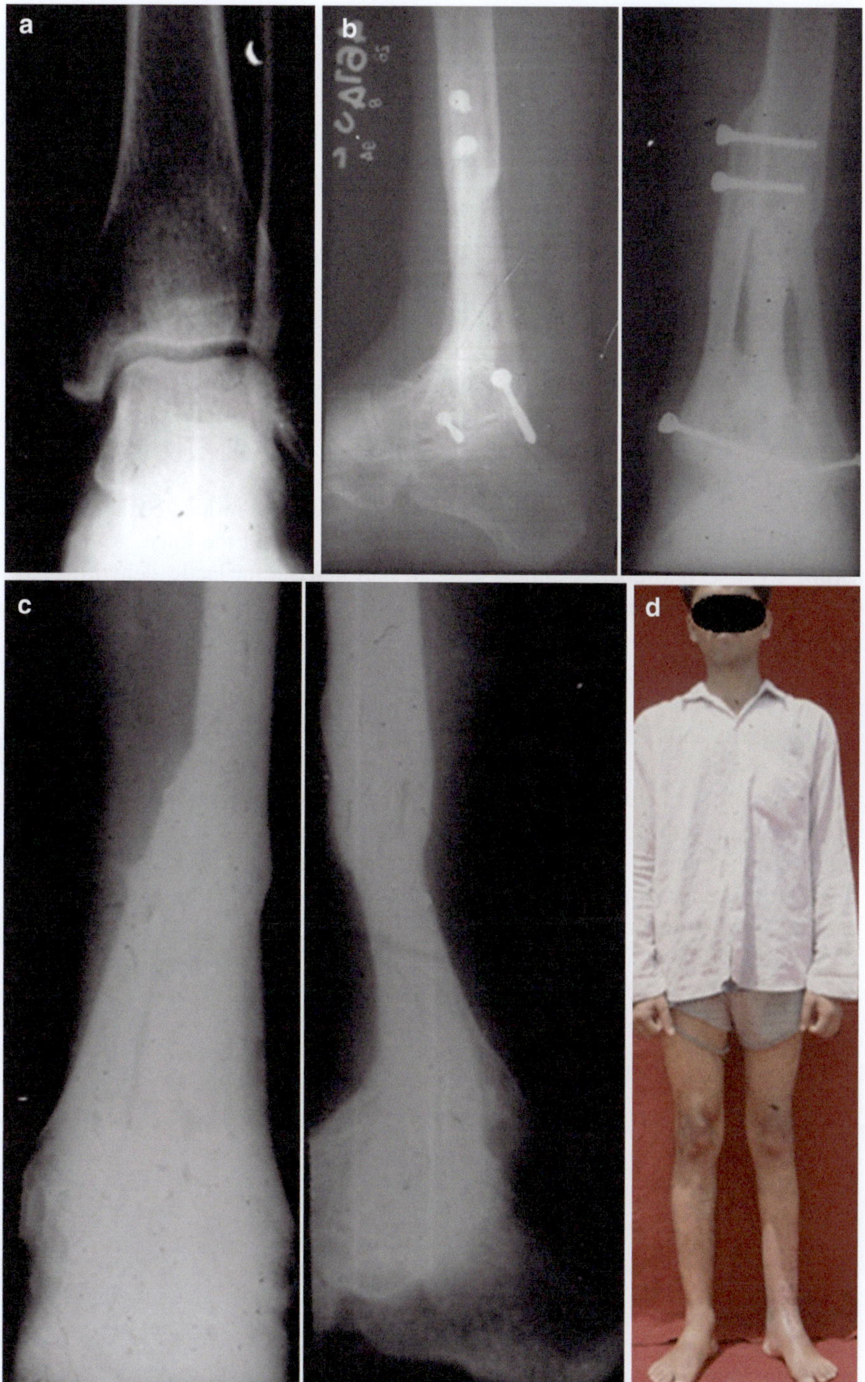

Fig. 6.31 (**a**) Roentgenogram reveals a GCT of the lower end of the right tibia. (**b**) Postoperative roentgenogram reveals three fibular struts fixed with screws. (**c**) Roentgenogram taken 1 year after surgery reveals complete healing and hypertrophy of the three struts with lateral union between the three struts. (**d**) Clinical picture of the patient

6.7 Osteosarcoma

Osteosarcoma is defined as a tumour in which malignant spindle cells produce bone. The more common osteosarcoma is called classic high-grade osteosarcoma or conventional osteosarcoma, and the other is called juxtacortical osteosarcoma. It accounts for approximately 20% of primary bone tumours. Some authors separate juxtacortical osteosarcomas into parosteal and periosteal osteosarcoma. Histologically, osteosarcomas are classified into osteoblastic, chondroblastic, fibroblastic, mixed and telangiectatic types. A radiograph of the chest should be obtained to observe for secondary metastases. The relation of osteosarcoma to the major neurovascular bundle must be determined. CT scan is performed because of a high incidence of patients presenting with pulmonary metastases. MRI is the best investigation to determine the anatomic extent of the lesion. Angiography has been important in certain cases, especially when there is a suggestion that the main blood vessels are encased by the tumour.

The patient is usually a teenager. Half of the lesions are located in the distal femur or proximal tibia. There is pain and a mass around the knee. An elevated serum alkaline phosphatase along with an elevated serum lactic dehydrogenase (LDH) has a bad prognosis.

Osteosarcomas should be resected with a wide surgical margin with suitable reconstruction. After en bloc resection, the gap is reconstructed with fibular grafts stabilized with long Kirschner wires (Figs. 6.32, 6.33a–h and 6.37a–f). At the hip and the knee, an L-plate has been used for fixation of the twin fibular grafts (Figs. 6.34a–e, 6.35a–d, 6.36a–c, 6.37, 6.38a–g). Preoperative and postoperative chemotherapy has been recommended. An amputation is indicated in cases of high-grade sarcoma with a grossly displaced pathological fracture and encasement of the neurovascular bundle. In rare cases, osteosarcoma has been observed at multiple sites. Most synchronous multifocal osteosarcomas have one dominant lesion with one to four more secondary lesions (Fig. 6.39a–c).

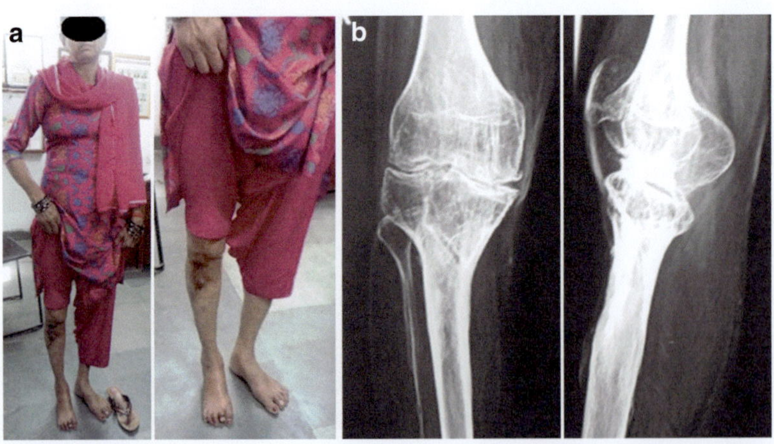

Fig. 6.32 (**a**) A 65-year-old lady had a GCT of the right proximal tibia. The lesion was excised, and reconstruction was done by twin fibular graft 40 years ago. (**b**) The recent radiograph reveals remodelling of the proximal tibia with no sign of the twin fibular graft. The knee reveals fibrous ankylosis

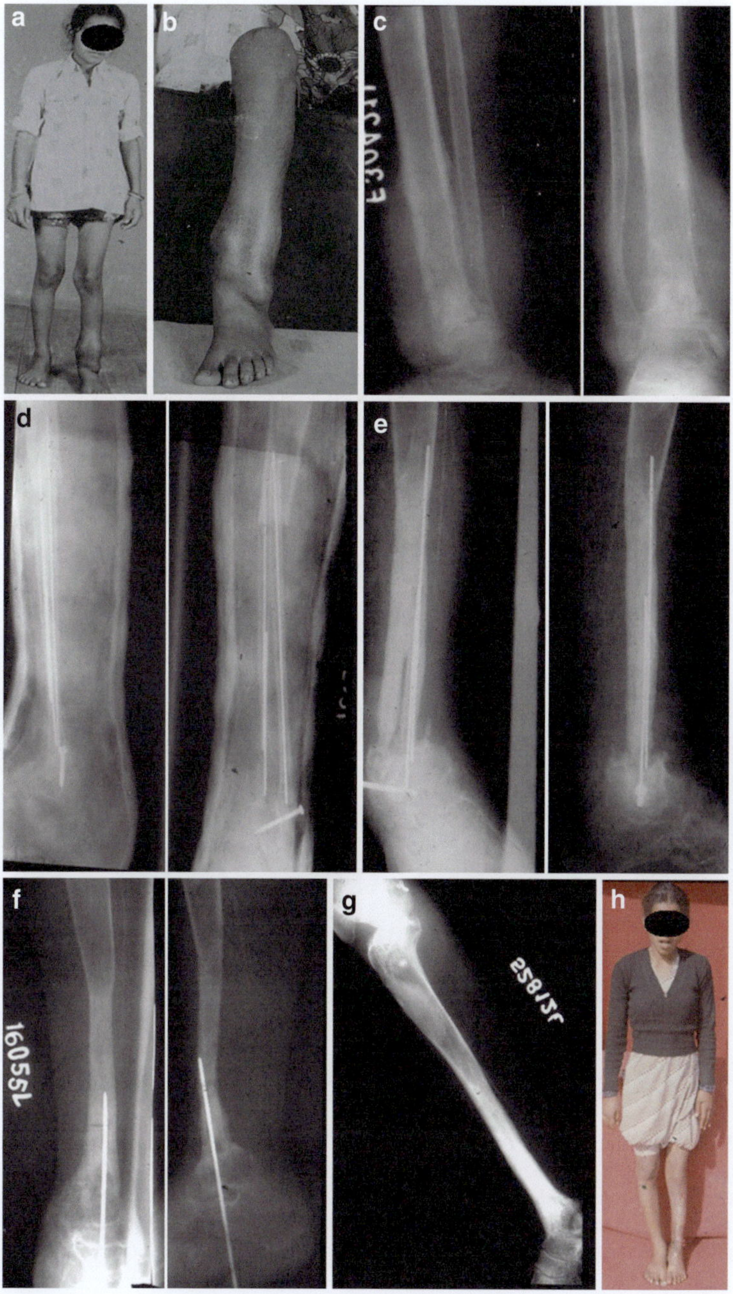

Fig. 6.33 (**a**, **b**) Conventional osteosarcoma of the distal end of the left tibia in a 16-year-old girl. (**c**) Radiograph revealing the extensive lesion with extension to the fibula. (**d**) Wide excision of the distal tibia and fibula. Twin-free fibular grafts have been stabilized with two Kirschner wires. (**e**) Subsequent radiograph shows non-union at the distal end. (**f**) Cancellous bone graft attempted with a 2.5-mm Kirschner wire through the calcaneus. (**g**) The final result with tibio-talar arthrodesis. (**h**) Clinical appearance of the patient after 1 year

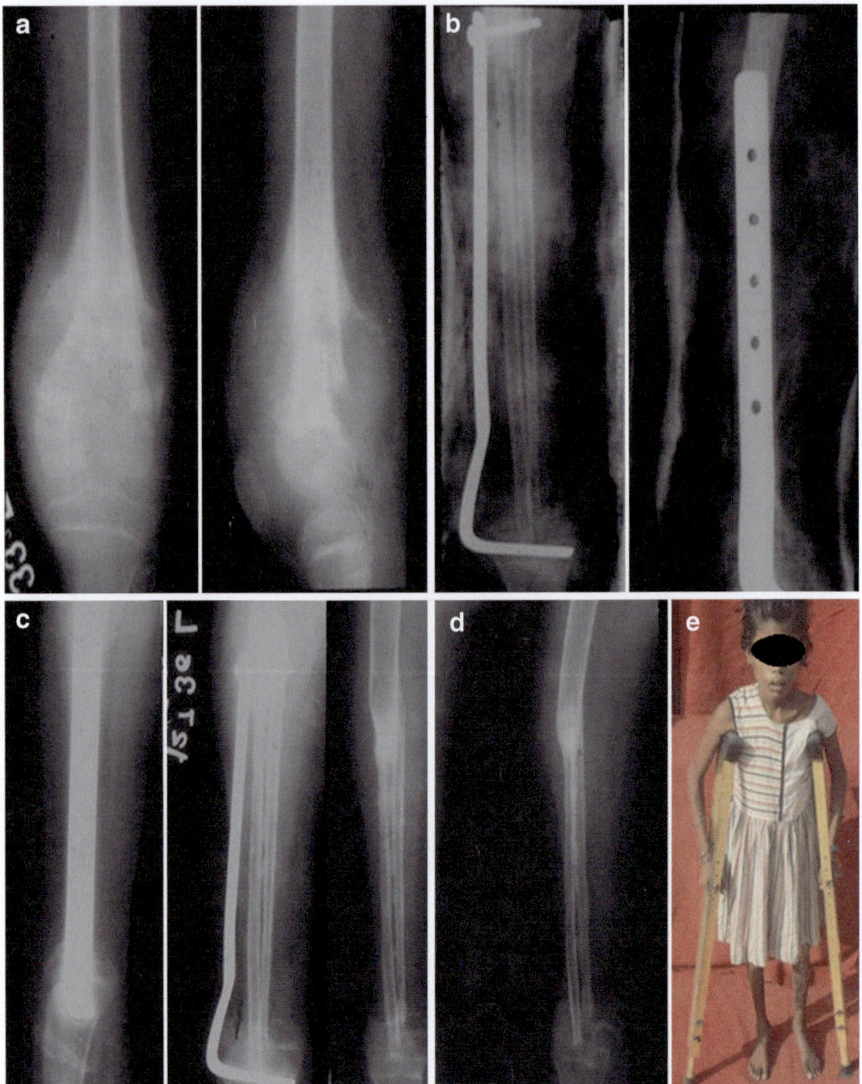

Fig. 6.34 (**a**) Osteosarcoma at the lower end of the femur. (**b**) Wide excision, double free fibular grafting fixed with an L-plate. (**c**) The graft in advanced stage of healing showing signs of lateral union. (**d**) The graft consolidates fully and the plate was removed. Note the onset of lateral union between the two fibular struts. (**e**) The patient walking with crutches after removal of the plaster. Although the limb was quite strong to bear weight, she died of chest metastases after 2 years

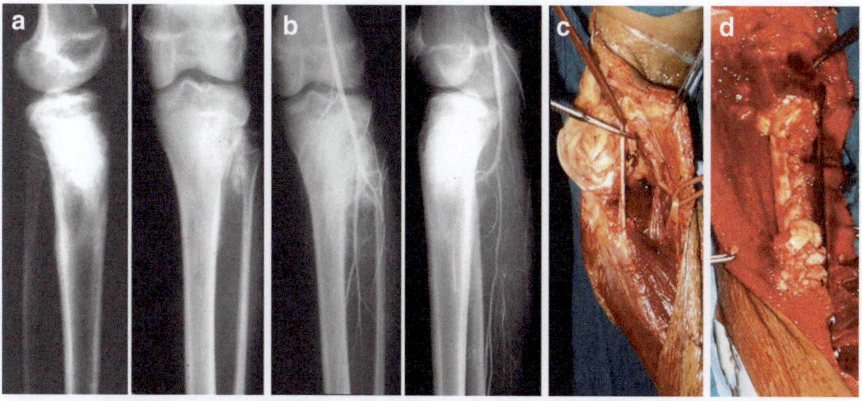

Fig. 6.35 (**a**) Osteosarcoma of the proximal tibia involving the proximal fibula. (**b**) Angiogram revealing the extension of the lesion to the fibular head. (**c**) Since the peroneal nerve could not be separated, it is seen being divided for a wide excision of the lesion. The head of the fibula also had to be excised. (**d**) Twin fibular grafts stabilized with an L-plate and covered with cancellous graft

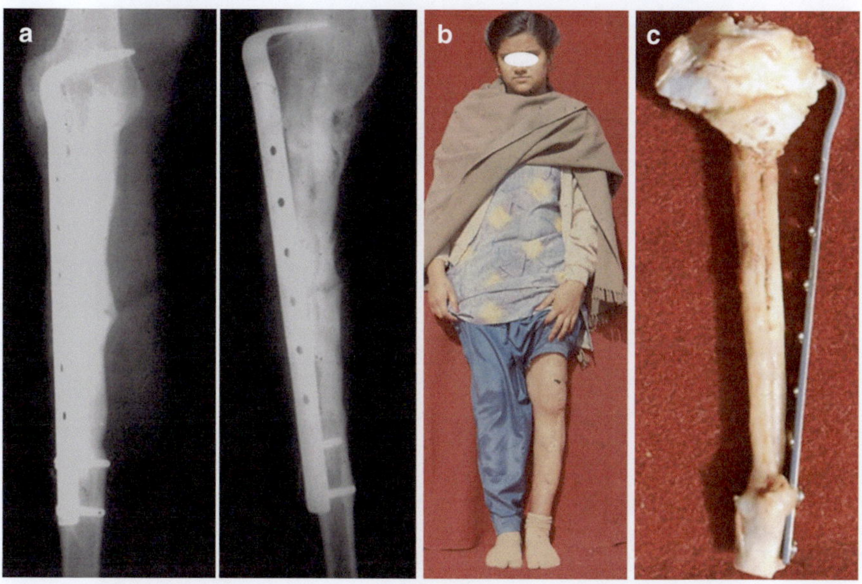

Fig. 6.36 (**a**) The graft fixed with an L-plate showing consolidation. (**b**) Patient with full weight-bearing. She died after 3 years with chest metastases. (**c**) Post-mortem specimen revealing lateral union of the twin fibular struts and complete consolidation with the parent bone, simulating the diameter of the tibia

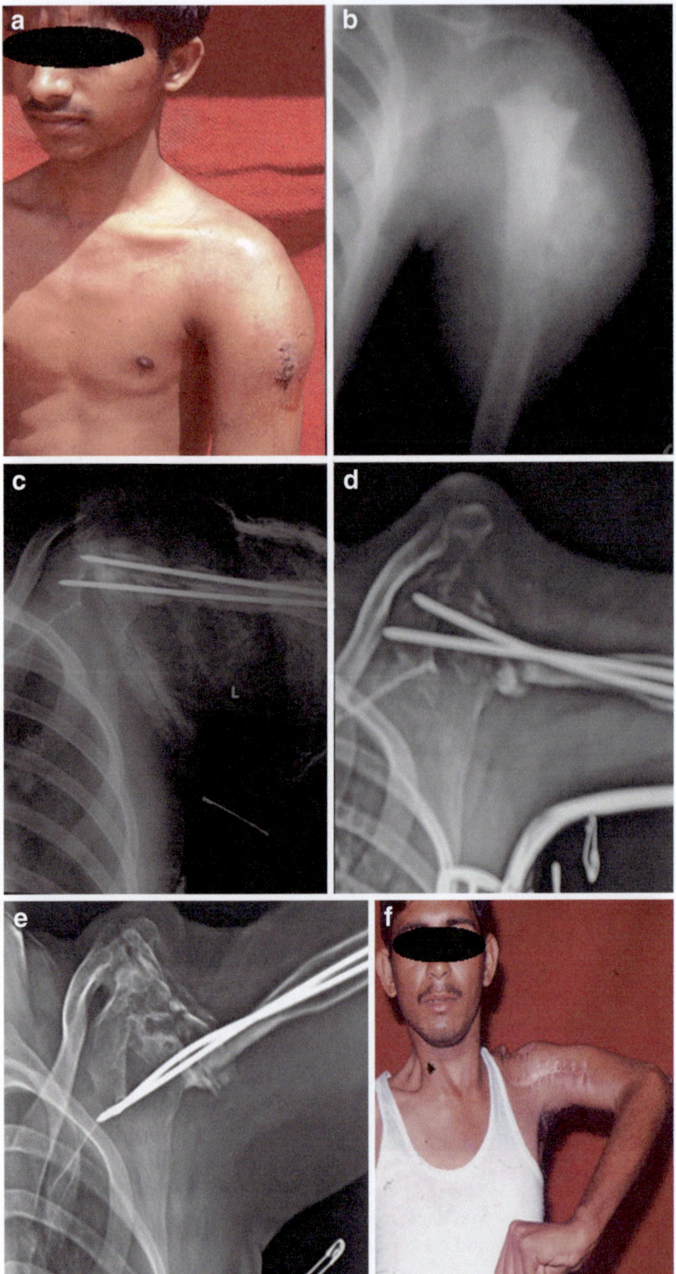

Fig. 6.37 (**a**) Osteosarcoma of the proximal humerus. Biopsy scar is seen. (**b**) Radiograph showing the lesion with typical appearance of an osteosarcoma. (**c, d**) Excision of the proximal humerus bridging the defect with twin fibular graft arthrodesing the shoulder joint. (**e**) Excision of the proximal humerus bridging the defect with twin fibular graft. (**f**) Dual fibular graft with arthrodesis of the shoulder. The patient showing the range of abduction of the arm at the scapulo-thoracic articulation

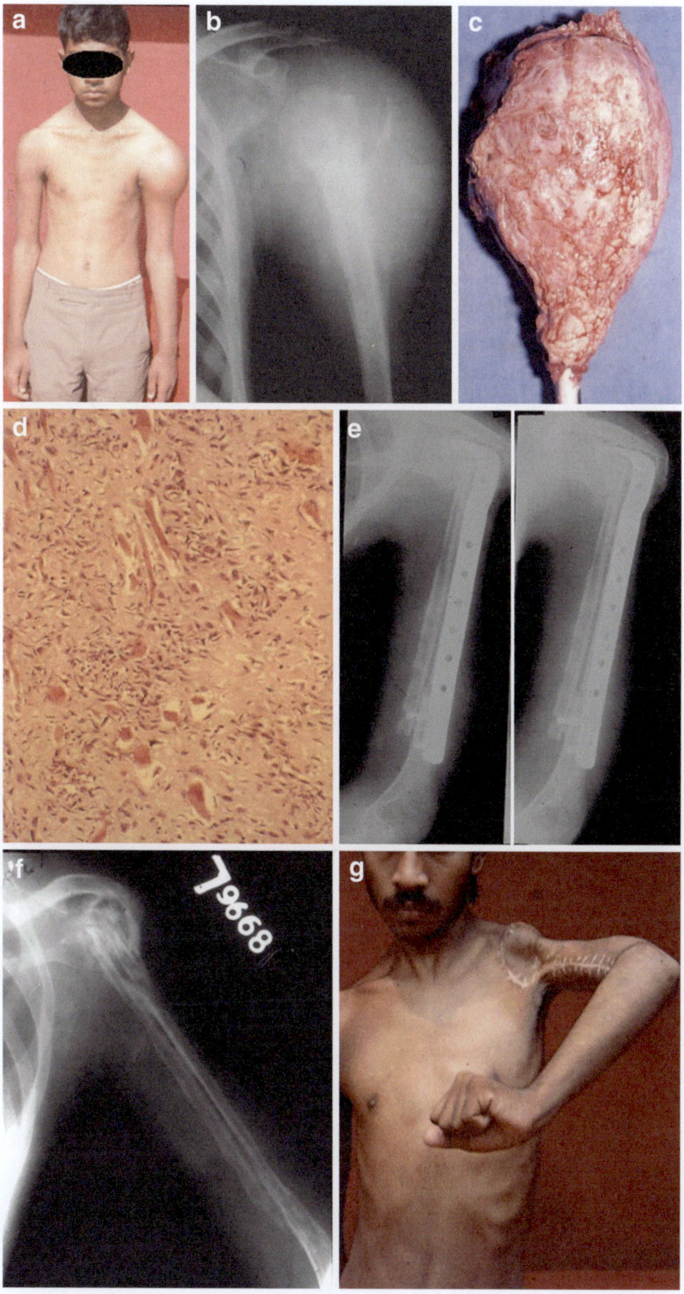

Fig. 6.38 (**a**) Large osteosarcoma of the proximal humerus. (**b**) Radiograph revealing the lesion involving the proximal humerus. (**c**). Excised specimen. (**d**) Histopathology of the lesion. (**e**) Twin fibular grafts stabilized with an L-plate arthrodesing the shoulder. (**f**). Radiograph shows consolidation of the graft with the host bone and arthrodesis of the shoulder. (**g**) Patient showing abduction of the arm at the scapulo-thoracic articulation after arthrodesis of the shoulder

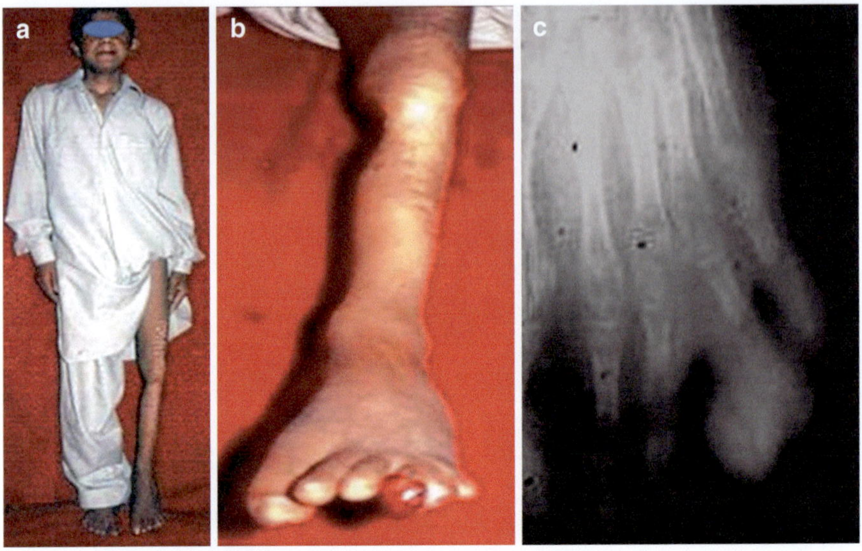

Fig. 6.39 (**a**, **b**) A previously treated case of osteosarcoma of the proximal tibia revealed a soft tissue lesion on the fourth toe after a span of 2 years. Biopsy from the toe revealed sarcomatous change. (**c**) Radiograph of the lesion. The toe was amputated

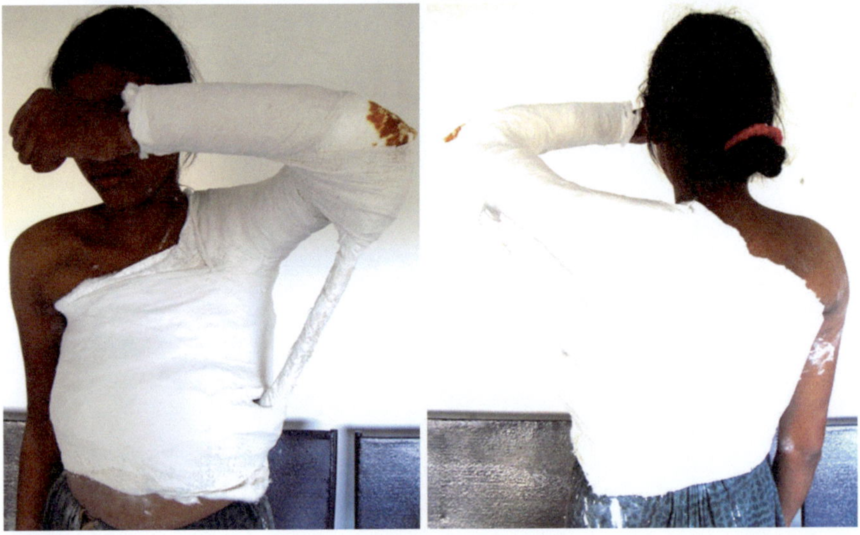

The front and back views of the POP shoulder spica

6.8 Telangiectatic Osteosarcoma

Telangiectatic osteosarcoma (TOS) is a rare and aggressive bone cancer that typically affects the long bones of adolescents and young adults. It most commonly occurs in the distal femur or proximal humerus, but it can also affect other long bones. Telangiectatic osteosarcoma is typically a purely lytic lesion with a permeative destructive growth pattern. This rapidly growing tumour often expands the contour of the bone and shows features of cortical disruption with minimal or no periosteal new bone formation (Fig. 6.40a–e).

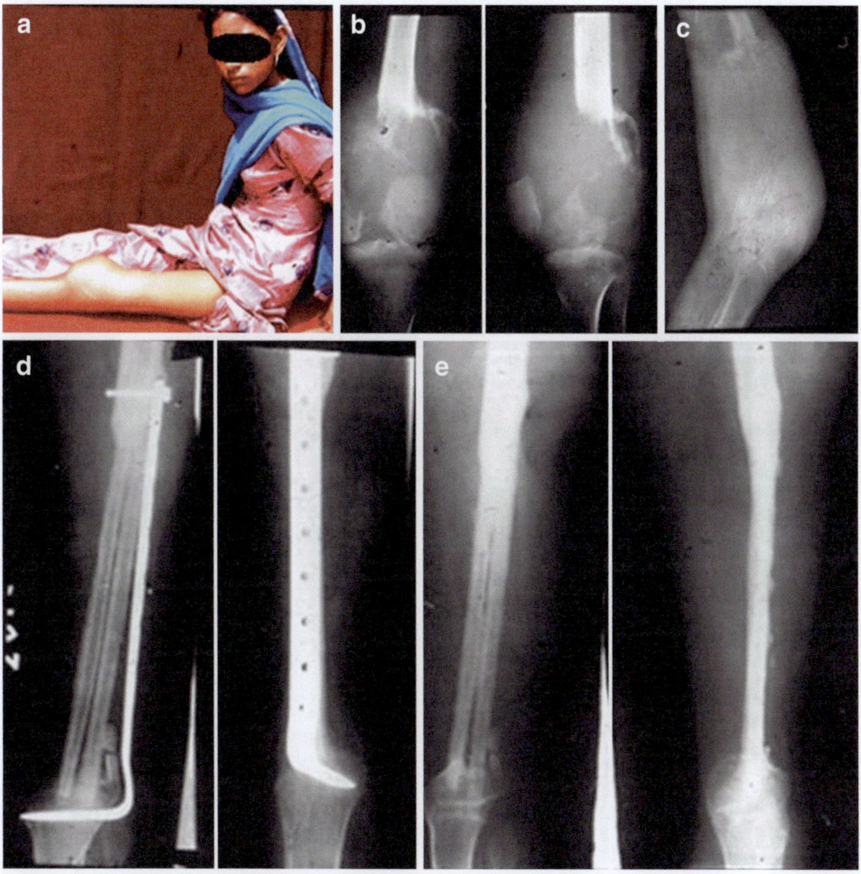

Fig. 6.40 (**a**) A 30-year-old lady with a rapidly increasing swelling of the left distal thigh. (**b**) Radiographs revealed a totally huge lytic lesion of the distal femur, suggesting telangiectatic osteosarcoma. (**c**) Radiograph of the same patient at the time of admission. (**d**) The lesion was widely excised, and twin fibular graft was performed to bridge the gap, stabilized with an L-plate. Note the beginning of the lateral union between the twin grafts. (**e**) The L-plate has been removed after complete lateral union between the fibular struts. The diameter of the construct is almost similar to that of the femur

6.9 Ewing Sarcoma

Patients with Ewing sarcoma initially complain of pain at the site. Males are affected at a 3:2 ratio over females, and most patients are between the age of 5 and 30 years. Any bone may be affected. The femur is the most common site of origin (20%); the pelvis, tibia and humerus are also common sites (Figs. 6.41a, 6.42a, b, 6.43a, b, 6.44, and 6.45). There is usually a soft tissue mass associated with the bone lesion (Fig. 6.44a, b). The mass is warm, firm and tender, and it may be pulsatile. There are no specific abnormal laboratory values diagnostic of Ewing sarcoma, but the sedimentation rate often is increased.

The typical plain radiograph of Ewing sarcoma reveals diffuse destruction of the bone, extension of the tumour through the cortex, a soft tissue component and a periosteal reaction. The periosteal reaction may produce a Codman triangle, an 'onion skin' appearance or a sunburst appearance. These suggest an aggressive lesion that has rapidly penetrated the cortex and elevated the periosteum. The extraosseous soft tissue mass and medullary canal involvement can be seen on CT and MRI scans.

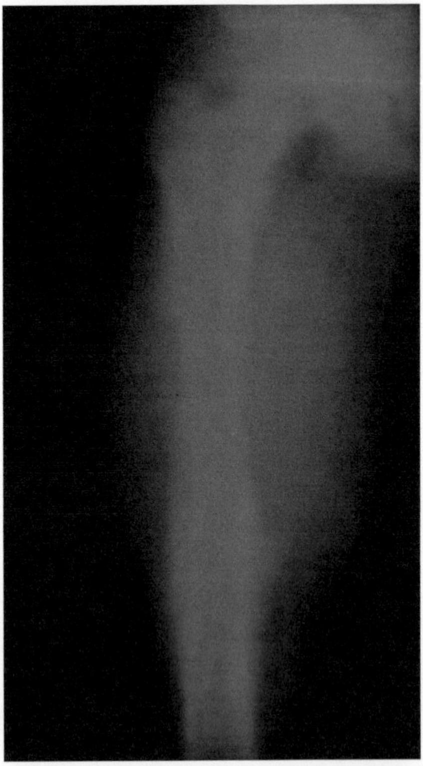

Fig. 6.41 (**a**) Radiograph reveals aggressive diaphyseal lesion of the femoral shaft. On biopsy, it was Ewing sarcoma. Note the large extraosseous component of this malignant tumour

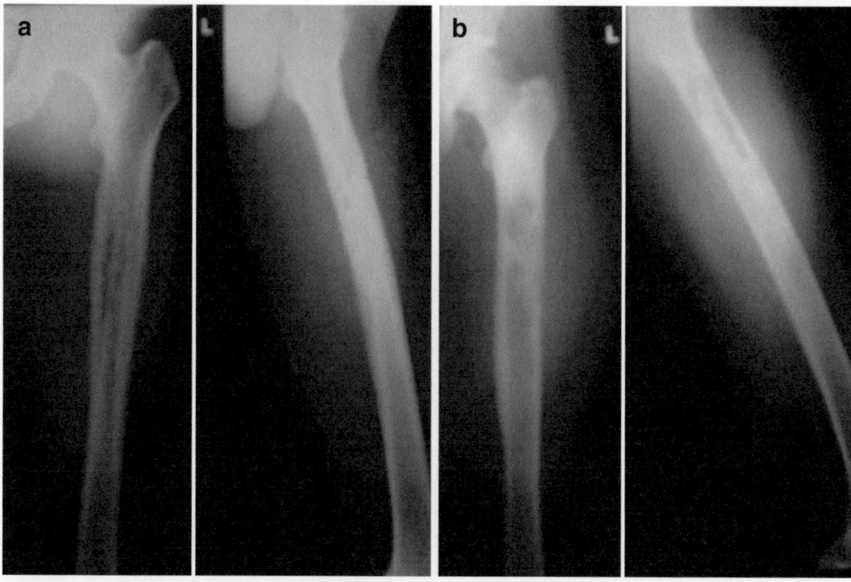

Fig. 6.42 (**a**) Ewing sarcoma of the femoral diaphysis. The radiograph simulates subacute osteomyelitis. (**b**) Ewing sarcoma involving the femoral shaft reveals bony destruction and large extraosseous component

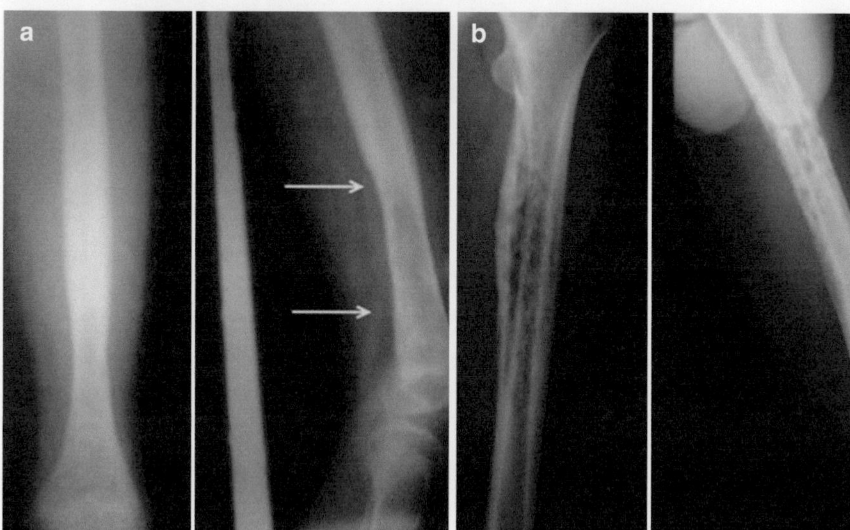

Fig. 6.43 (**a**) AP and lateral radiograph showing an aggressive femoral lesion. Note the lamellated periosteal reaction and broad zone of transition. (**b**) Ewing sarcoma of the femoral diaphysis. The radiograph simulates subacute osteomyelitis

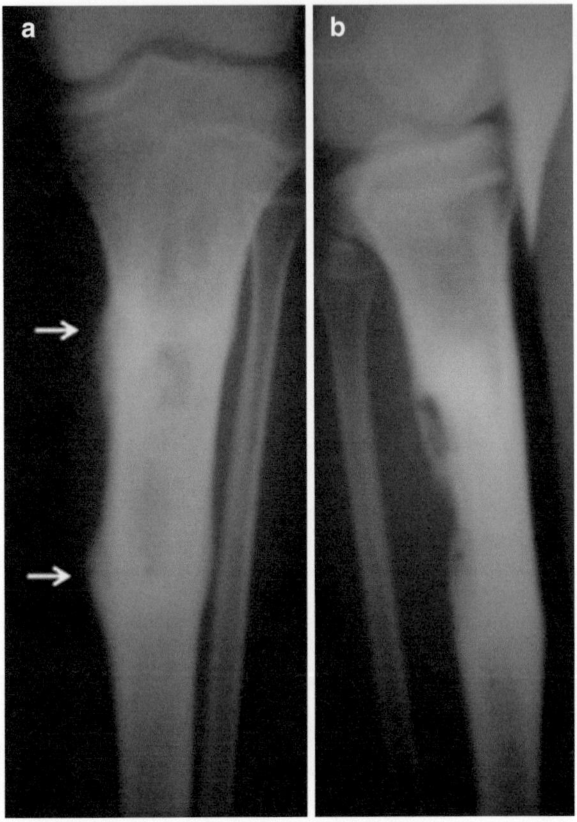

Fig. 6.44 (**a**) Roentgenogram revealing an aggressive proximal tibial lesion. Note the laminated periosteal reaction and broad zone of transition. (**b**) An advanced case of Ewing sarcoma showing destruction of the cortex and sclerotic medulla

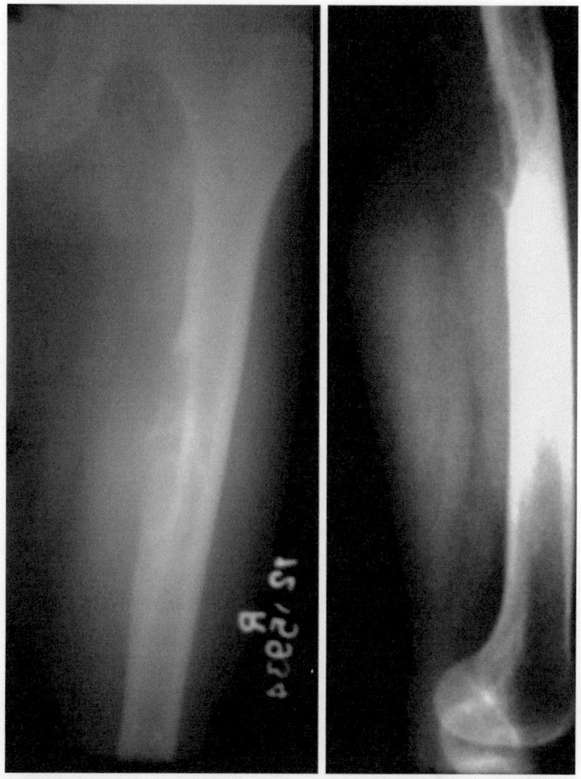

Fig. 6.45 Radiograph reveals confirmed Ewing sarcoma with destruction of the shaft of the femur with a huge soft tissue swelling

MRI has proved to be more accurate in determining the intramedullary extent of Ewing sarcoma than the CT scan. The technetium bone scan is most useful in finding occult bone metastasis. Approximately 5% of the patients present with pulmonary metastasis. More recent therapeutic protocols start with two or four courses of multidrug chemotherapy regimen and then irradiation or a surgical resection followed by more chemotherapy. Despite the lack of data to indicate that a surgical resection is better than irradiation, surgeons increasingly have resected the residual abnormal tissues after preoperative chemotherapy (Figs. 6.46a–g and 6.47a–j).

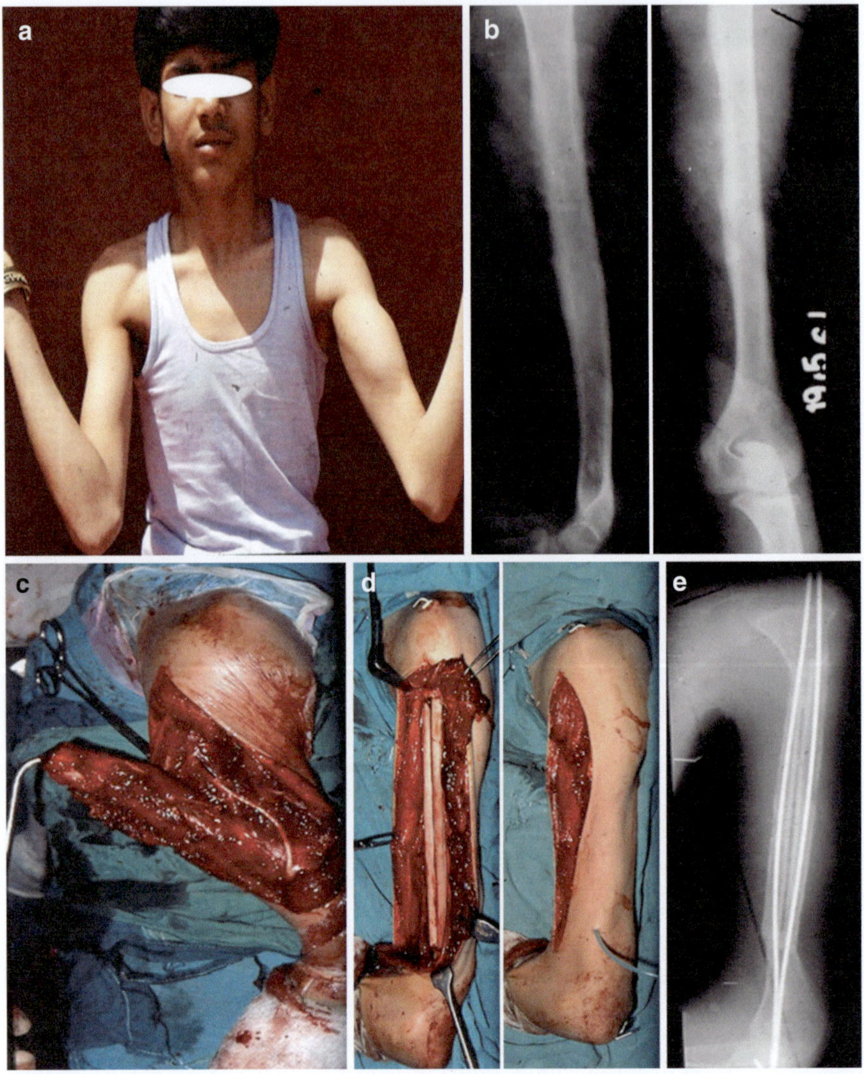

Fig. 6.46 (**a**) This 14-year-old boy had gradually increasing swelling over the left arm. (**b**) Radiograph reveals Ewing sarcoma which was confirmed on biopsy. (**c**) Intraoperative pictures during the excision. The radial nerve can be seen in the operative field. (**d**) Reconstruction was attempted with twin fibular grafts stabilized with Kirschner wires. Note the bent Kirschner wires on top and below. (**e**) Postoperative radiograph reveals the construct showing lateral union between the fibular struts. (**f**) Healing of the construct with lateral union between the fibular struts, simulating the humeral shaft. The wires have been removed. (**g**) Clinical picture of the patient showing abduction at the shoulder after 1 year. The patient had been treated with chemotherapy

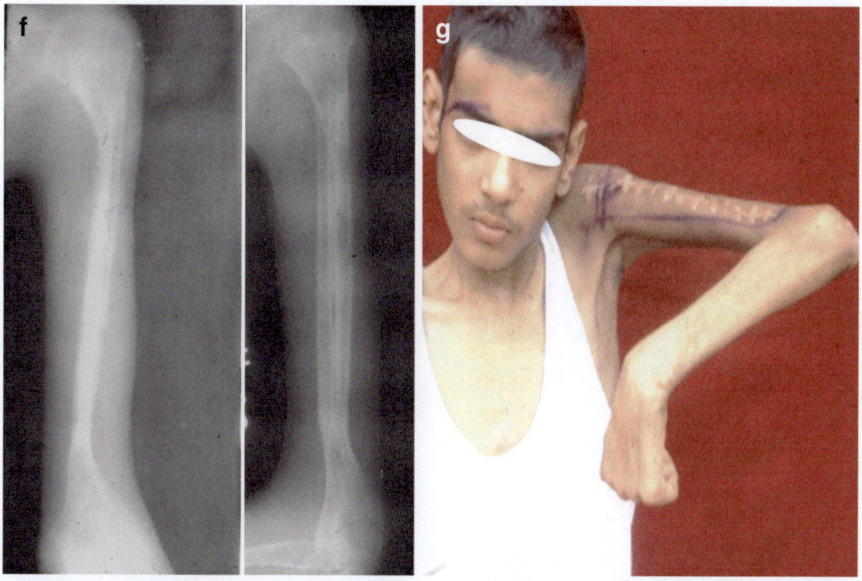

Fig. 6.46 (continued)

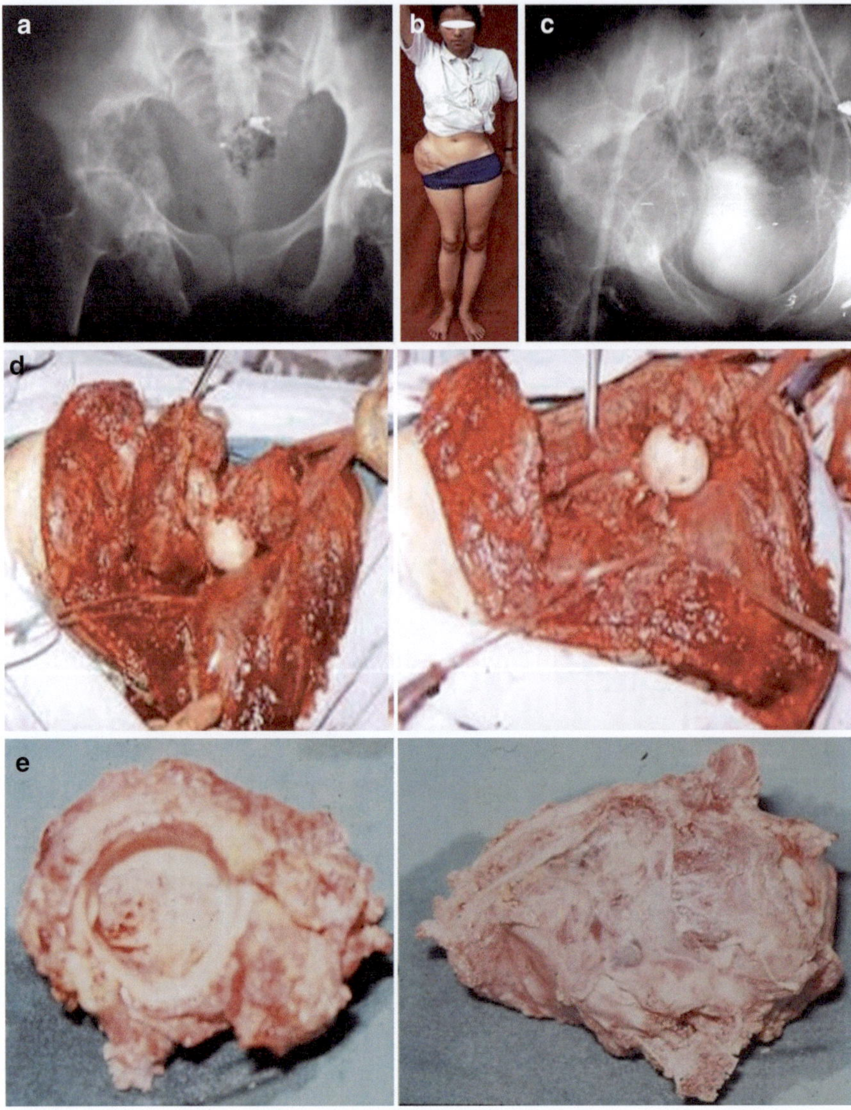

Fig. 6.47 (**a**) Roentgenogram revealing Ewing sarcoma of the right ilium and ischium after radiation. (**b**) Clinical picture of the patient. (**c**) An angiogram showing the vascularity of the lesion. (**d**) Intraoperative photographs after excision of the lesion. (**e**) The anterior and posterior views of the excised specimen. (**f**) The immediate postoperative picture showing the incision line. (**g**) Postoperative roentgenogram revealing the twin fibular graft stabilized with Kirschner wires between the head of the femur and the spine. One Kirschner wire was fixed between the remaining ischium and the neck of the femur. The patient was put in a spica cast. (**h**) Postoperative picture of the patient in hip spica cast. (**i**) Postoperatively, the patient had a right-sided foot drop for which she was given an orthosis. (**j**) The clinical picture of the patient 8 months after surgery

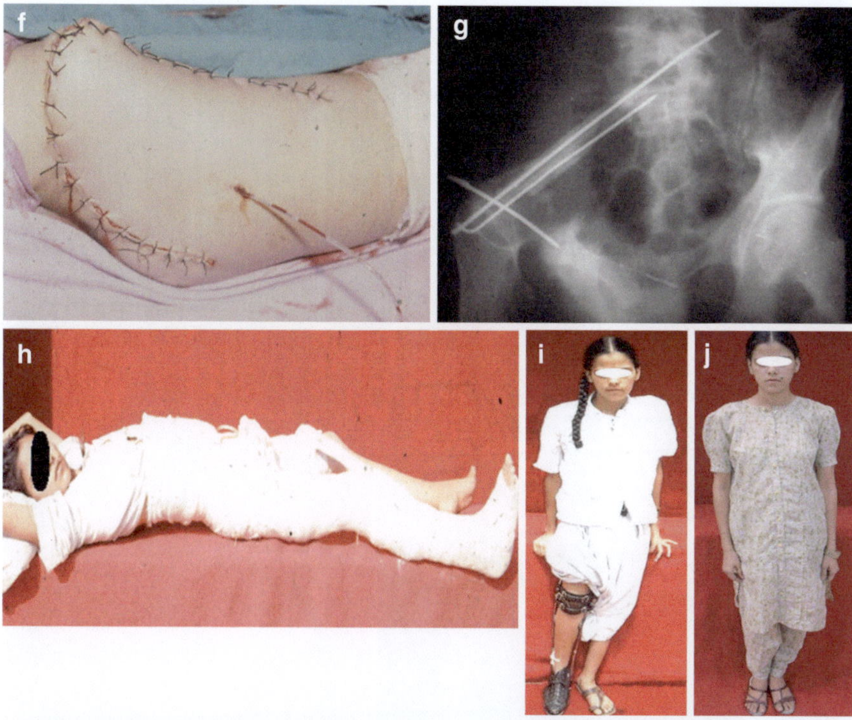

Fig. 6.47 (continued)

6.10 Malignant Fibrous Histiocytoma (MFH)

Malignant fibrous histiocytoma (MFH) is a tumour that can occur in the bone as well as soft tissues. Earlier, these tumours were diagnosed as rhabdomyosarcoma. MFH of the bone is uncommon, but it occurs in adults usually after the age of 50 years. It is usually firm but without other typical characteristics. On radiograph, only a soft tissue density is seen. MRI is the diagnostic test of choice.

The treatment of soft tissue and bone MFH is a wide surgical resection with bony reconstruction (Fig. 6.48a–e). Adjuvant chemotherapy has been suggested particularly in cases where a wide margin cannot be achieved without an amputation. The most likely site of distance spread is the lung. The overall survival rate is 52–60%.

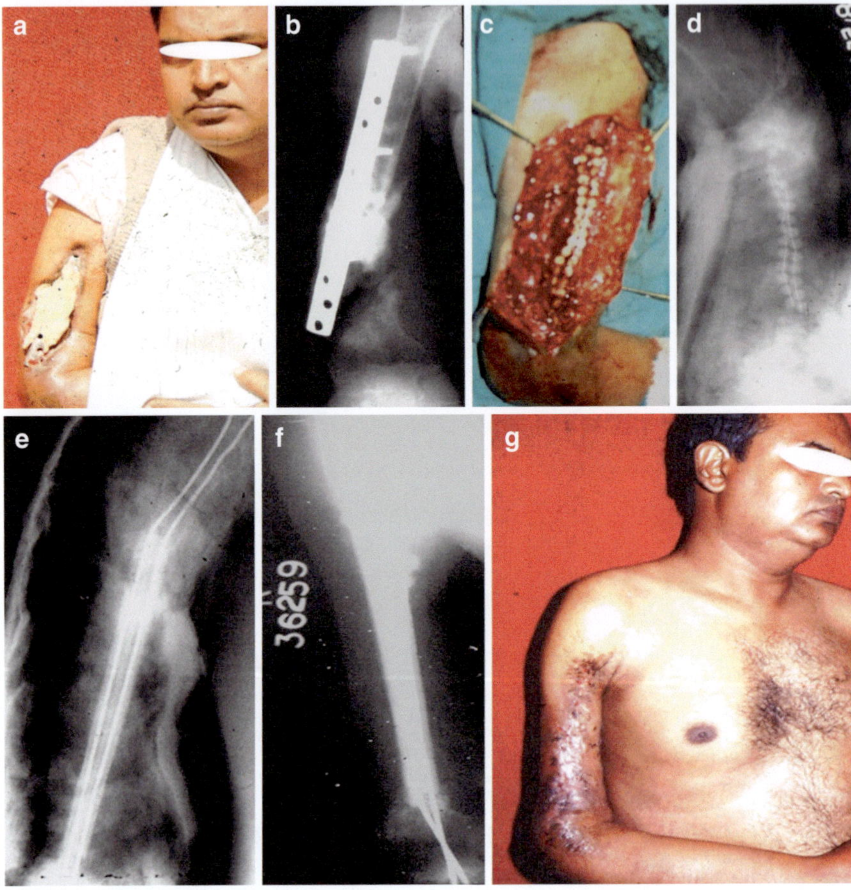

Fig. 6.48 (**a**) This naval officer had come to us in this condition. He was previously operated elsewhere for malignant fibrous histiocytosis of the right humeral shaft with excision, plating and cementation which was exposed. (**b**) Radiograph of the construct as described above. The bone was highly osteoporotic. (**c**) The plate and cement were removed along with the shell of the osteoporotic bone, and thorough cleaning was attempted. A twin row of gentamicin beads was placed in the centre not only to provide local antibiotics but also to preserve a space for a future procedure where a twin fibular grafts can be attempted. (**d**) Radiograph showing the gentamicin beads. (**e**) As proposed, a twin fibular graft was stabilized with Kirschner wires after removal of the gentamicin beads. (**f**) The radiograph reveals complete healing of the construct with lateral union and union at both ends which simulated the shaft of the humerus. (**g**) Clinical picture of the patient with the healed wound

6.11 Adamantinoma

Adamantinoma is a very rare, slow-growing malignant tumour of uncertain histogenesis that histologically resembles adamantinoma (ameloblastoma) of the jaw. The tumour occurs in the diaphysis of long bones, particularly the tibia and fibula; in some cases, both bones are involved. The tumour arises mainly in young and middle-aged adults. Males and females are affected equally. There is often a long history of pain and swelling (Fig. 6.49a–e).

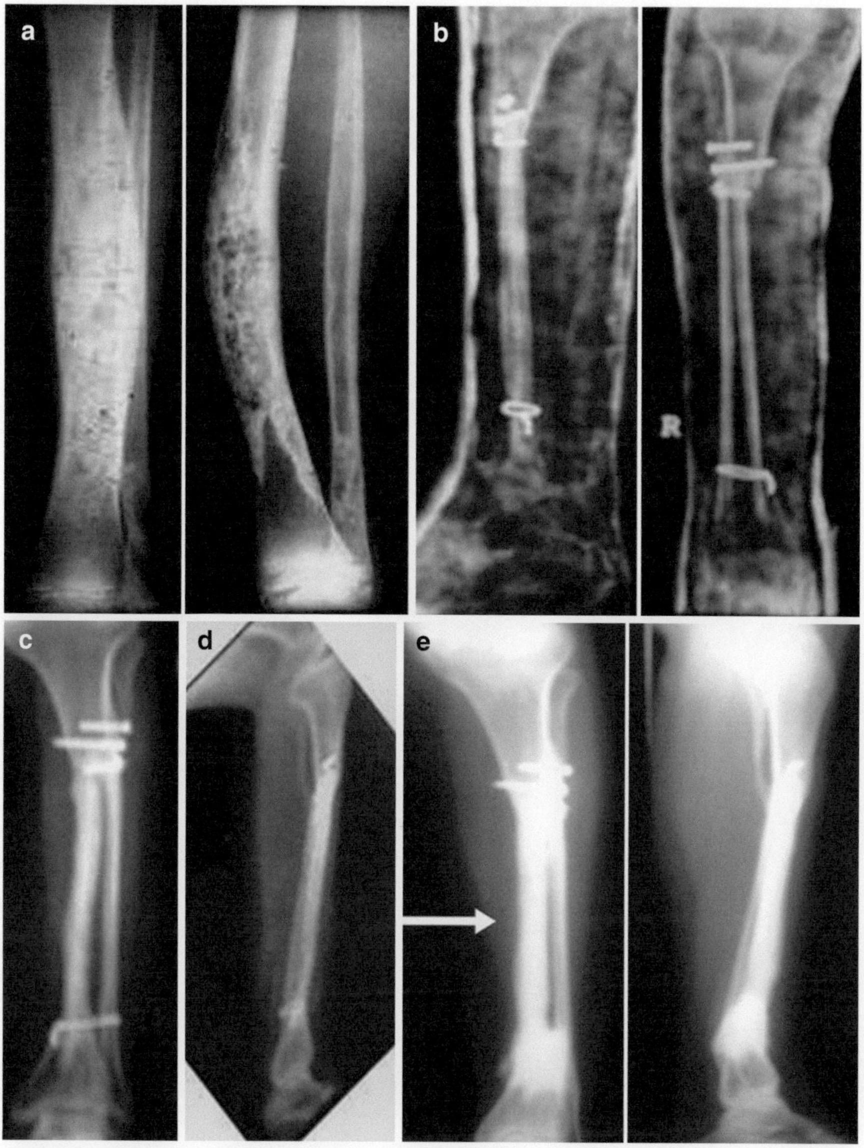

Fig. 6.49 (**a**) Radiograph of a case of adamantinoma of the left tibia. (**b**) Postoperative AP and lateral radiograph after excision and reconstruction by medialization of the fibula, along with a fibular strut taken from the contralateral side, fixed proximally with screws and distally with wiring. (**c**, **d**) AP and lateral radiograph after 28 weeks showing hypertrophy of the construct, more in the fibular strut transferred from the contralateral side, which reveals that the fibular strut has been viable. (**e**) The radiograph taken after 1 year reveals further hypertrophy of the transplanted fibular strut in comparison to the medialized fibula

The lesion is usually an eccentric, well-defined, osteolytic defect which is multilobulated and cystic. Prominent bone sclerosis is often present around the lesion and between cystic areas (Fig. 6.50a–h). Most lesions are found in the diaphysis, but large lesions may extend into the metaphysis. Both the cortex and medulla are usually involved; in a minority of cases, the tumour is confined to the cortex. A bowing deformity may be seen in the affected bone.

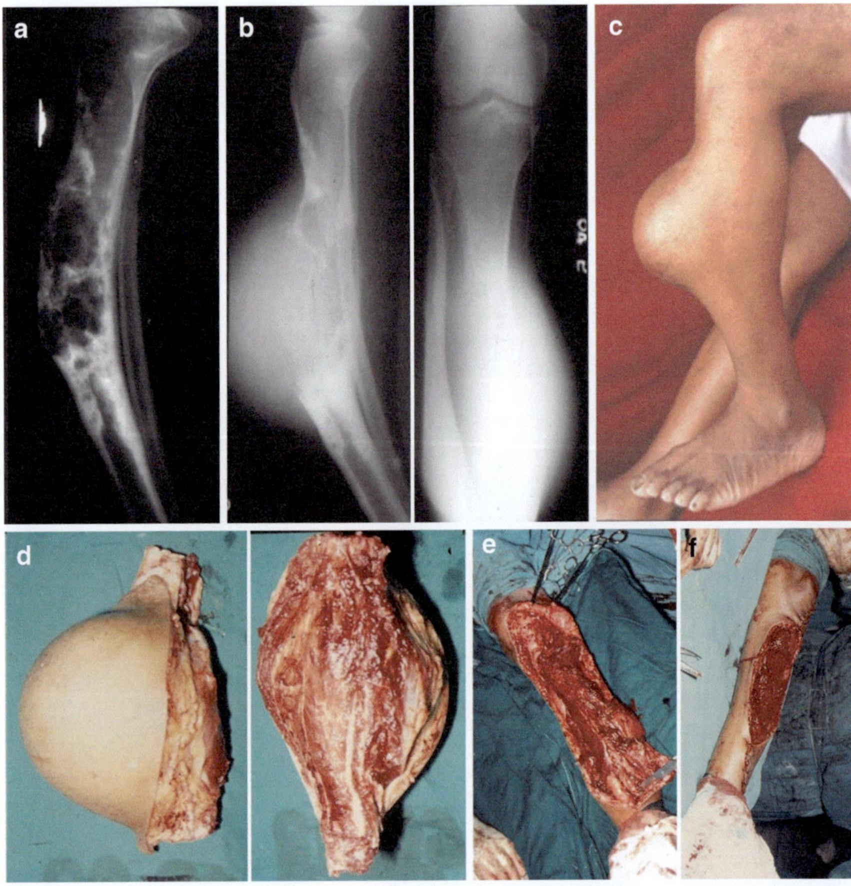

Fig. 6.50 (**a**) Radiograph of the tibia showing mid-diaphyseal adamantinoma with anterior bowing of the left tibia. (**b**) The same patient came later with a huge lesion after 10 months. AP and lateral radiograph of the patient in the advanced stage with a huge aggressive lesion involving the entire mid-shaft of the tibia. (**c**) Clinical picture of the patient with advanced lesion at the time of admission. (**d**) AP and lateral views of the excised lesion with mid-shaft of the tibia. (**e**) Intraoperative photographs after excision of the lesion. Lateral skin release incision was made to cover the wound anteriorly. After healing, tibialization of the fibula was performed to bridge the gap. (**f**) Postoperative radiograph showing healing after tibialization of the fibula. (**g**) Radiograph taken at 8 months reveals healing. (**h**) Clinical picture of the patient after 1 year

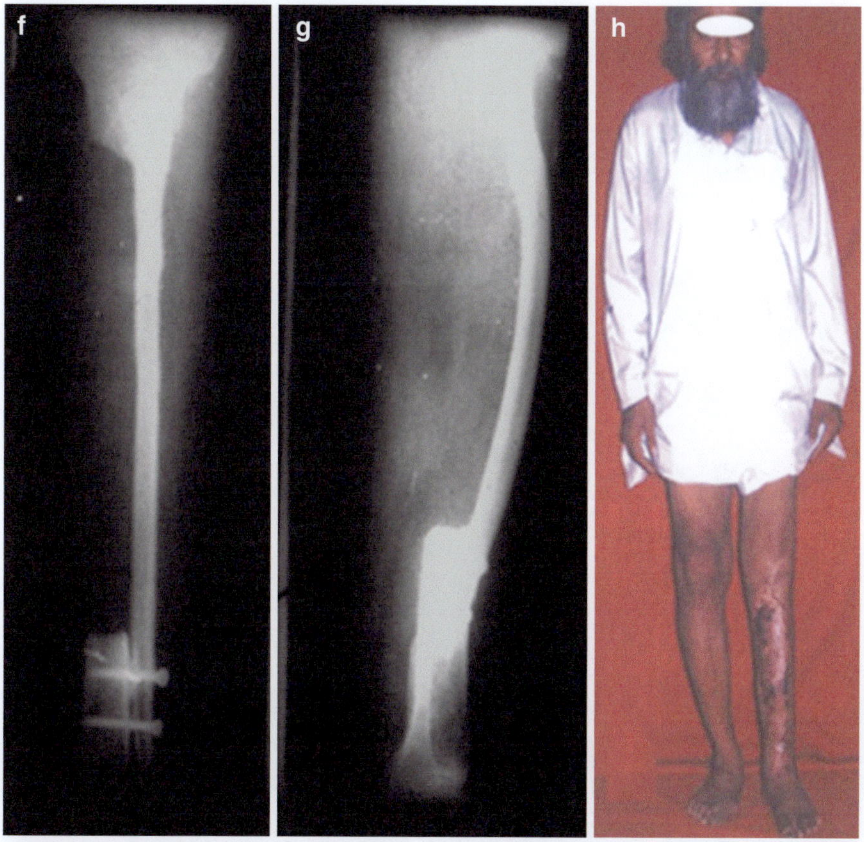

Fig. 6.50 (continued)

6.12 Chondrosarcoma

Chondrosarcoma is a cartilage-forming cell tumour, and its incidence is nearly 20% of primary bone sarcomas. The lesion is subdivided into central when it is situated in the medullary cavity and peripheral when it arises from the surface. Some distinct morphological variants of this tumour are mesenchymal, dedifferentiated and clear cell chondrosarcoma. It usually occurs in patients above the age of 30 years (Figs. 6.51a–d and 6.52a–d). Patients complain of painful swelling over the site, which may rarely result in a pathological fracture (Fig. 6.53a, b). It mainly involves the diaphysis and the metaphysis. There is usually 'popcorn' calcification irregularly all over. The cortex may be thin with scalloping. A peripheral chondrosarcoma is usually large and lobulated with a cartilage cap which can be best appreciated on CT and MRI.

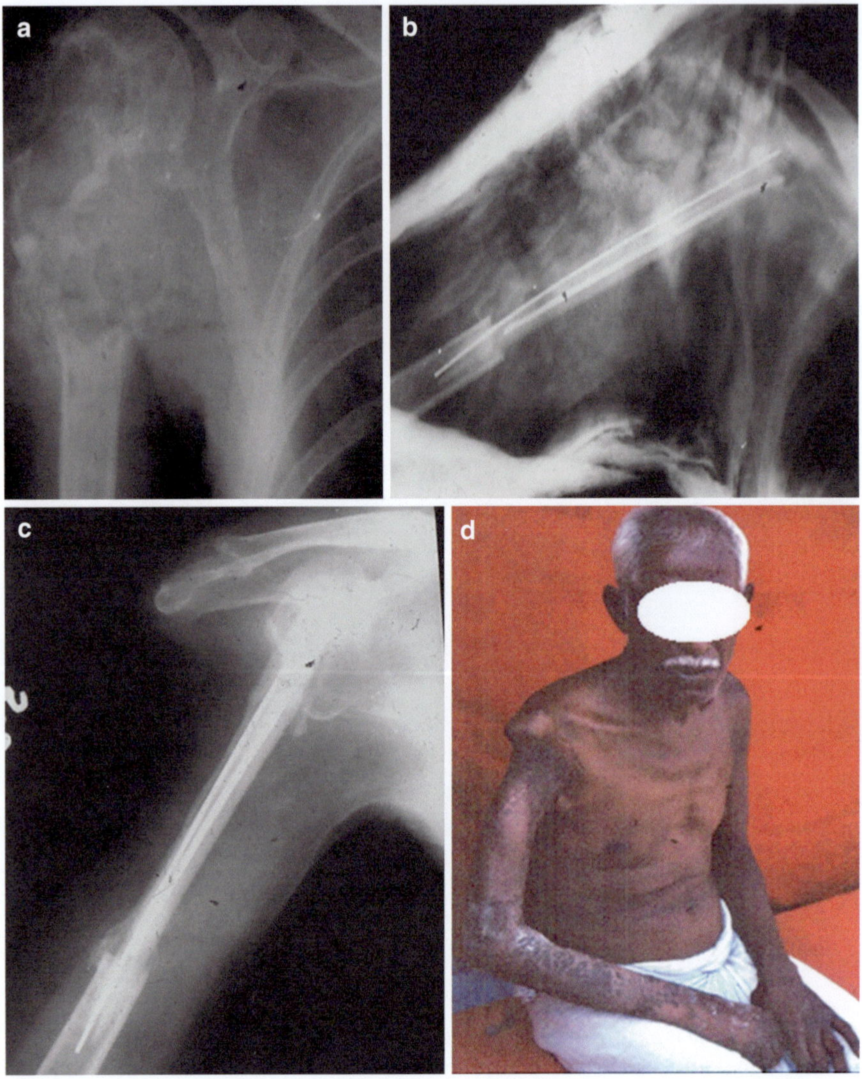

Fig. 6.51 (**a**) A large chondrosarcoma of the proximal end of the right humerus. (**b**) After excision of the lesion, the radiograph reveals a twin fibular graft stabilized with two Kirschner wires further supported by a spica cast. The shoulder was arthrodesed. (**c**) Radiograph reveals complete healing of the graft at both ends and reveals hypertrophy; the proximal end shows healed arthrodesis. (**d**) The patient after removal of the plaster

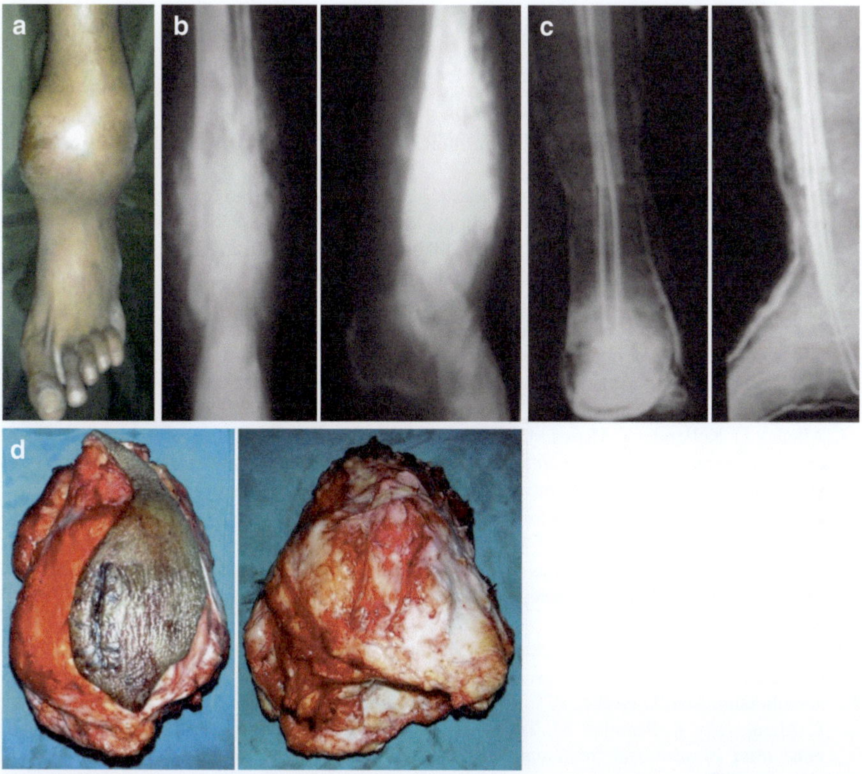

Fig. 6.52 (**a**) An advanced case of chondrosarcoma at the lower end of the tibia. (**b**) The radiograph reveals an extension to the lower end of the fibula. (**c**) Excision of the lower end of the tibia and fibula was carried out, and the gap was bridged by a twin fibular graft stabilized by two long Kirschner wires and ankle arthrodesis. (**d**) The anterior and posterior views of the excised specimen. The lesion recurred within 6 months, and a below-knee amputation was carried out

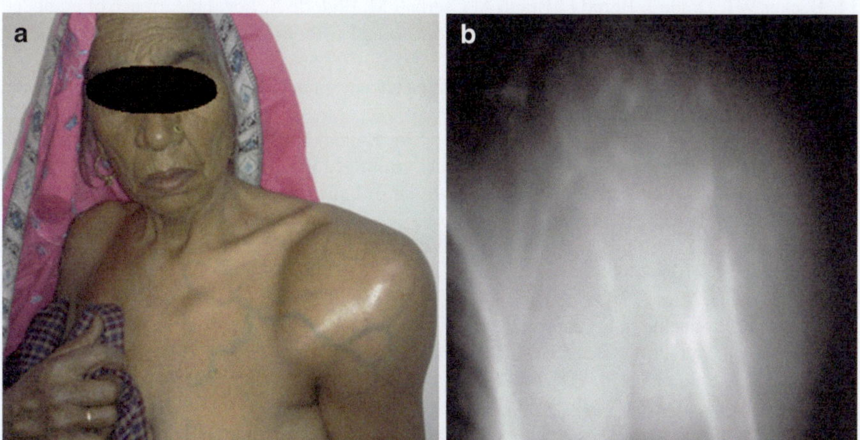

Fig. 6.53 (**a**) A large chondrosarcoma of the proximal end of the humerus. Note the shiny skin and the presence of dilated veins. (**b**) Radiograph reveals total destruction of the proximal humerus with huge soft tissue swelling. The patient was treated with a fore-quarter amputation

Suggested Readings

1. Rock MG, Pritchard DJ, Unni KK. Metastases from histologically benign giant cell tumour of bone. J Bone Joint Surg. 1984;66A:269–74.
2. Peimer CA, Schiller AL, Mankin HJ, Smith RJ. Multicentric giant cell tumour of bone. J Bone Joint Surg. 1980;62A:652–6.
3. Potter HG, Schneider R, Ghelman B, et al. Multiple giant cell tumors and Paget disease of bone. Radiographic and clinical correlations. Radiology. 1991;180:261–4.
4. Merkow RL, Bansal M, Inglis AE. Giant cell reparative granuloma in the hand. Report of three cases and review of the literature. J Hand Surg. 1985;10:733–9.
5. Picci P, Baldini N, Sudanese A, et al. Giant cell reparative granuloma and other giant cell lesions of the bones of the hands and feet. Skeletal Radiol. 1986;15:415–21.
6. Algawahmed H, Turcotte R, Farrokhyar F, Ghert M. High-speed burring with and without the use of surgical adjuvants in the intralesional management of giant cell tumor of bone: a systematic review and meta-analysis. Sarcoma. 2010;2010:586090.
7. Alkalay D, Kollender Y, Mozes M, Meller I. GCT with intraarticular fracture. Two stages local excision, cryosurgery and cementation in 5 patients with distal femoral tumor followed for 2-4 years. Acta Orthop Scand. 1996;67:291–4.
8. Andreas FM, Vasileios GI, Panayiotis DM, Georgios NP, Panayiotis JP, Panayotis S. Giant cell tumour of bone revisited. SICOT J. 2017;3:54.
9. Anract P, De Pinieux G, Cottias P, Pouillart P, Forest M, Tomeno B. Malignant giant-cell tumours of bone. Clinico-pathological types and prognosis: a review of 29 cases. Int Orthop. 1998;22(1):19–26.
10. Anshul Sobti DNB, Pranshu Agrawal MS, Sanjay Agarwala MS, Manish Agarwal MS. Giant cell tumor of bone – an overview. Arch Bone Joint Surg. 2016;4(1):2–9.
11. Knochentumoren A, Becker WT, Dohle J, Bernd L, Braun A, Cserhati M, Enderle A, Hovy L, Matejovsky Z, Szendroi M, Trieb K, Tunn PU. Local recurrence of giant cell tumor of bone after intralesional treatment with and without adjuvant therapy. J Bone Joint Surg. 2008;90:1060–7.
12. Balke M, Schremper L, Gebert C, Ahrens H, Streitbuerger A, Koehler G, Hardes J, Gosheger G. Giant cell tumor of bone: treatment and outcome of 214 cases. J Cancer Res Clin Oncol. 2008;134:969–78.
13. Balke M, Ahrens H, Streitbuerger A, Koehler G, Winkelmann W, Gosheger G, Hardes J. Treatment options for recurrent giant cell tumors of bone. Cancer Res Clin Oncol. 2009;135:149–58.
14. Becker WT, Dohle J, Bernd L, Braun A, Cserhati M, Enderle A. Local recurrence of giant cell tumor of bone after intra-lesional treatment with and without adjuvant therapy. J Bone Joint Surg. 2008;90:1060–7.
15. Bertoni F, Bacchini P, Staals EL. Malignancy in giant cell tumor of bone. Cancer. 2003;97:2520–9.
16. Blackley HR, Wunder JS, Davis AM, White LM, Kandel R, Bell RS. Treatment of giant-cell tumors of long bones with curettage and bone-grafting. J Bone Joint Surg. 1999;81:811–20.
17. Bini SA, Gill K, Johnston JO. Giant cell tumour of bone: curette and cement reconstruction. Clin Orthop. 1995;321:245–50.
18. Campanacci M, Baldini N, Boriani S, Sudanese A. Giant-cell tumor of bone. J Bone Joint Surg. 1987;69:106–14.
19. Carrasco CH, Murray JA. Giant cell tumors. Orthop Clin North. 1989;20:395–405.
20. Cheng JC, Johnston JO. Giant cell tumor of bone. Prognosis and treatment of pulmonary metastases. Clin Orthop Relat Res. 1997;338:205–14.
21. Cheng CY, Shih HN, Hsu KY, Hsu RW. Treatment of giant cell tumour of the distal radius. Clin Orthop Relat Res. 2001;383:221–8.
22. Chen TH, Su YP, Chen WM. Giant cell tumors of the knee: subchondral bone integrity affects the outcome. Int Orthop. 2005;29:30–4.

23. Chakarun CJ, Forrester DM, Gottsegen CJ, Patel DB, White EA, Matcuk GR Jr. Giant cell tumor of bone review, mimics and new developments in treatment. Radiographics. 2013;33:197–211.
24. Cory Julian B, Erika LG, Wood J, Therese B. Two cases of sarcoma arising in giant cell tumor of bone treated with Denosumab. Case Rep Med. 2015;2015:767198.
25. Cooper KL, Beabout JW, Dahlin DC. Giant cell tumour: ossification in soft tissue implants. Radiology. 1984;153:597–602.
26. Dahlin DC, Caldwell Lecture. Giant cell tumor of bone: highlights of 407 cases. AJR Am J Roentgenol. 1985;144:955–60.
27. Deheshi BM, Jaffer SN, Griffin AM, Ferguson PC, Bell RS, Wunder JS. Joint salvage for pathological fracture of giant cell tumor of the lower extremity. Clin Orthop Relat Res. 2007;459:96–104.
28. Durr HR, Maier M, Jansson V, Baur A. Refior HI phenol as an adjuvant for local control in the treatment of giant cell tumour of the bone. Eur J Surg Oncol. 1999;25:610–8.
29. Errani C, Ruggieri P, Asenzio MA, Toscano A, Colangeli S, Rimondi E, Rossi G, Longhi A, Mercuri M. Giant cell tumor of the extremity: a review of 349 cases from a single institution. Cancer Treat Rev. 2010;36(1):1–7.
30. Fain JS, Unni KK, Beabout JW, Rock MG. Nonepiphyseal giant cell tumor of long bones. Cancer. 1993;71:3514.
31. Malek F, Krueger P, Hatmi ZN, Malayeri AA, Faezipour H, O'Donnell RJ. Local control of long bone giant cell tumour using curettage, burring and bone grafting without adjuvant therapy. Int Orthop. 2006;30(6):495–8.
32. Gupta AK, Nath R, Mishra MP. Giant cell tumour of bone; multimodal approach. Indian J Orthop. 2007;41:115–20.
33. Yadav SS. Bridging of large skeletal defects by Twin fibular grafts supported by L-Plate fixation. Orthop Int Edition. 1995;3:213–21.

Chapter 7
Pelvic Reconstruction with Non-vascularized Twin Fibular Grafts Stabilized with Kirschner Wires After Excision of Bone Tumour

7.1 Pelvic Reconstruction with Non-vascularized Twin Fibular Grafts Stabilized with Kirschner Wires After Excision of Bone Tumours

Primary bone tumours of the pelvic ring occur in about 10–15% of cases. Internal hemipelvectomy followed by reconstruction of the pelvic ring has been a standard procedure after excision of malignant bone tumours. However, it is a surgical challenge to achieve a negative tumour margin at this site. Various methods of reconstruction of the pelvis have been described. Non-vascularized fibular grafts have been used with success. Vascularized fibular grafts for reconstruction of gaps after excision of tumours have also been described with improved results. Other techniques may involve the use of prostheses, allografts, autoclaved grafts and tumours treated with liquid nitrogen.

Earlier authors who have used non-vascularized and vascularized fibular grafts have advocated the procedure they have adopted for reconstruction. However, there has been no standard and accepted technique, as the results of most of them have been almost similar. The reported methods of reconstruction of the pelvic ring using

S. S. Yadav, *Non-Vascularised Fibular Grafts in Orthopaedic Practice*,
https://doi.org/10.1007/978-981-95-1794-7_7

fibular grafts include direct wedging of the fibular struts into the host bone, tension-band wiring, screw fixation and plate fixation. This may be the first report of fixing twin fibular struts with Kirschner wires in the pelvic region. In the beginning, it appeared that fixation of the grafts with Kirschner wires may not be adequate at this site. However, in due course of time, this biological construct with lateral union has proved stable. With more and more experience in such fixations, the technique has been improved, leading to better stability and encouraging results (Figs. 7.1a–f and 7.2a–f). Three-point fixation has proved advantageous in fixing the struts. However, a spica cast is required for 2 weeks. If the technique is followed adequately, the construct has proven to be quite stable and acceptable (Fig. 7.3a–h).

The literature reveals that whenever double fibular struts have been used, the upper strut usually fails to unite and the lower graft sustains the reconstruction. The advantage of the technique advocated in the present series is that placing the two struts together results in 'lateral union' that occurs throughout the length of the grafts and allows simultaneous incorporation into the host bone. It is because of this biological construct that none of the grafts have resulted in non-union, there has been no fatigue fracture and healing has been achieved in a relatively short time (Figs. 7.4a–f and 7.5a–g). Union has been observed between 12 and 36 weeks with a mean of 20.4 weeks. However, full weight-bearing had been possible only after radiological union. No patient had required additional surgery (Figs. 7.6a, b, 7.7a–e, and 7.8). The mean MSTS rating score in our cases has been 81.2% at the time of postoperative rehabilitation. If there are no complications, the score improves during the course of rehabilitation (Figs. 7.9a, b, 7.10, 7.11a–f, 7.12a–h, and 7.13a–d).

7.2 Chondrosarcoma

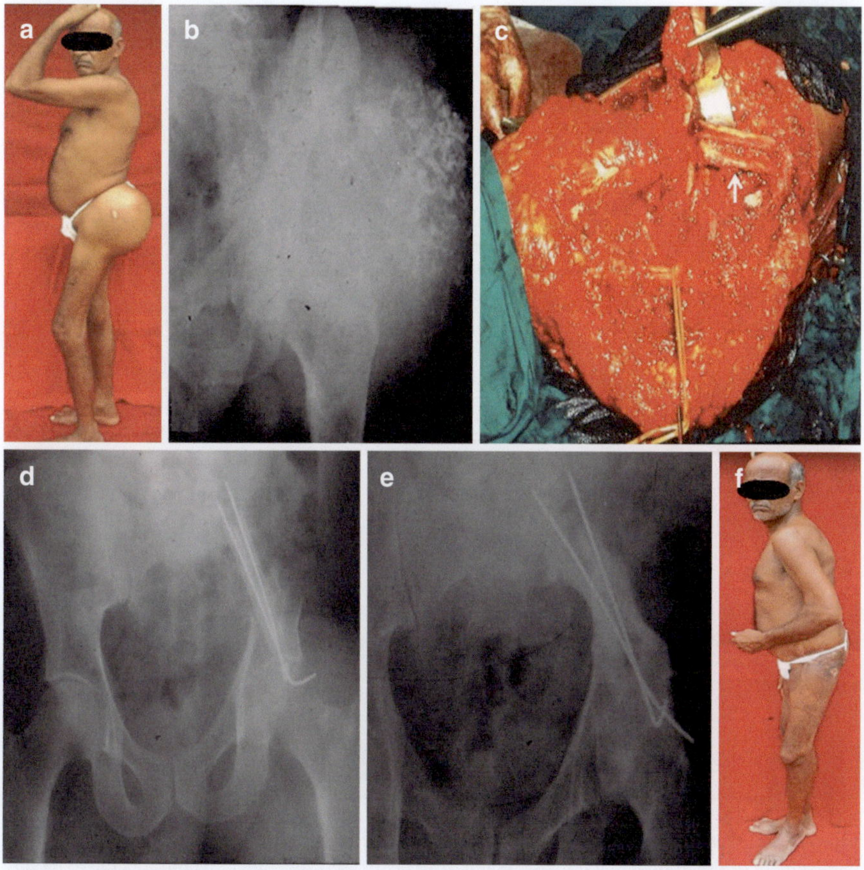

Fig. 7.1 (**a**) A massive osteochondroma of the left buttock. (**b**) The radiograph reveals a huge classical chondrosarcoma involving the whole of the left ilium. (**c**) Intraoperative picture after excision of the lesion and bridging the gap with twin non-vascularized fibular struts (arrow). Note the sciatic nerve has been retracted. (**d**) Postoperative radiograph revealing the twin fibular graft stabilized by two Kirschner wires. (**e**) A follow-up radiograph after 2 years reveals lateral union and hypertrophy of the graft. The pelvic ring is maintained. (**f**) Clinical picture 2 years postoperative with 3 cm shortening

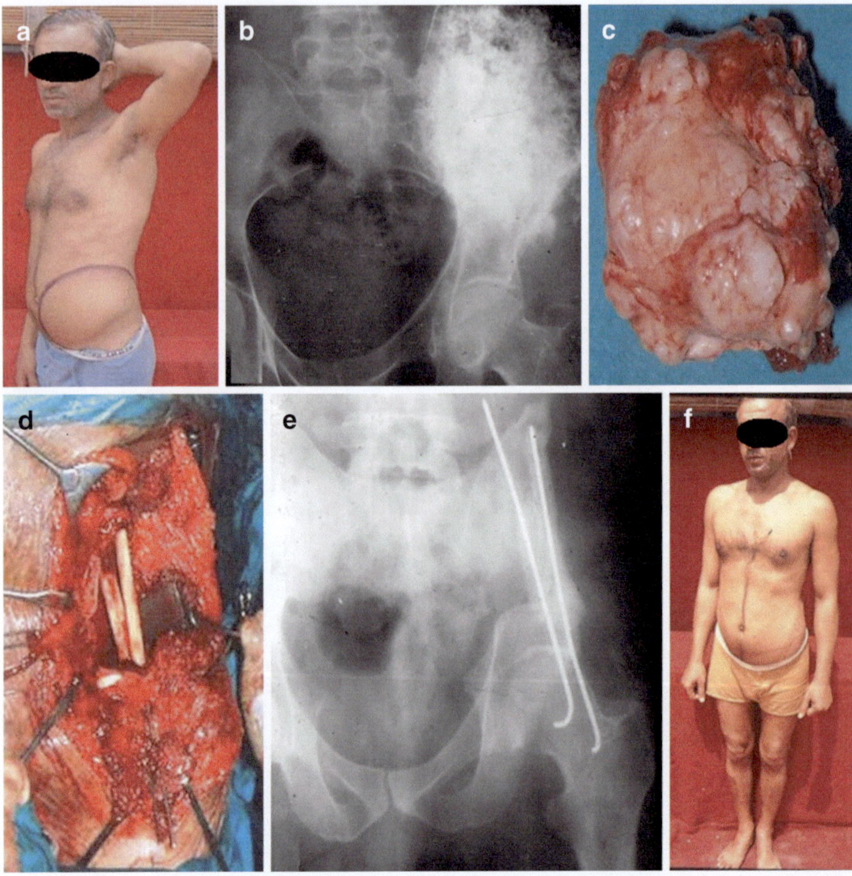

Fig. 7.2 (**a**) A case of massive chondrosarcoma of the left ilium. (**b**) Radiograph reveals total involvement of the ilium and the sciatic notch. (**c**) The excised specimen. (**d**) Intraoperative picture after excision and reconstruction with a twin non-vascularized fibular graft stabilized with Kirschner wires. (**e**) Roentgenogram with hypertrophy of the graft taken after 2 years. (**f**) The patient had 2 cm shortening

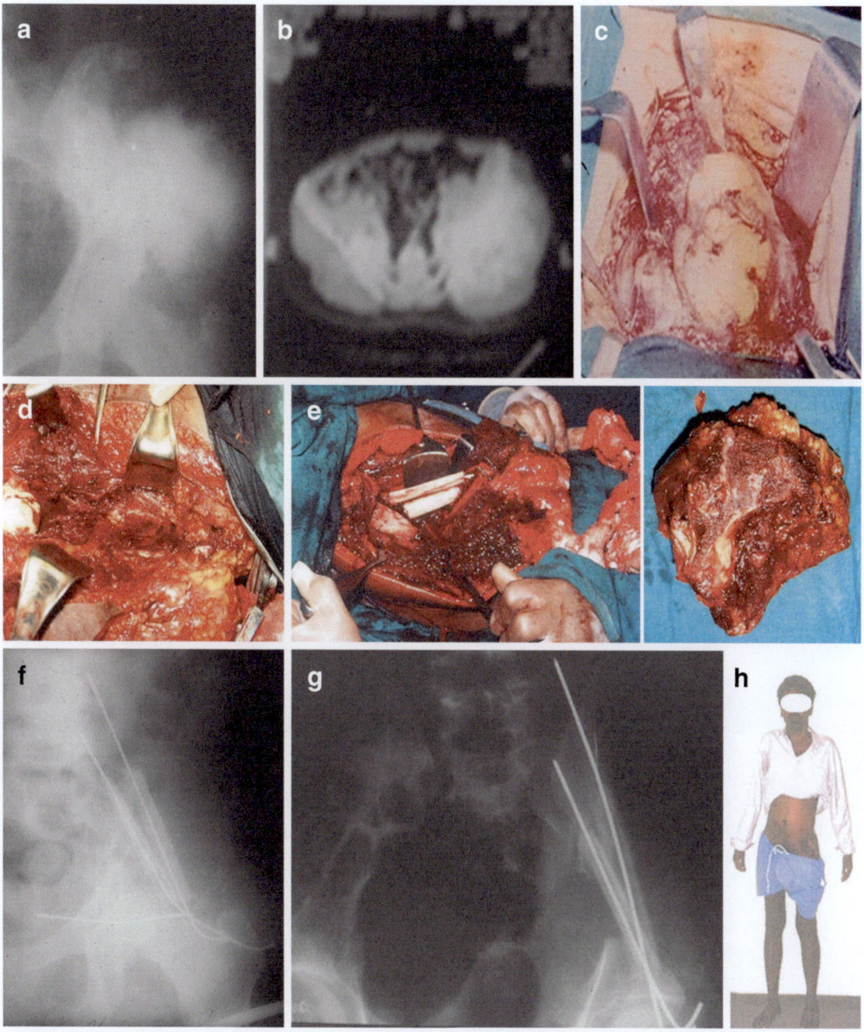

Fig. 7.3 (**a**) Radiograph revealing chondrosarcoma arising from the outer table of the left ilium. (**b**) MRI reveals the extent of the tumours. (**c**) Intraoperative picture during excision. (**d**) Intraoperative picture after excision of the tumour. (**e**) Reconstruction by twin fibular struts stabilized by Kirschner wires. The excised specimen. (**f**) Postoperative radiograph. (**g**) Radiograph revealing healing of the twin graft after 6 months, showing complete union of the construct. (**h**). Clinical picture of the patient bearing weight on both sides after 6 months

7.3 Giant Cell Tumour of the Pelvis

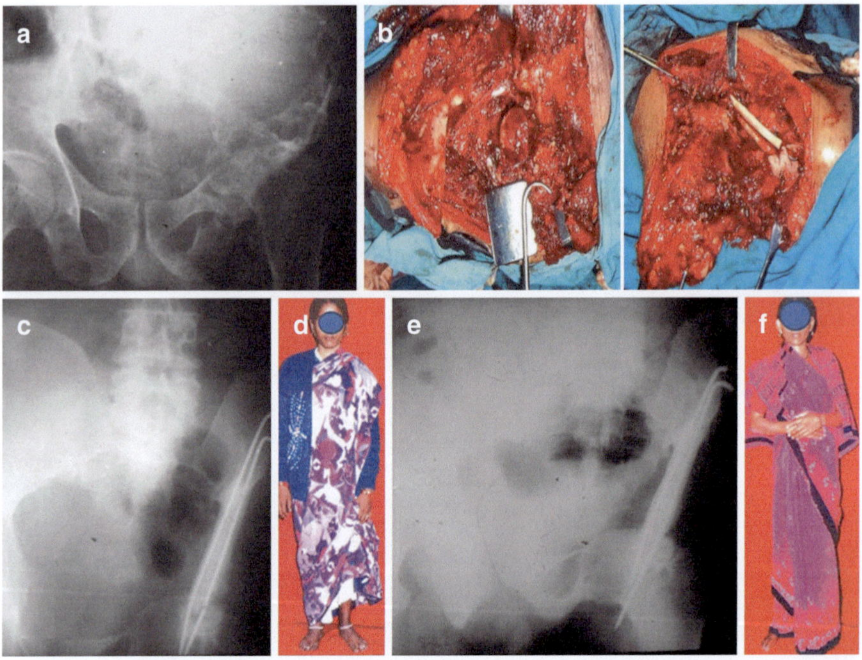

Fig. 7.4 (**a**) Radiograph showing a massive giant cell tumour of the left ilium. (**b**) Intraoperative pictures after excision of the lesion and reconstruction with twin fibular grafts fixed with Kirschner wires. (**c**) Roentgenogram taken 2 years after surgery shows lateral union and hypertrophy of the twin grafts resulting in a sheet of bone. (**d**) The patient with 2 cm shortening. (**e**, **f**) The radiograph of the same patient at the last follow-up after 5 years, showing total hypertrophy of the construct. The patient is able to carry out all the activities of daily living in a near-normal fashion

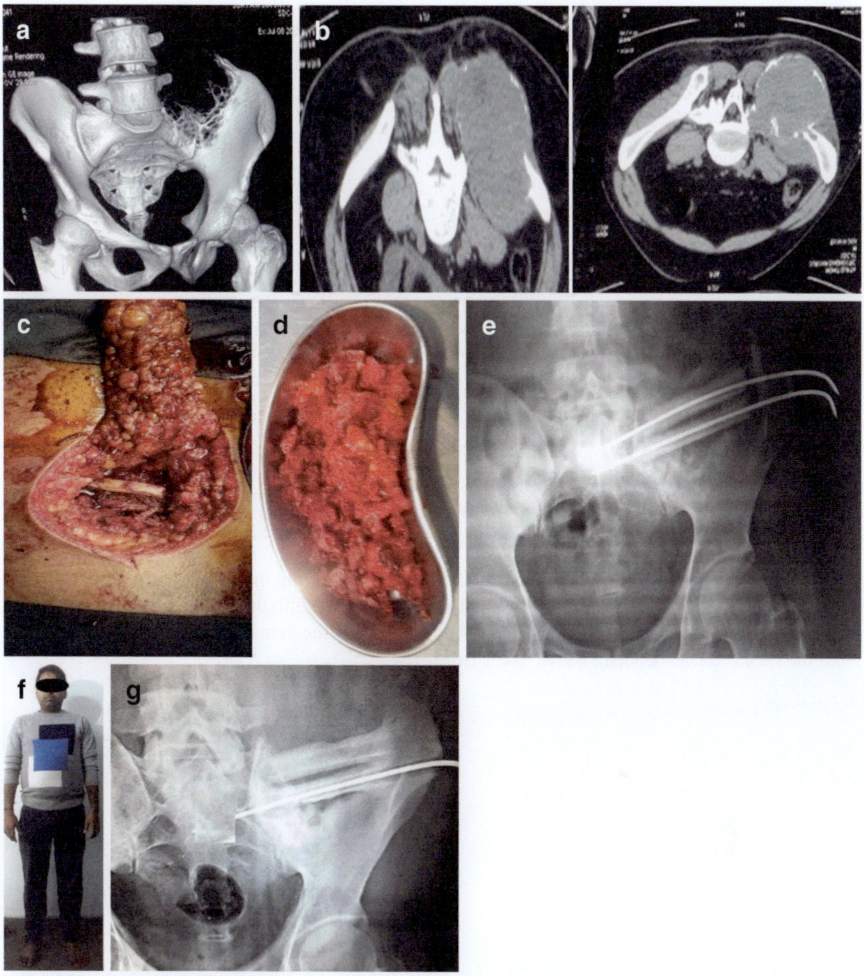

Fig. 7.5 (**a**) CT scan of a large giant cell tumour of the left ilium involving the sacro-iliac joint and the sacrum. (**b**) CT Scan revealing a clear demarcation of the lesion with intact sciatic notch. (**c**) Intraoperative picture showing the twin fibular graft bridging the gap after thorough curettage. (**d**) The curetted material. (**e**) Postoperative roentgenogram after curettage and reconstruction with dual struts stabilized with Kirschner wires. (**f**) The patient could bear weight 8 weeks after surgery. (**g**) Roentgenogram 20 weeks after excision and reconstruction. Note the wires have been removed after healing. Lateral union between the struts has developed

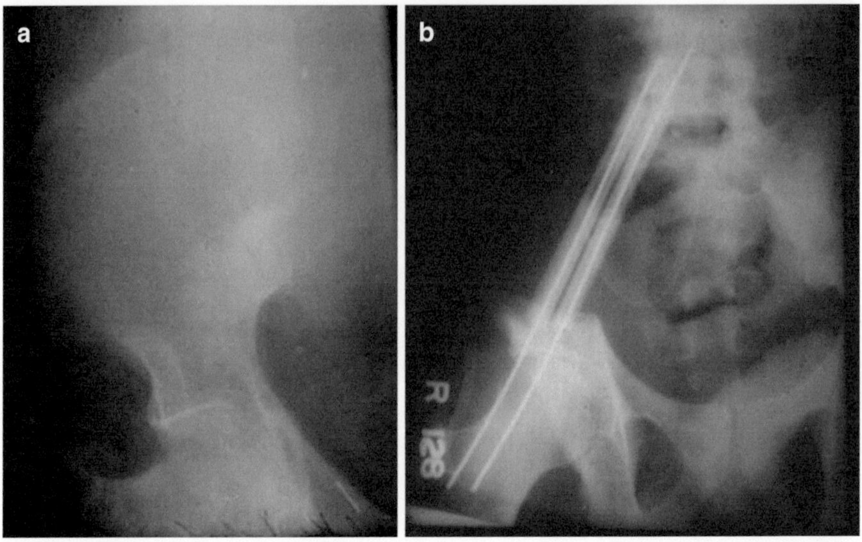

Fig. 7.6 (**a**) Radiograph reveals a huge chondrosarcoma involving the whole of the ilium. (**b**) The lesion was excised and reconstruction was attempted with twin fibular grafts stabilized with long Kirschner wires between the body of the L4 vertebra and the remaining supra-acetabular area. Note the lateral union between the fibular struts

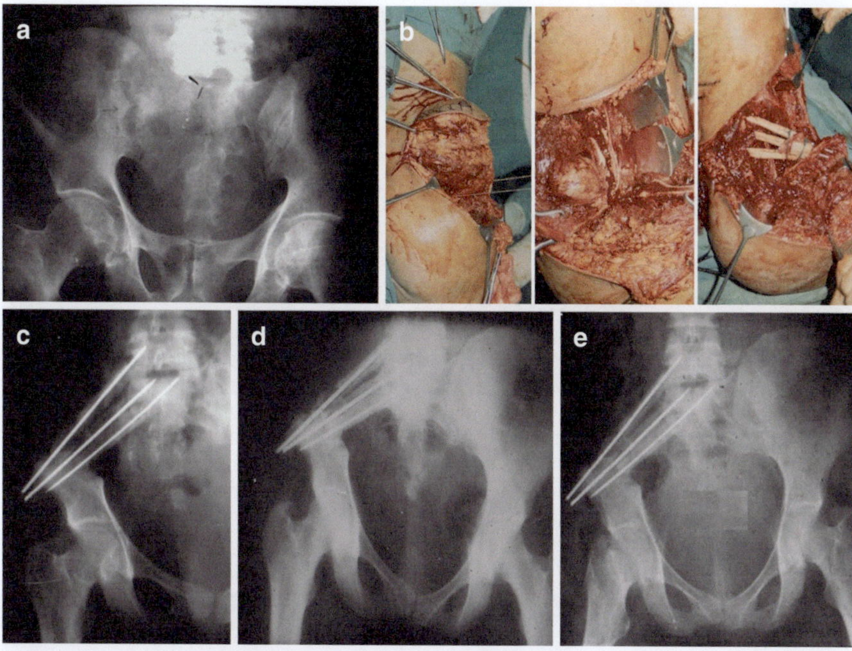

Fig. 7.7 (**a**) Radiograph revealing a massive chondrosarcoma of the right ilium involving the sacro-iliac joint. (B) The intraoperative pictures showing excision of the lesion and three fibular struts fixed between the spine (L-4) and the remaining ilium distally. (**c**) The postoperative radiograph taken after 16 weeks showing lateral union between the three struts. (**d**) Roentgenogram taken after 32 weeks. The fibular struts have shown complete union at both the host-graft junctions and reveal lateral union. (**e**) The final roentgenogram taken after 1 year which reveals complete healing at both ends. The middle and the lower struts have united after lateral union, and the union between the top and middle one is in progress. Note the boundaries of the pelvis are normal

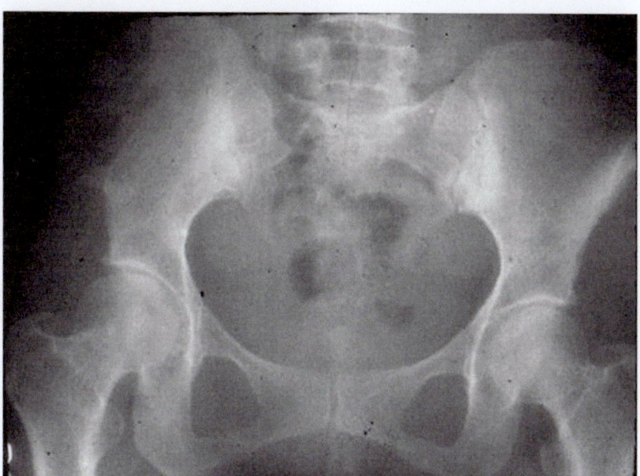

Fig. 7.8 Radiograph of the pelvis revealing chondrosarcoma of the right ilium with posterior extension. The involved ilium was removed

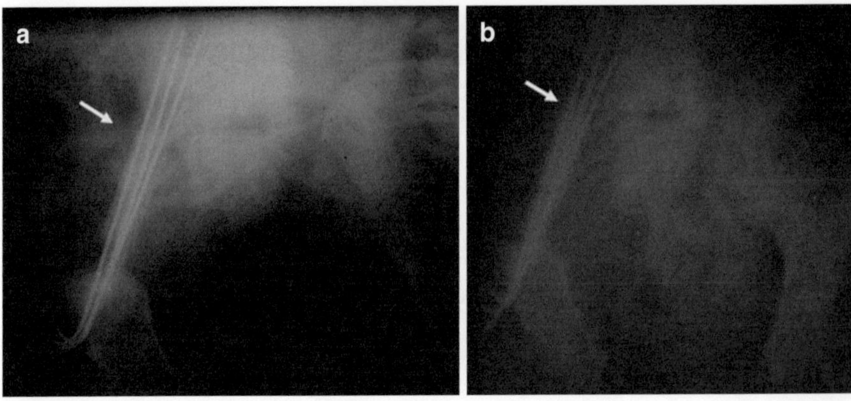

Fig. 7.9 (**a**) Radiograph revealing triple fibular struts used to bridge the gap stablized with three Kirschner wires (arrow). The struts extend covering the excised gap, and the wires only go beyond fixing the grafts to the L4 vertebra. (**b**) Radiograph taken 6 months later revealed complete union between the fibular struts and at both ends of the construct

Fig. 7.10 Angiogram showing a displaced iliac arterial trunk in a case of massive chondrosarcoma of the right ilium. Though invasive, the investigation is very useful to the surgeon during excision of the lesion

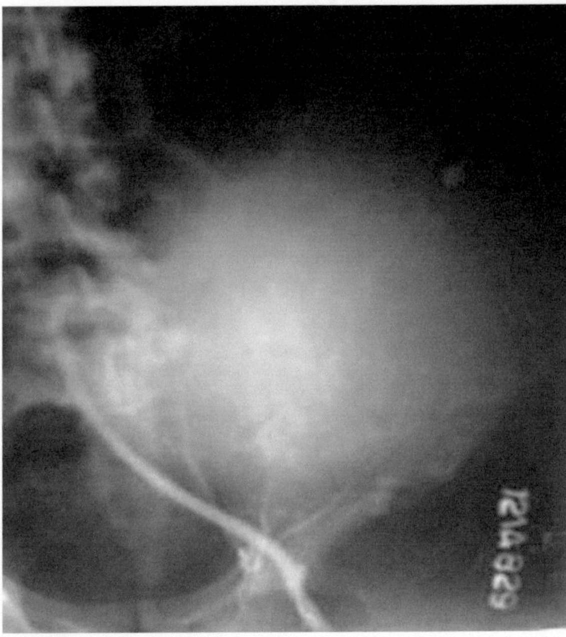

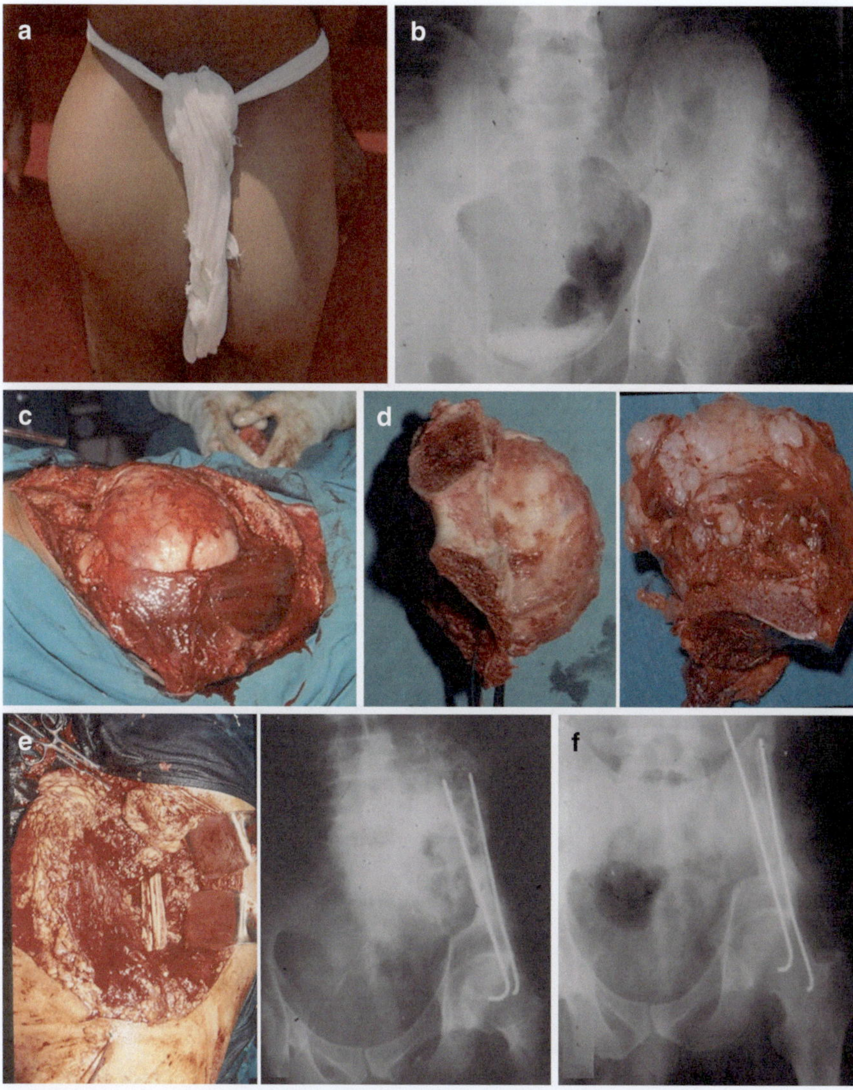

Fig. 7.11 (**a**) A large chondrosarcoma of the left ilium. (**b**) Radiograph reveals the lesion from the outer crest of the bone. (**c**) Intraoperative picture during excision. (**D**) The excised specimen. (**E**) Radiograph taken after 6 months reveal the twin fibular grafts fixed to the remaining bone with twin Kirschner wires. Note the construct shows healing, bridging the defect. (**F**) Radiograph 1 year after the surgery shows recurrence. The patient was put on chemotherapy

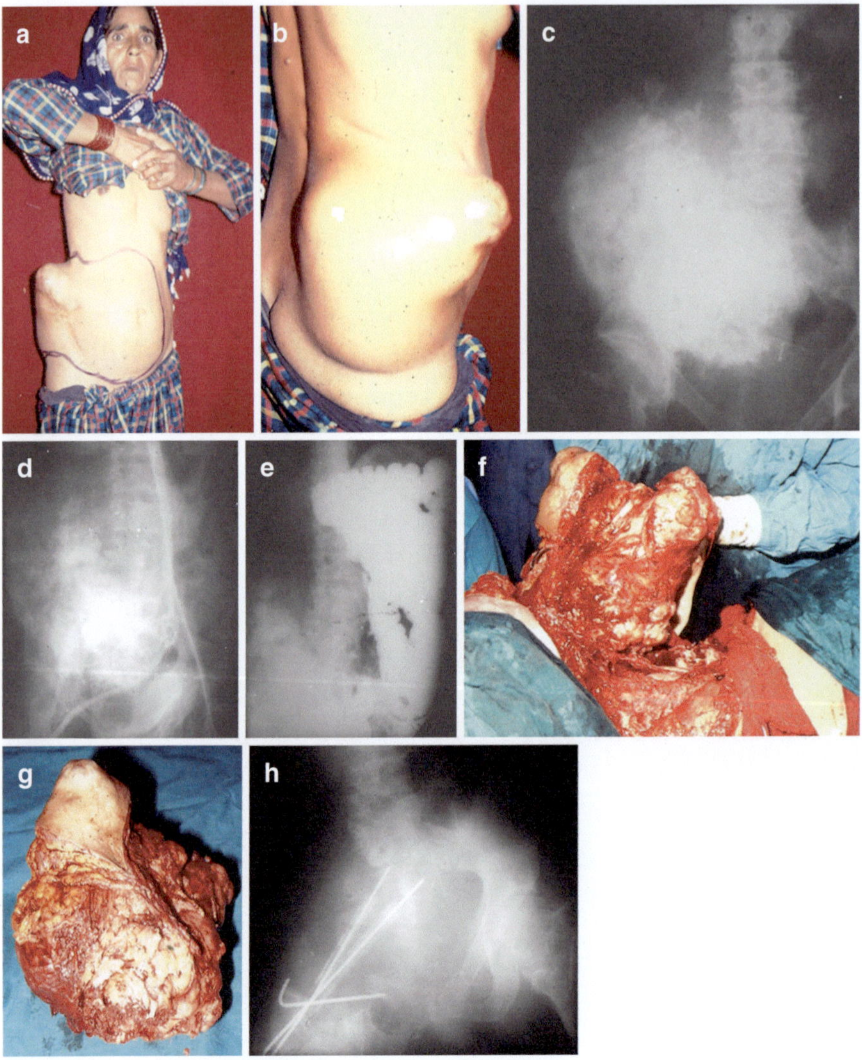

Fig. 7.12 (**a**, **b**) Massive bony swelling in the right iliac region in a 43-year-old lady. (**c**) Radiograph revealed a huge chondrosarcoma of the ilium. (**d**) Angiogram revealing severe displacement of the common iliac arterial trunk and the right iliac artery. (**e**) Barium enema shows displacement of the intra-abdominal contents on the left side. (**f**) Intraoperative picture during excision of the lesion. (**g**) The excised specimen. (**h**) Radiograph after excision of the lesion and reconstruction with twin fibular grafts with Kirschner wires stabilizing the pelvis

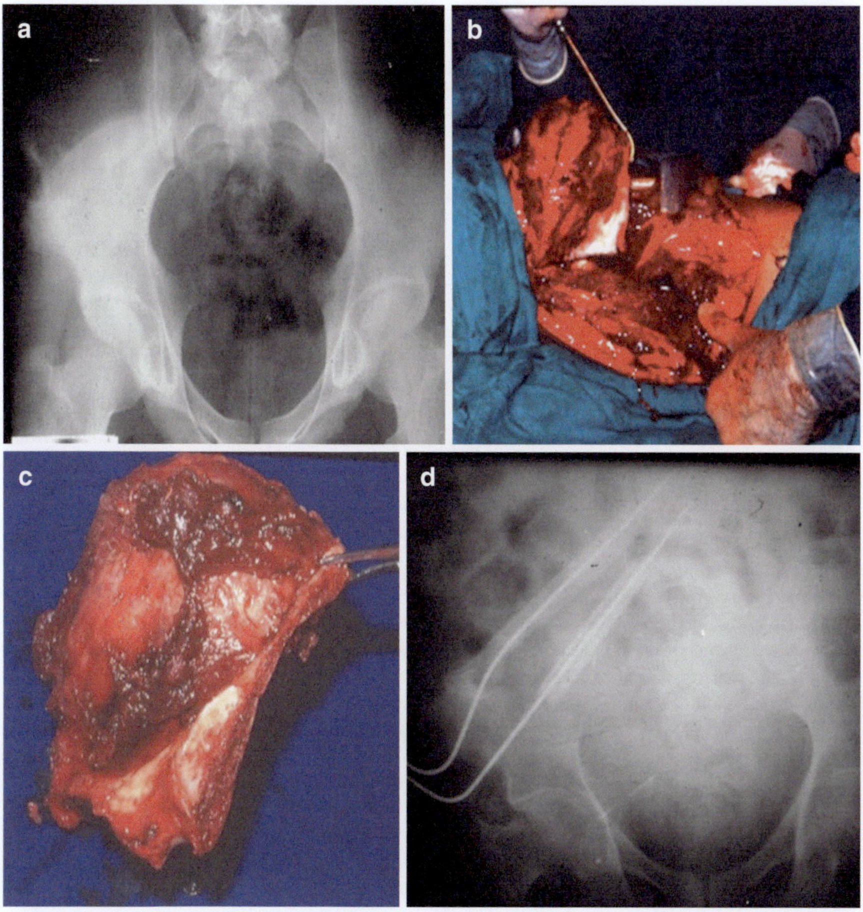

Fig. 7.13 (**a**) Roentgenogram reveals chondrosarcoma involving the posterior aspect of the right ilium. (**b**) Intraoperative picture showing the removal of the lesion and reconstruction with twin fibular grafts stabilized with Kirschner wires. (**c**) The excised specimen. (**d**) Roentgenogram revealing the twin grafts bridging the gap and stabilized with twin Kirschner wires. Note the healing of both host-graft junctions and the lateral union between the fibular struts. The inlet of the pelvis is near-normal

Suggested Reading

1. Akiyama T, Clark JC, Miki Y, Choong PF. The non-vascularised fibular graft: a simple and successful method of reconstruction of the pelvic ring after internal hemipelvectomy. J Bone Joint Surg. 2010;92:999–1005.
2. Aboulafia AJ, Buck R, Mathews J, Li W, Malawer MM. Reconstruction using the saddle prosthesis following excision of primary and metastatic Periacetabular Tumors. Clin Orthop Relat Res. 1995;314:203–13.
3. Bell RS, Davis AM, Wunder JS, et al. Allograft reconstruction of the acetabulum after resection of stage-IIB sarcoma. Intermediate-term results. J Bone Joint Surg. 1997;79:1663–74.
4. Beadel GP, McLaughlin CE, Aljassir F, et al. Iliosacral resection for primary bone tumors: is pelvic reconstruction necessary? Clin Orthop Relat Res. 2005;438:22–9.
5. Chang DW, Fortin AJ, Oates SD, Lewis VO. Reconstruction of the pelvic ring with vascularised double-strut fibular flap following internal hemipelvectomy. Plast Reconstr Surg. 2008;121:1993–2000.
6. Enneking WF, Dunham WK, Gebhardt MC, Malawar M, Pritchard DJ. A system for the functional evaluation of reconstructive procedures after surgical treatment of tumors of the musculoskeletal system. Clin Orthop Relat Res. 1993;286:241–6.
7. Enneking WF, Dunham WK. Resection and reconstruction for primary neoplasms involving the innominate bone. J Bone Joint Surg. 1978;60:731–46.
8. Erikson U, Hjelmstedt A. Limb saving radical resection of chondrosarcoma of the pelvis. J Bone Joint Surg. 1976;58:568–70.
9. Harrington KD. The use of hemipelvic allografts or autoclaved grafts for reconstruction after wide resections of malignant tumors of the pelvis. J Bone Joint Surg. 1992;74:331–41.
10. Hilmann A, Hoffmann C, Gosheger G, et al. Tumours of the pelvis: complications after reconstruction. Arch Orthop Trauma Surg. 2003;123:340–4.
11. Hsu RW, Wood MB, Sim FH, Chao EY. Free vascularised fibular grafting for reconstruction after tumour resection. J Bone Joint Surg. 1997;79:36–42.
12. Johnson JT. Reconstruction of the pelvic ring following tumor resection. J Bone Joint Surg. 1978;60:747–51.
13. Krieg AH, Lenze U, Gaston MS, Hefti F. The outcome of pelvic reconstruction with non-vascularised fibular grafts after resection of bone tumours. J Bone Joint Surg. 2010;92:1568–73.
14. Krieg AH, Hefti F. Reconstruction with non-vascularised fibular grafts after resection of bone tumours. J Bone Joint Surg. 2007;89:215–21.
15. Kojimoto H, Yasui N, Goto T, Matsuda S, Shimomura Y. Bone lengthening in rabbits by callus distraction: the role of periosteum and endosteum. J Bone Joint Surg. 1988;70:543–9.
16. Leggon RE, Zlotecki R, Reith J, Scarborough MT. Giant cell tumor of the pelvis and sacrum: 17 cases and analysis of the literature. Clin Orthop Relat Res. 2004;423:196–207.
17. Balke M, Streitbuerger A, Budny T, Henrichs M, Gosheger G, Hardes J. Treatment and outcome of giant cell tumors of the pelvis. Acta Orthop. 2009;80(5):590–6.
18. Nagoya S, Usui M, Wada T, Yamashita T, Ishii S. Reconstruction and limb salvage using a free vascularised fibular graft for periacetabular malignant bone tumours. J Bone Joint Surg. 2000;82:1121–4.
19. Osaka S, Toriyama S. Surgical treatment of giant cell tumours of the pelvis. Clin Orthop. 1980;222:123–31.
20. O'Connor MI, Sim FH. Salvage of the limb in the treatment of malignant pelvic tumors. J Bone Joint Surg. 1989;71:481–94.
21. Ozaki T, Hillmann A, Lindner N, Blasius S, Winkelmann W. Chondrosarcoma of the pelvis. Clin Orthop Relat Res. 1997;337:226–39.
22. Pacifico MD, Floyd D, Wood SH. Tibial stress fracture as a complication of free fibula vascularised graft for mandibular reconstruction. Br J Plast Surg. 2003;56:832–4.
23. Pant R, Moreau P, et al. Pelvic limb-salvage surgery for malignant tumors. Int Orthop. 2001;24(6):311–5.

24. Ray RD. Vascularization of bone grafts and implants. Clin Orthop Relat Res. 1972;87:43–8.
25. Sakuraba M, Kimata Y, Iida H, et al. Pelvic ring reconstruction with the vascularized fibular free flap double-barreled. Plast Reconstr Surg. 2005;116(5):1340–5.
26. Springfield S. Autograft reconstruction. Ortho Clin Am. 1996;27:483–92.
27. Parker T, Urbaniak JR, Durham NC. Donor-site morbidity with use of vascularized autogenous fibular grafts. J Bone Joint Surg. 1996;78:204–11.
28. Taylor GI, Miller GD, Ham FJ. The free vascularized bone graft: a clinical extension of microvascular techniques. Plast Reconstr Surg. 1975;55(5):533–44.
29. Tuli SM. Bridging of bone defects by massive bone grafts in tumorous conditions and in osteomyelitis. Clin Orthop. 1972;87:60–73.
30. Uchida A, Myoui A, Araki N, et al. Prosthetic reconstruction for periacetabular malignant tumors. Clin Orthop Relat Res. 1996;326:238–45.
31. Yadav SS. Bridging of large skeletal defects by twin fibular grafts supported by L-plate fixation. Orthop Int Edition. 1995;3:213–21.
32. Yadav SS. Dual-fibular grafting for massive bone gaps in the lower extremity. J Bone Joint Surg. 1990;72:486–94.

Chapter 8
Post-infective Massive Bone Loss of Long Bones That Require Bridging

8.1 Post-infective Massive Bone Loss of Long Bones That Require Bridging

Large diaphyseal defects of long bones after post-infective sequestration continue to be a challenge for the surgeon. Chronic osteomyelitis and persistent sepsis often result in loss of diaphysis of long bones, more so in children. It may follow massive segmental bone death, wrongly timed sequestrectomy or a radical bone debridement (Figs. 8.1a–g and 8.2a–e). Such a situation is also associated with severe fibrosis and poor vascularity in the soft tissue envelope. This makes the tissues less

S. S. Yadav, *Non-Vascularised Fibular Grafts in Orthopaedic Practice*,
https://doi.org/10.1007/978-981-95-1794-7_8

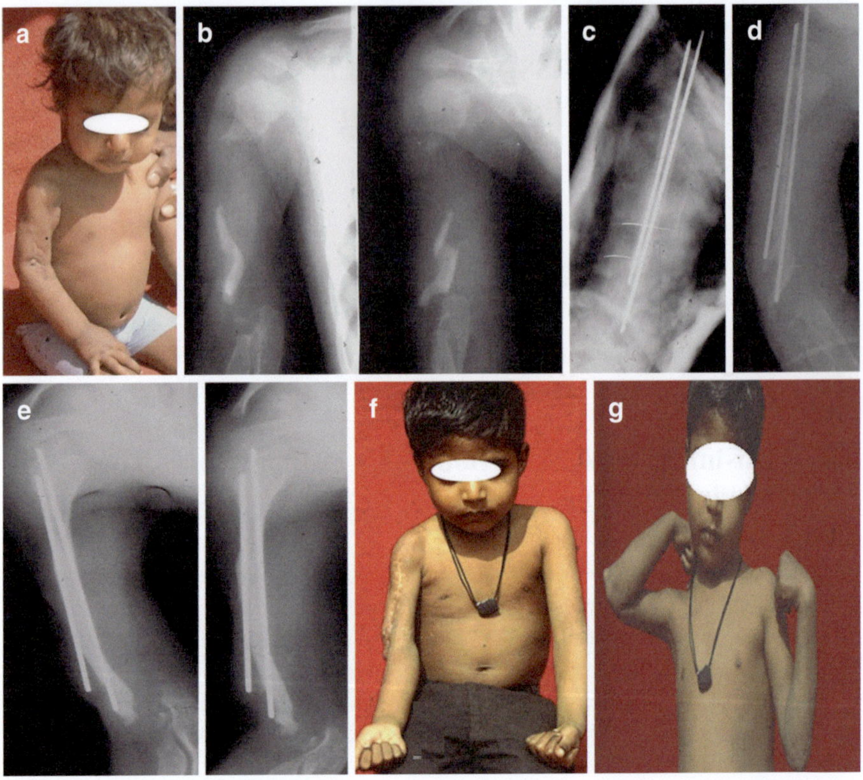

Fig. 8.1 (**a**) A child with a history of acute osteomyelitis of the right humerus was brought with a short right arm and healed scars. (**b**) Radiograph revealed post-infective severe diaphyseal loss of the right humerus with the head of the humerus and distal end deformed. It has been a challenge to manage this case. (**c**) Post-operative radiograph illustrates twin fibular strut grafts stabilized by twin Kirschner wires between the head of the humerus and the remaining distal end, further supported with a POP cast. (**d**) Note the healing of the fibular struts with lateral union. (**e**) Note the final healing with lateral union that simulates the humeral shaft. The final radiograph illustrates the lengthening of the humerus that has occurred (the Kirschner wires appear short). (**f, g**) The clinical pictures reveal the lengthening of the arm. Note the movements at the elbow and shoulder and the function of the right hand

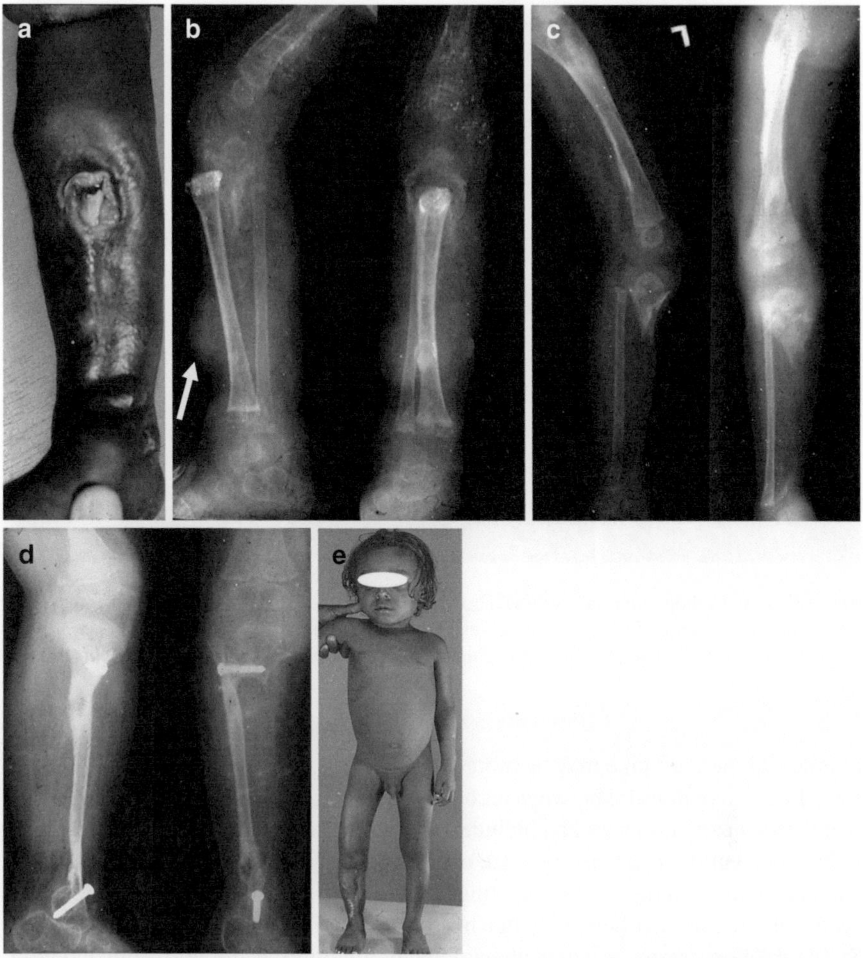

Fig. 8.2 (**a**) A 3-year-old child with acute osteomyelitis of the tibial shaft on the right side. The leg was swollen and drained pus. Note the abscess at the distal leg and ankle (arrow). (**b**) The roentgenogram revealed separated diaphyseal ends at the metaphyseal level. (**c**) While dressing, the whole separated diaphysis came out, leaving behind a small tibial end proximally. The distal end of the tibia was almost missing. (**d**) After the wounds healed, the entire fibular shaft was medialized and fixed to the proximal tibial end with a screw. Since the distal end of the tibia was not available, the fibular end was wedged into the body of the talus and also fixed with a screw. The roentgenogram taken 6 months after fixation revealed complete union at both ends and hypertrophy of the fibular shaft. (**e**) Clinical picture of the patient bearing weight on the right leg. Note the scaring on the anteromedial aspect of the right leg

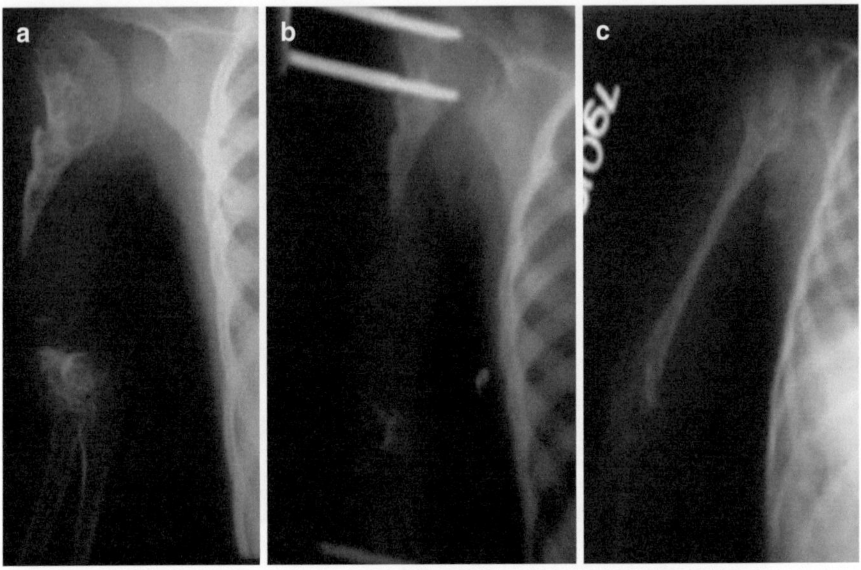

Fig. 8.3 (**a–c**) Radiograph of a 7-year-old boy showing post-infective diaphyseal gap with a short right arm. Lengthening of the arm was achieved by gradual distraction. The gap was bridged with single fibular strut stabilized by a long Kirschner wire that resulted in formation of the right humerus

pliable and the graft take may be more difficult (Figs. 8.3a–c and 8.4a–g). In severe bone loss, the options lie between reconstruction and even amputation. The modalities for reconstruction vary and include the use of non-vascularized graft and vascularized bone graft. The construct also offers a better mechanical advantage for early and dependable union and remodelling. Twin fibular grafts not only provide added graft volume but also help in better host-graft fixation (Figs. 8.5a–d and 8.6a–e). Stable fixation creates a better physiological condition at the host-graft junction,

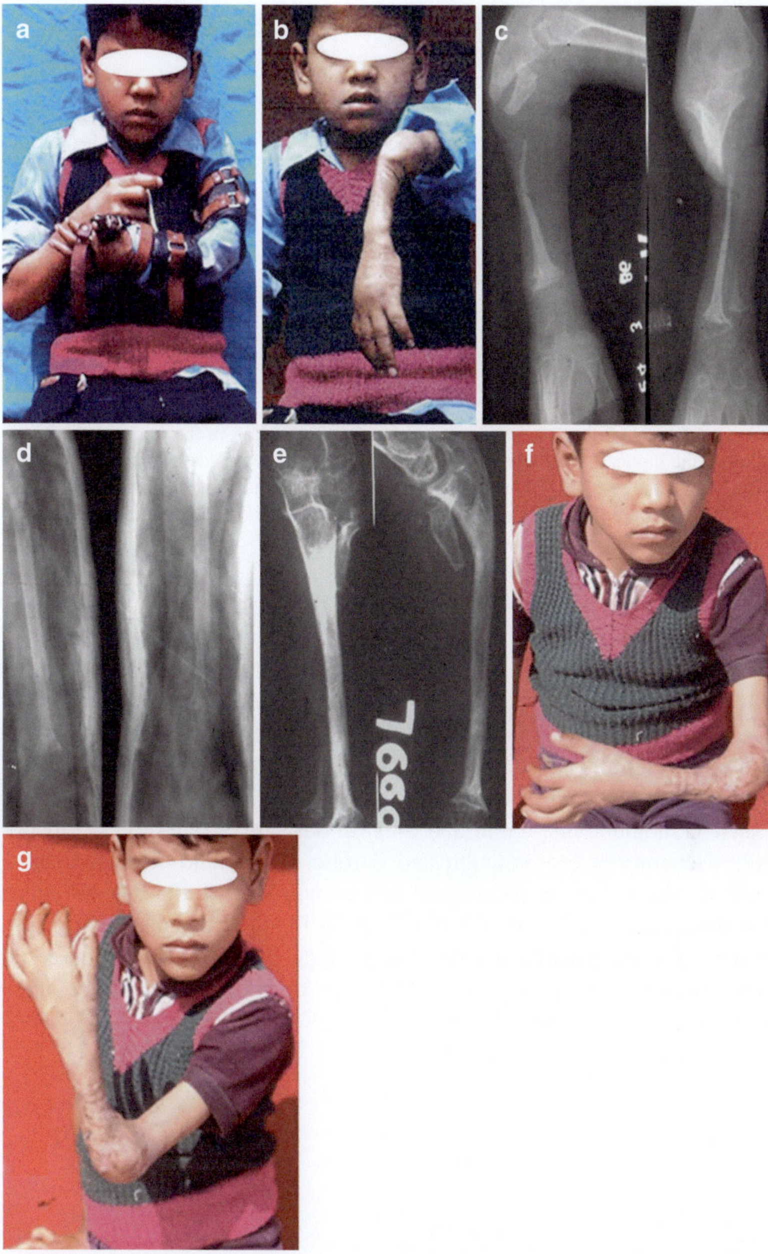

Fig. 8.4 (**a–e**) A 7-year-old boy came with an orthotic appliance of the left forearm. The left forearm was unstable. Radiograph revealed a post-infective large bone gap non-union of the left radius and ulna. Roentgenogram revealed gap non-union of the radius and ulna. A single bone forearm was reconstructed by a single fibular strut stabilized by a Kirschner wire between the ulna proximally and radius distally. Union had taken place at both ends and the single bone forearm. Note the hypertrophy of the fibular strut. (**f, g**) The forearm has been stable and functional

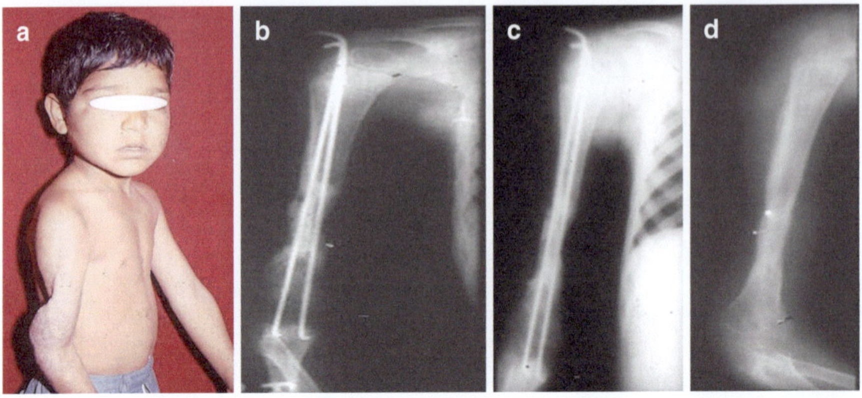

Fig. 8.5 (**a**) Clinical picture of the right arm showing angulation in the middle, consistent with non-union of the humeral shaft (the first radiograph could not be made available). (**b**) The radiograph illustrates bridging with twin fibular grafts stabilized with long Kirschner wires. (**c**) The radiograph reveals complete healing. (**d**) The wires have been removed. Note the hypertrophy of the twin fibular grafts which simulates the shaft of the humerus

resulting in early lateral union, and minimizes the period of immobilization of the extremity.

Our results have revealed that these fibular struts have united to the host bone without undergoing the classical degenerative changes, described earlier in non-vascularized grafts (Figs. 8.7a–e, 8.8a–c, and 8.9a, b). Enhanced quality and quantity of these strut grafts have also the advantage that 'lateral union' between the two struts has resulted in a sheet of bone with a diameter similar to that of the parent bone such as the humerus, femur and tibia. In post-infective cases, the host bed is relatively ischemic or less vascular and fibrotic. In late and neglected cases, the extremity is short, can be lengthened and a twin strut grafts can be attempted (Figs. 8.10a–c, 8.11a–c, 8.12a–d, 8.13a–d, and 8.14a–d). Immediate transplantation of the non-vascularized fibular struts retains their cellular activity and results in enhanced osteogenesis which further adds to the strength of the construct during the period of graft incorporation (Fig. 8.15a–f).

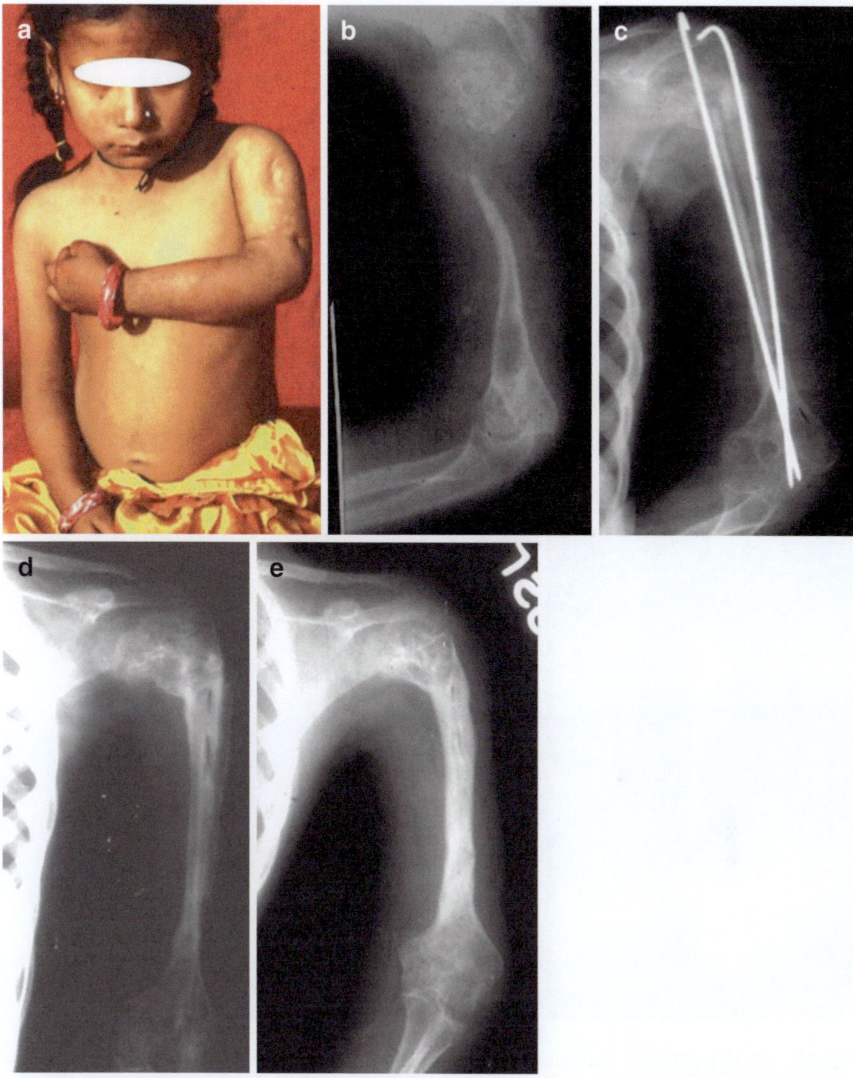

Fig. 8.6 (**a**) A 7-year-old girl had osteomyelitis of the left humerus which resulted in bone gap and shortening of the arm. (**b**) Radiograph revealing the bone gap. (**c**) A twin fibular graft stabilized with long Kirschner wires was attempted to bridge the bone gap. (**d**) Radiograph reveals healing of the construct. (**e**) The final picture of the twin grafts which simulate the diaphysis of the humerus

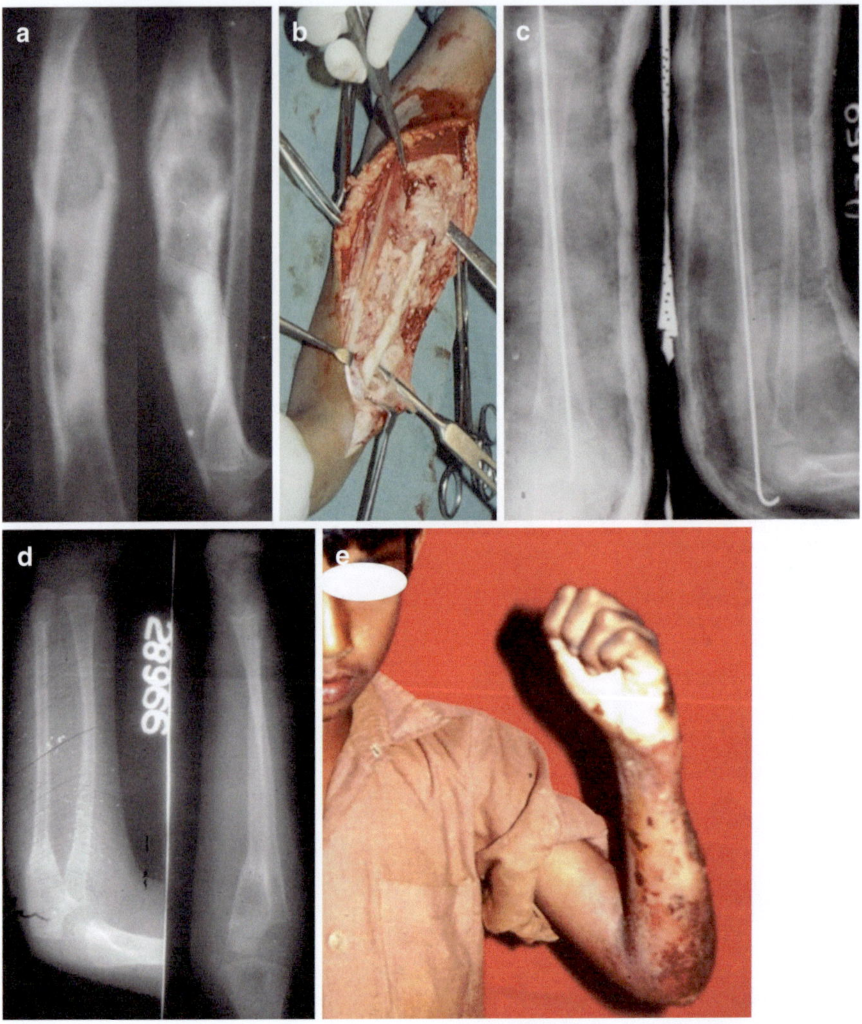

Fig. 8.7 (**a**) AP and lateral radiograph of chronic osteomyelitis of the left ulna with huge diaphyseal thickening, multiple lytic and sclerotic areas and cloacae discharging pus at multiple sites for the last 5 years. A diaphyseal excision in such cases is recommended. (**b**) Intraoperative picture after total ulnar diaphysectomy and a long fibular strut graft has been stabilized with a long Kirschner wire between both ends of the ulna. (**c**) AP and lateral postoperative radiographs reveal the fibular graft stabilized at both ends by a Kirschner wire. (**d**) The final AP and lateral roentgenogram showing union of the graft which simulates the ulnar shaft. (**e**) Clinical picture of the patient after removal of the POP cast. Note the function of the hand

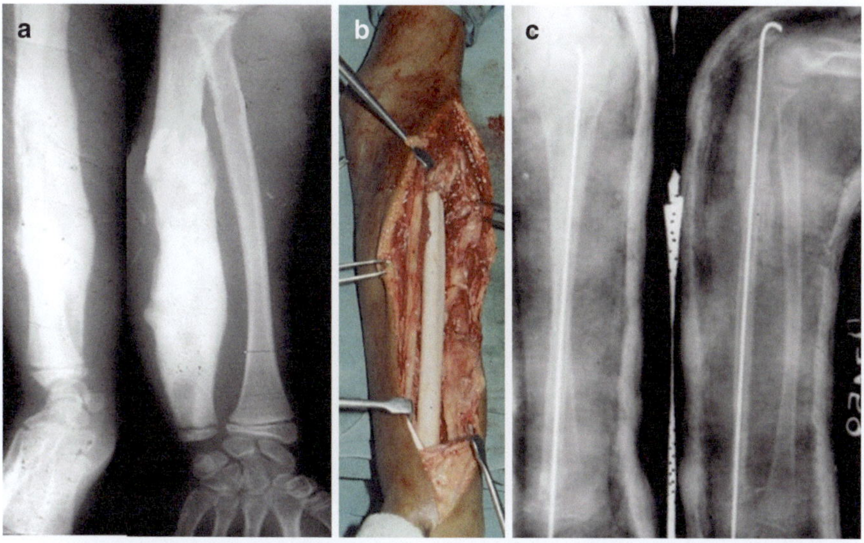

Fig. 8.8 (**a**) AP and lateral roentgenogram of a case of chronic sclerosing osteomyelitis of the left ulnar shaft discharging pus at multiple sites for the last 2 years. Note the huge irregular thickening of the diaphysis. (**b**) Intraoperative photograph of the fibular graft after excision of the ulnar diaphysis. (**c**) Postoperative radiograph showing the fixation of the fibular strut between the remaining ends of the ulna

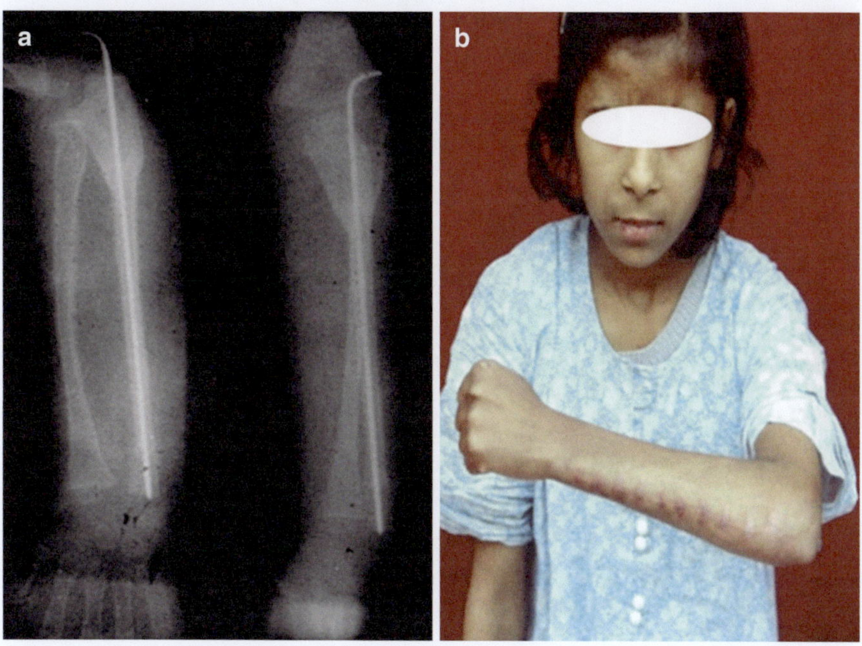

Fig. 8.9 (**a**) The final radiograph of the healed graft that simulates an ulnar shaft. (**b**) The clinical picture of the patient. Note the shape of the forearm, the stitch line and the function of the hand

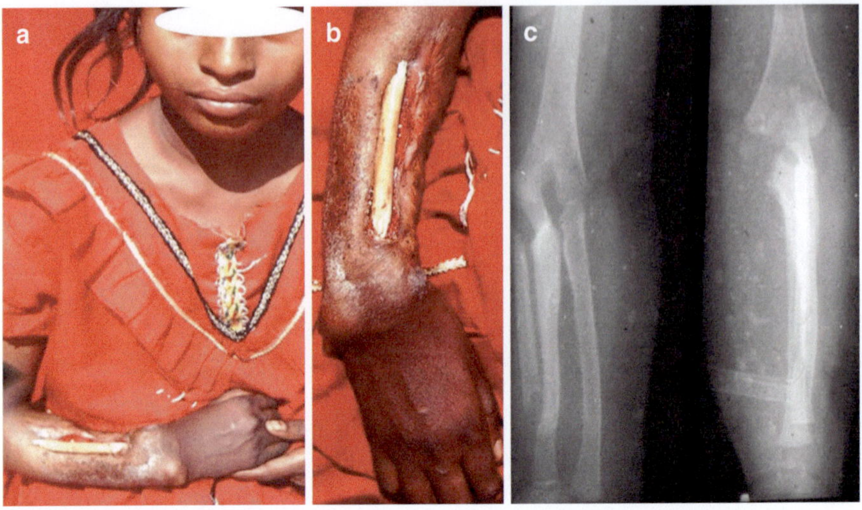

Fig. 8.10 (**a, b**) A 10-year-old girl shows an exposed diaphyseal sequestrum of the right ulna. (**c**) Roentgenogram reveals a long diaphyseal sequestrum with fully formed long involucrum united at both ends. The large diaphyseal sequestrum reveals a sclerotic appearance. The long sequestrum was removed and the wound healed

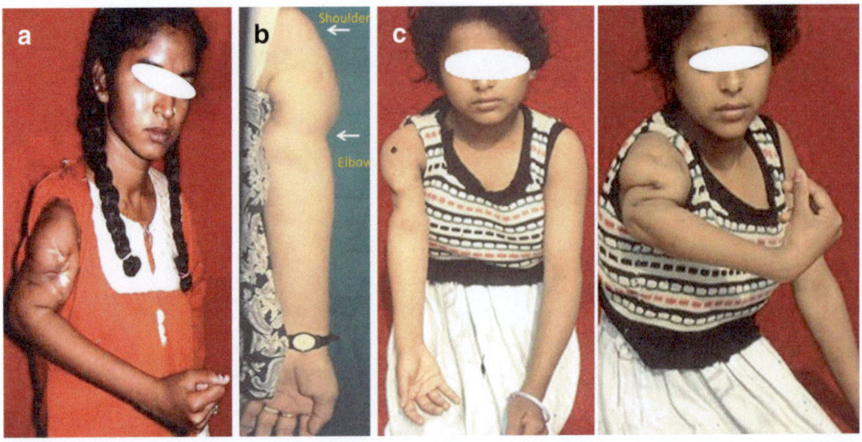

Fig. 8.11 (**a–c**) It was a coincidence that three lady patients came within a week with post-infective shortening of the arm with diaphyseal bone loss

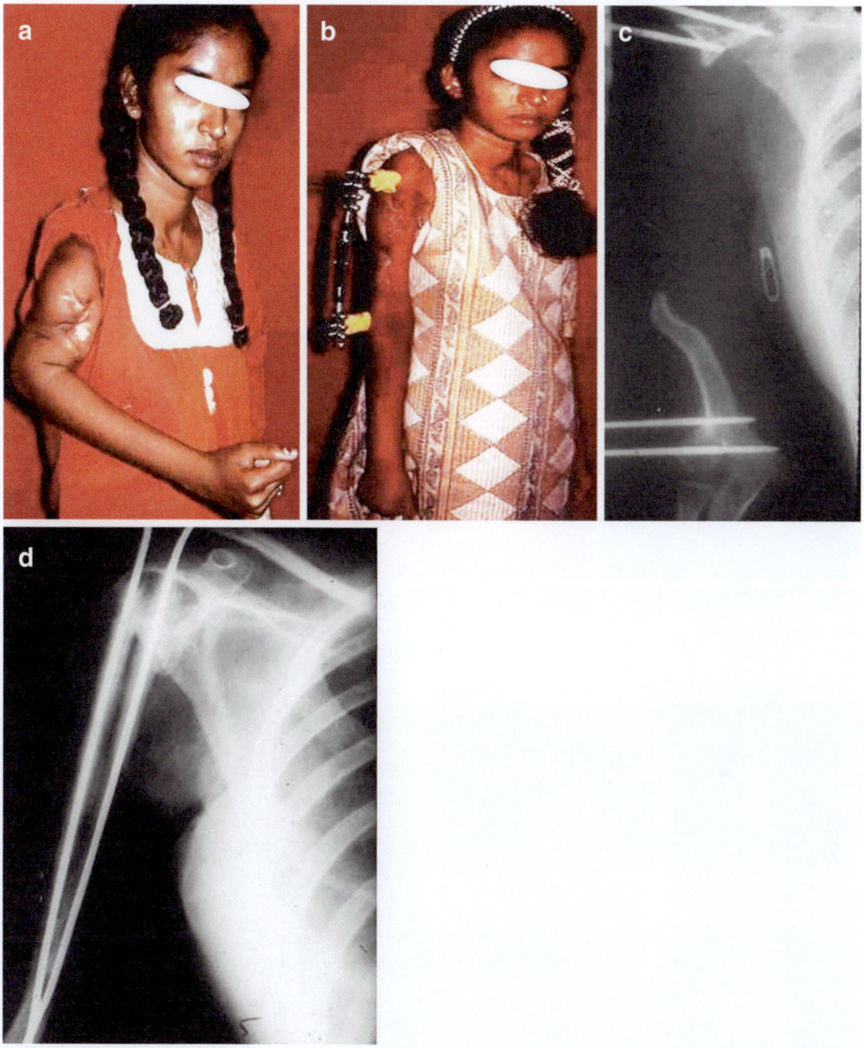

Fig. 8.12 **(a–d)** A 22-year-old girl had chronic osteomyelitis of the right humerus with a shortened arm. Large diaphyseal sequestration resulted in the shortening. Gradual lengthening of the arm was achieved using an external fixator along the full length of the arm. Twin fibular struts were stabilized with long twin Kirschner wires fixed to the host bone ends, resulting in union at both ends of the graft. Note the early lateral union between the struts

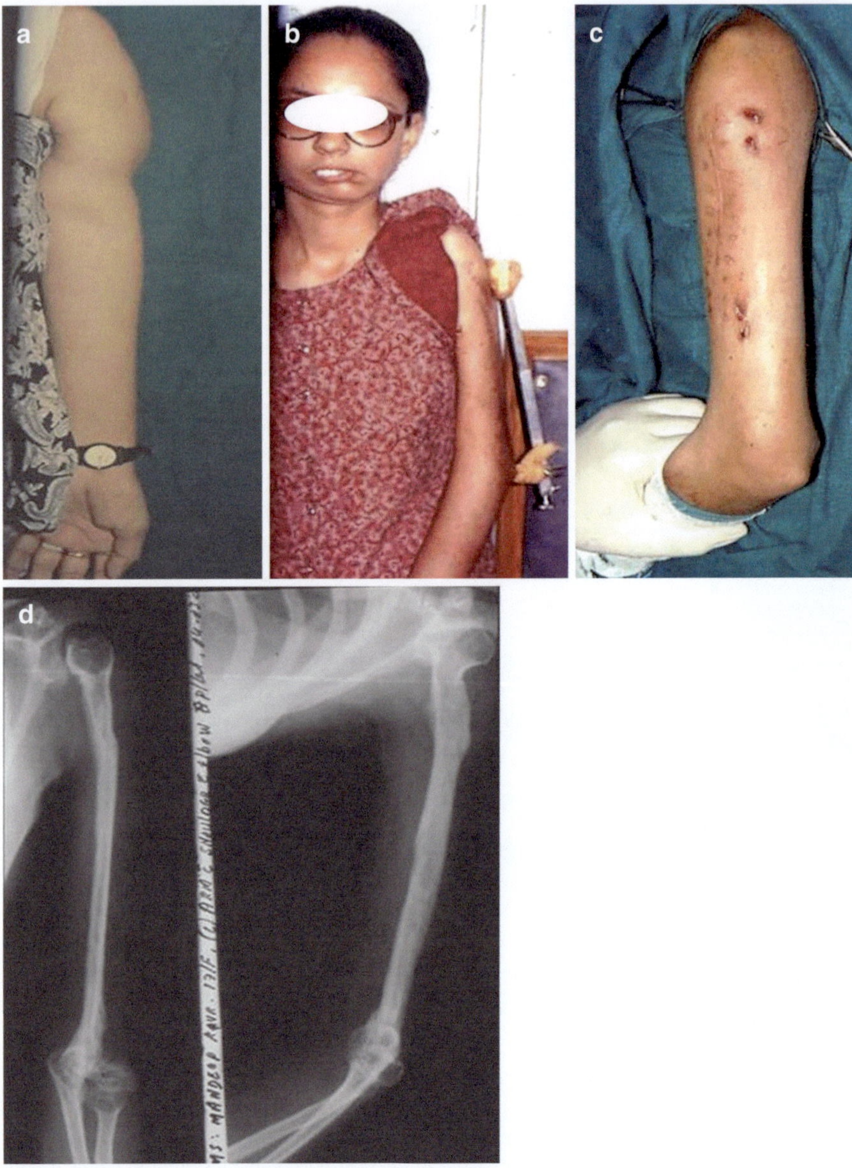

Fig. 8.13 (**a**) An 18-year-old girl had chronic osteomyelitis of the left humerus. Large diaphyseal sequestration resulted in a shortened arm (arrows). The first radiograph could not be made available. However, the bone ends could be felt. (**b**) Gradual lengthening of the arm was attempted using an external fixator, and the full length of the arm was achieved. (**c**) Twin fibular struts were stabilized using long twin Kirschner wires between the host bone ends which resulted in complete lateral union between the struts. (**d**) A roentgenogram taken 2 years after surgery revealed union and remodelling of the shaft simulating the humerus

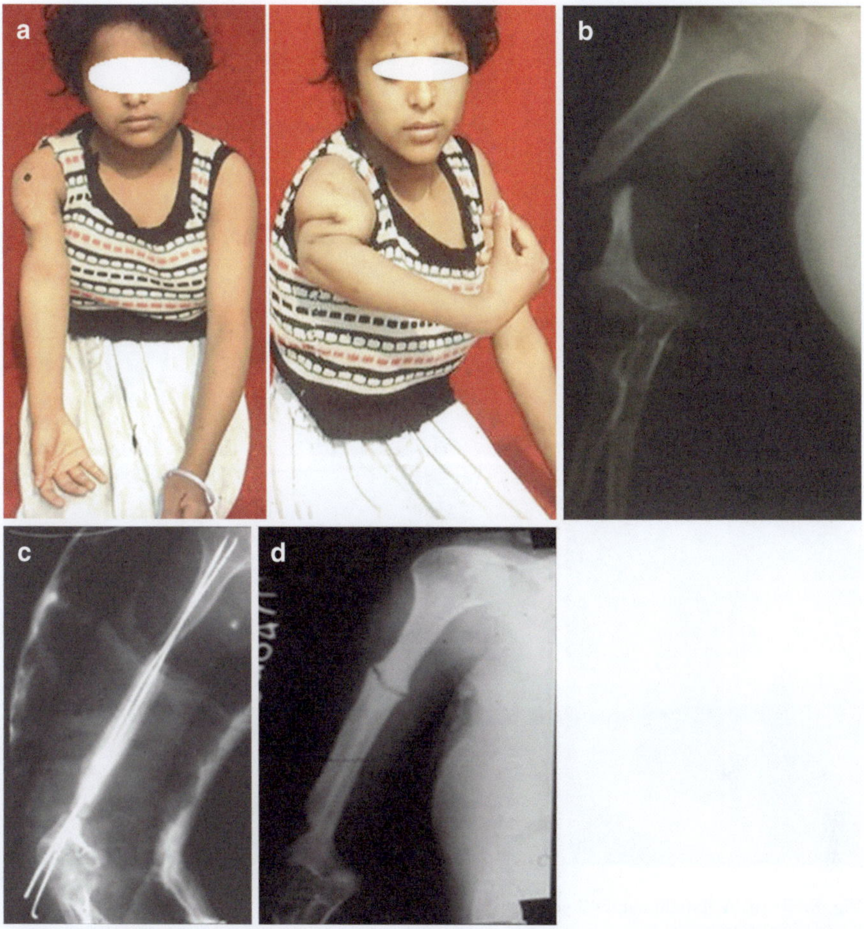

Fig. 8.14 (**a**) A 20-year-old girl had osteomyelitis of the right humerus and had premature diaphyseal sequestration which resulted in a very short arm. (**b**) Radiograph of the short arm showing gradual lengthening with an external fixator, which led to lengthening of the arm. (**c**) Twin fibular grafts were stabilized with long Kirschner wires. (**d**) Radiograph reveals non-union at the proximal end of the graft which needed additional cancellous bone graft surgery

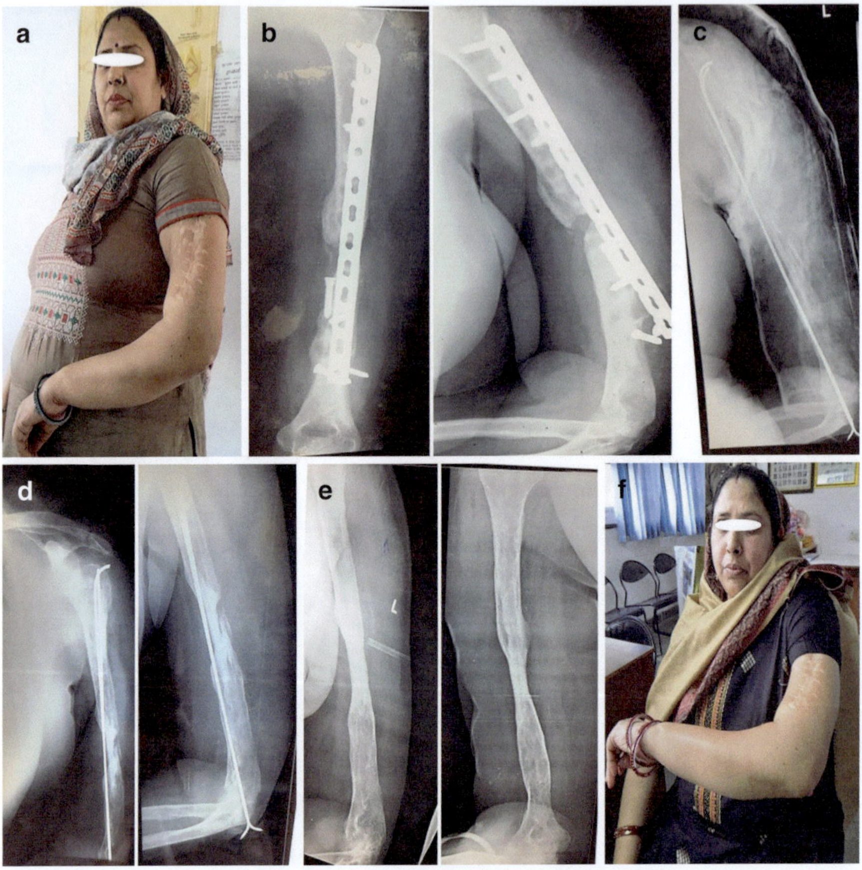

Fig. 8.15 (**a**) A female aged 40 years sustained fracture of the shaft of the left humerus. (**b**) She was operated many times in other centres and came to us with the present radiograph revealing gap non-union with failed plating. (**c**) She was operated, the plate was removed and twin fibular grafts were stabilized with twin long Kirschner wires along with additional cancellous bone grafting. (**d**) The roentgenogram reveals early healing. Note the bent wires above and below securing the construct. (**e**) The final radiograph illustrates complete healing and remodelling of the twin grafts after 18 months. (**f**) The clinical picture of the patient with a stable arm after the treatment

Suggested Readings

1. Arai K, Toh YM, Okamoto Y, Harata S. One bone forearm formation using vascularized fibula graft massive bone defect of the forearm with infection: case report. J Reconstr Microsurg. 2001;17:151–3.
2. Steinlechner CWB, Mkandawire NC. Non-vascularised fibular transfer in the management of defects of long bones after sequestrectomy in children. J Bone Joint Surg. 2005;87(9):1259–63.
3. Lew DP, Waldvogel FA. Osteomyelitis. Lancet. 2004;364:369–79.
4. Al-Zharani S, Halting MG, Kremli M, et al. Free fibular graft still has a place in treatment of bone defects. Injury. 1993;24:551–4.
5. Enneking WF, Eady JL, Burchardt H. Autogenous cortical bone grafts in the reconstruction of segmental skeletal defects. J Bone Joint Surg Am. 1980;62(7):1039–58.
6. Yadav SS. Dual fibular grafting for massive bone gaps in the lower extremity. J Bone Joint Surg. 1990;72:484–94.
7. Yadav SS. Bridging of large skeletal defects by twin fibular grafts supported by L-plate fixation. Orthop Int Edition. 1995;3:213–21.
8. Krieg AH, Hefti F. Reconstruction with non-vascularised fibular grafts after resection of bone tumours. J Bone Joint Surg Br. 2007;89:215–21.
9. Schuh R, Panotopoulos J, Puchner SE, Willegger M, Hobusch GM, Windhager R, Funovics PT. Vascularisd or non-vascularised autologous fibular grafting for the reconstruction of a Diaphyseal bone defect after resection of a musculoskeletal tumour. Bone Joint J. 2014;96:1258–63.
10. Soucacos PN, Korompilias AV, Vekris MD, Zoubos A, Beris AE. The free vascularized fibular graft for bridging large skeletal defects of the upper extremity. Microsurgery. 2011;31:190–7.
11. Cannada LK. Viable bone and circulatory factors required for survival of bone grafts. Orthop Clin North Am. 2010;41(1):5–13.
12. Ray RD. Vascularization of bone grafts and implants. Clin Orthop. 1972;87:43–8.
13. Urist MR. Bone transplant and implants. In: Fundamental and clinical bone physiology. Philadelphia: J. B. Lippincott; 1980. p. 331.
14. Arai K, Toh S, Tsubo K, et al. Complications of vascularized fibula graft for reconstruction of long bones. Plast Reconstr Surg. 2002;109:2301–6.
15. Davis OK, Mazug JM, Coloman GN. A torsional strength comparison of vascularised and non-vascularised bone grafts. J Biomech. 1982;15:875–80.
16. Kocaoglu M, Eralp L, Tomak Y. Treatment of humerus shaft non-unions by the Ilizarov method. Int Orthop. 2001;25:396–400.
17. Beris AE, Lykissas MG, Korompilias AV, et al. Vascularized fibula transfer for/lower limb reconstruction. Microsurgery. 2011;31:205–11.
18. Shaffer JM, Field GS, Goldberg VM, Davy DT. Fate of vascularised and non-vascularised autograft. Clin Orthop. 1985;197:34–43.

Chapter 9
Post-traumatic Bone Loss of Long Bones Replaced with NVFG

9.1 Post-traumatic Bone Loss of Long Bones Replaced with NVFG

High-velocity injuries mostly due to road traffic accidents may result in post-traumatic bone loss. Such mutilating injuries of the extremities need careful assessment, thorough evaluation and early management. Extrusion of a diaphyseal fragment of a long bone of the extremity has been a challenge for the treating surgeon (Fig. 9.1a–e). The commonly suggested procedures to bridge such a bone loss are autologous fibular grafts—both non-vascularized and vascularized—bone transport, the Ilizarov technique and allografts.

In case the major extruded bone fragment in a compound fracture is available at the accident site, it is advisable to clean and wash it with antiseptic solution and then boil it for 20–30 min or sterilize it by any other technique. It can then be successfully replaced with suitable fixation. In case the extruded fragment is not available or the bone is crushed, the use of non-vascularized autogenous fibular strut bone graft is an option to bridge such a segmental loss (Fig. 9.2a–d). However, it has been a challenge to bridge such gaps.

In early and clean cases, single or twin fibular (NVFG) struts have been used (Fig. 9.3a, b). Stabilization of the graft to the host bone ends by Kirschner wires or screws has been described. In late presentations and infected cases, an attempt should be made to maintain the length of the bony defect for future surgery. A secondary procedure is required in late and infected cases, depending on the specifics of each case (Fig. 9.4a–c). Bridging the bone defects with NVFG in such cases has also proven useful once the infection has subsided (Figs. 9.5 and 9.6a, b).

S. S. Yadav, *Non-Vascularised Fibular Grafts in Orthopaedic Practice*,
https://doi.org/10.1007/978-981-95-1794-7_9

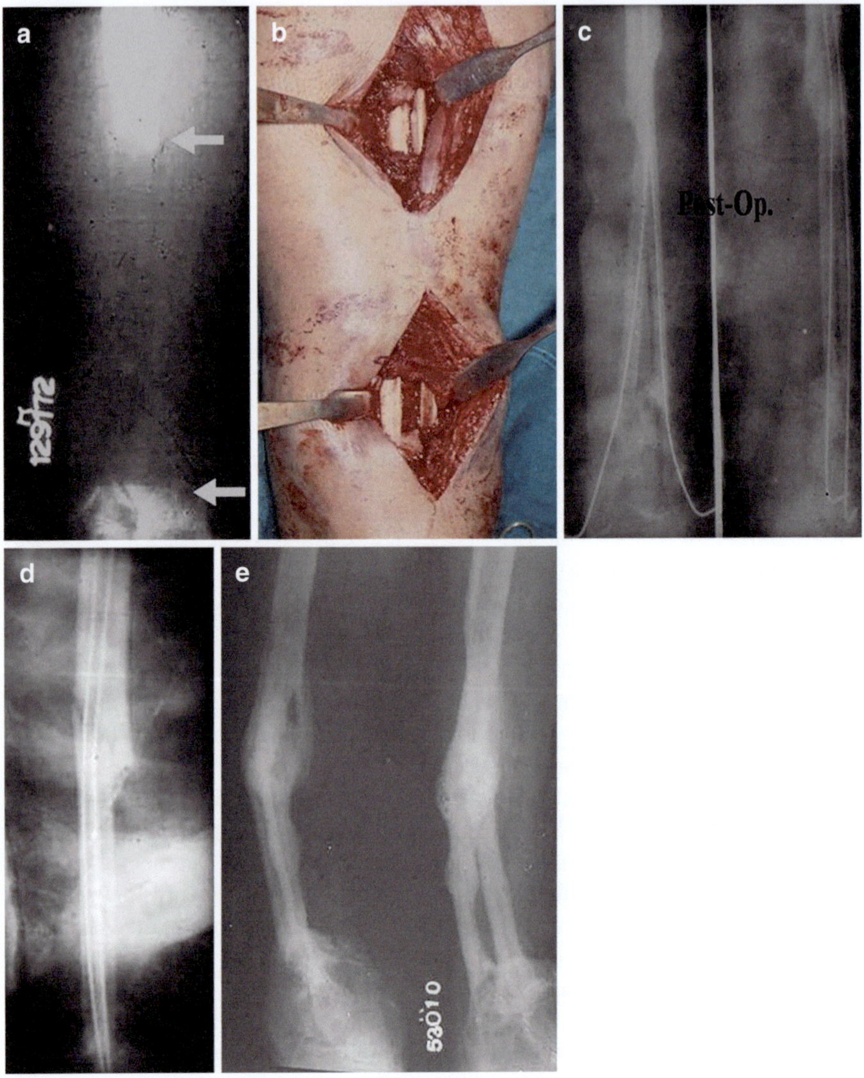

Fig. 9.1 (**a**) Roentgenogram of a 35–year-old veterinary surgeon who had a compound fracture of the distal half of the right femur 4 hours ago. A 9-inch segment of the distal diaphysis was missing. However, the condyles were intact (arrows). Under the circumstances, it appeared difficult to save the extremity. (**b**) Intraoperative picture demonstrates submuscular twin fibular grafting, stabilized with twin long Kirschner wires between the distal end of the available femur and the condyles. Since the gap was long, the contralateral fibula was also used. (**c**) AP and lateral postoperative roentgenograms reveal the twin fibular struts bridging the massive bone gap. (**d**) Roentgenogram taken after a year showed complete healing of the fibular struts with lateral union and healing at both host-graft junctions. (**e**) The patient had a fall and fractured one strut of the construct that had healed in a POP cast. The extremity has been short by 6 cm which had been compensated by a shoe raise. However, he is able to carry out his normal duties. Roentgenogram taken 35 years later shows sound healing and hypertrophy of the fibular struts

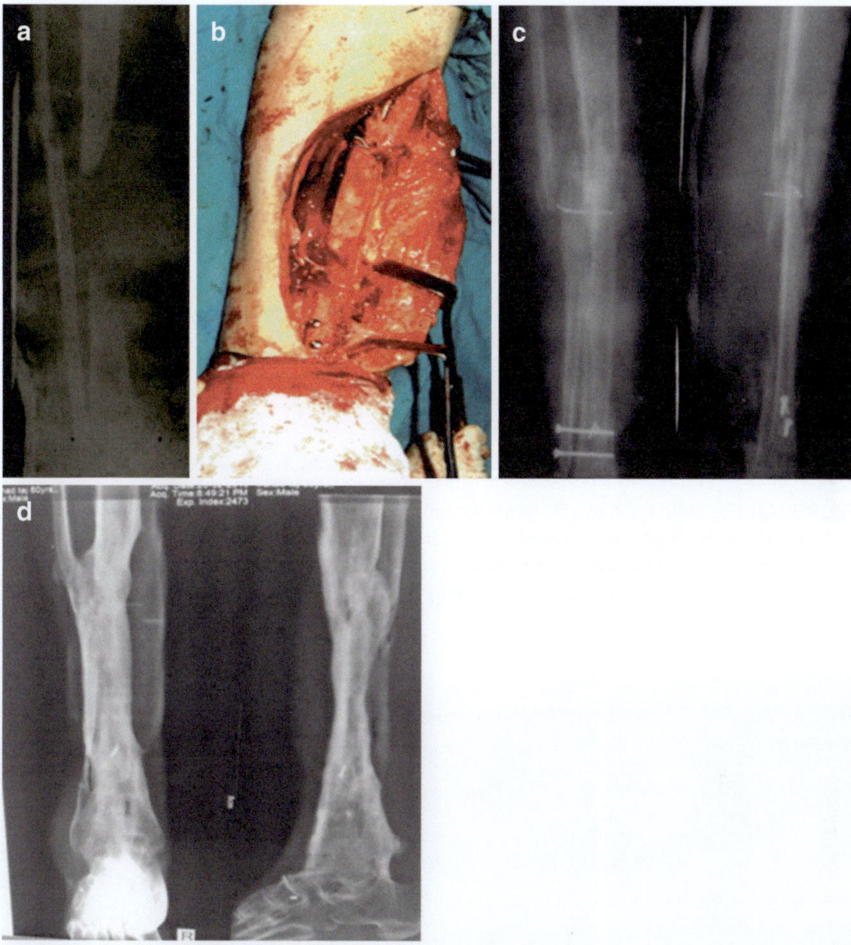

Fig. 9.2 (**a**) A 39-year-old male patient had a bomb-blast injury to his right leg where he had lost a 10-cm segment of the distal tibia. He also had a fracture of the fibular shaft. (**b**) Intraoperative picture reveals fixation of twin fibular graft bridging the gap. One of the struts was wedged into the tibial ends. The proximal ends of the graft were fixed with circumferential wiring and the distal ends stabilized with a pair of screws. (**c**) Postoperative AP and lateral radiographs show the fibular struts further stabilized in a plaster of Paris cast. (**d**) AP and lateral radiographs taken after 1 year reveal complete healing, consolidation and remodelling of the graft, simulating the shaft of the tibia

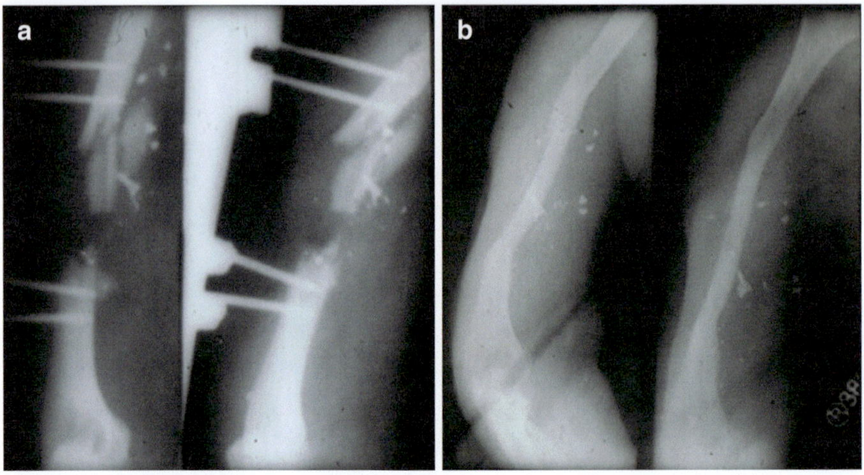

Fig. 9.3 (**a**) The radiograph of a 31-year-old male who sustained a bomb-blast injury of the right humerus where the diaphysis was crushed. The arm was stabilized with an external fixator. A twin fibular graft was stabilized with long Kirschner wires (radiograph not available). (**b**) A radiograph taken after 12 months revealed complete healing and remodelling of the fibular struts. The blast pellets can be seen

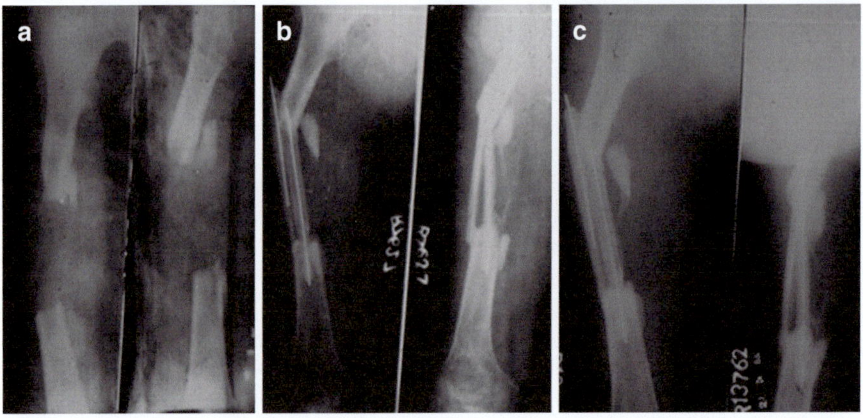

Fig. 9.4 (**a**) AP and lateral radiographs of a 48-year-old male who had a car accident and sustained a compound fracture with a 15-cm loss of the femoral diaphysis. (**b**) AP and lateral radiographs reveal twin fibular struts grafts stabilized with Kirschner wires. One of the struts was wedged into the femoral ends. The construct was further supported by a plaster of Paris cast. (**c**) AP and lateral radiographs taken after 10 months revealed complete healing with lateral union, though with slight angulation at the proximal end of the construct. Note the fibular construct simulates the diaphysis of the femur

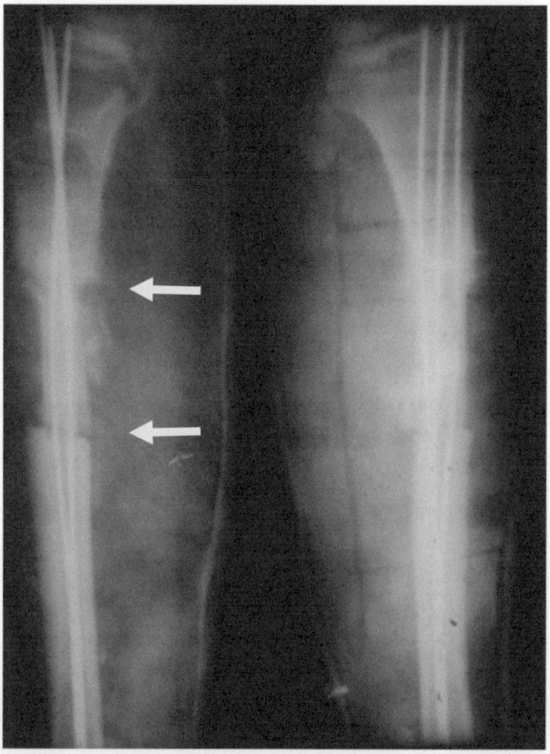

Fig. 9.5 AP and lateral radiographs of a challenging non-union of the proximal tibia which was excised and reconstructed with three fibular struts stabilized using suitable long inlay Kirschner wires (arrows). Note the healing of the gap after 8 months

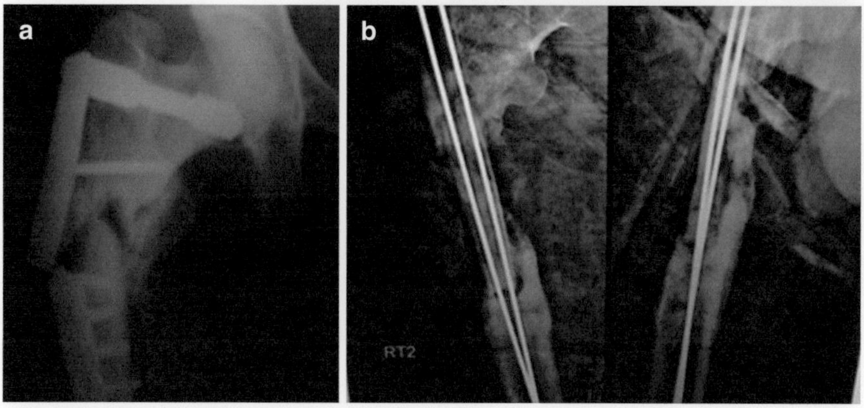

Fig. 9.6 (**a**) An ununited subtrochantric fracture with failed metallic implant. (**b**) After excision of the fibrous tissue, the gap was bridged by twin fibular grafts stabilized with Kirschner wires, resulting in union after 5 months

Suggested Readings

1. Al-Zharani S, Halting MG, Kremli M, et al. Free fibular graft still has a place in treatment of bone defects. Injury. 1993;24:551–4.
2. Enneking WF, Eady JL, Burchardt H. Autogenous cortical bone grafts in the reconstruction of segmental skeletal defects. J Bone Joint Surg. 1980;62(7):1039–58.
3. Yadav SS. Bridging of large skeletal defects by twin fibular grafts supported by L-plate fixation. Orthop Int Edition. 1995;3:213–21.
4. Krieg AH, Hefti F. Reconstruction with non-vascularised fibular grafts after resection of bone tumours. J Bone Joint Surg. 2007;89:215–21.
5. Schuh R, Panotopoulos J, Puchner SE, Willegger M, Hobusch GM, Windhager R, Funovics PT. Vascularisd or non-vascularised autologous fibular grafting for the reconstruction of a Diaphyseal bone defect after resection of a musculoskeletal tumour. Bone Joint J. 2014;96:1258–63.
6. Soucacos PN, Korompilias AV, Vekris MD, Zoubos A, Beris AE. The free vascularized fibular graft for bridging large skeletal defects of the upper extremity. Microsurgery. 2011;31:190–7.
7. Cannada LK. Viable bone and circulatory factors required for survival of bone grafts. Orthop Clin North Am. 2010;41(1):5–13.
8. Ray RD. Vascularization of bone grafts and implants. Clin Orthop. 1972;87:43–8.
9. Urist MR. Bone transplant and implants. In fundamental and clinical bone physiology. Philadelphia: J. B. Lippincott; 1980. p. 331.
10. Davis OK, Mazug JM, Coloman GN. A torsional strength comparison of vascularised and non-vascularised bone grafts. J Biomech. 1982;15:875–80.
11. Kocaoglu M, Eralp L, Tomak Y. Treatment of humerus shaft non-unions by the Ilizarov method. Int Orthop. 2001;25:396–400.
12. Beris AE, Lykissas MG, Korompilias AV, et al. Vascularized fibula transfer for/lower limb reconstruction. Microsurgery. 2011;31:205–11.
13. Shaffer JM, Field GS, Goldberg VM, Davy DT. Fate of vascularised and non-vascularised autograft. Clin Orthop. 1985;197:34–43.

Chapter 10
NVFG Used for Filling Bony Cavities After Curettage

10.1 NVFG Used for Filling Bony Cavities After Curettage

Curettage is a commonly performed procedure. The leftover cavity if small will heal. However, a large cavity does require a filler to avoid a pathological fracture. An autologous cancellous graft is the best material to fill such cavities, but because of its well-known disadvantage of limited availability, the cavity is not adequately filled. We have used NVFG as cavity filler after curettage (Fig. 10.1a–g). It can be used as single, double or even in multiple pieces (Fig. 10.2). The graft is easily available and has proven useful in healing and remodelling such cavities (Fig. 10.3).

S. S. Yadav, *Non-Vascularised Fibular Grafts in Orthopaedic Practice*,
https://doi.org/10.1007/978-981-95-1794-7_10

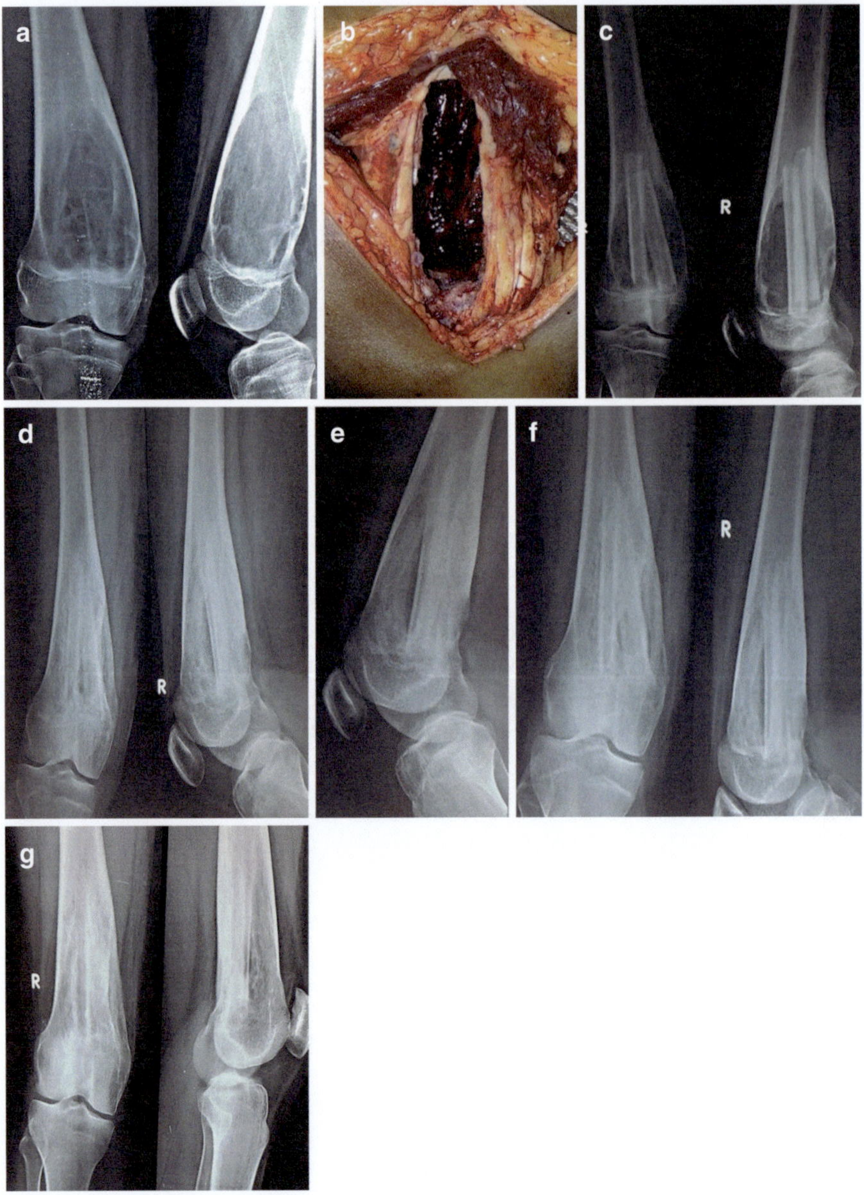

Fig. 10.1 (**a**) AP and lateral radiographs of a huge ABC of the distal end of the femur. (**b**) Intraoperative picture during curettage showing the haemorrhagic field in the cavity. (**c**) Radiograph reveals twin fibular struts of appropriate size stabilized within the cavity. (**d**, **e**) The struts have healed and are merging with the parent bone. (**f**) The twin fibular grafts have completely united with the parent bone. (**g**) Note the remodelling of the bone and the cavity after healing

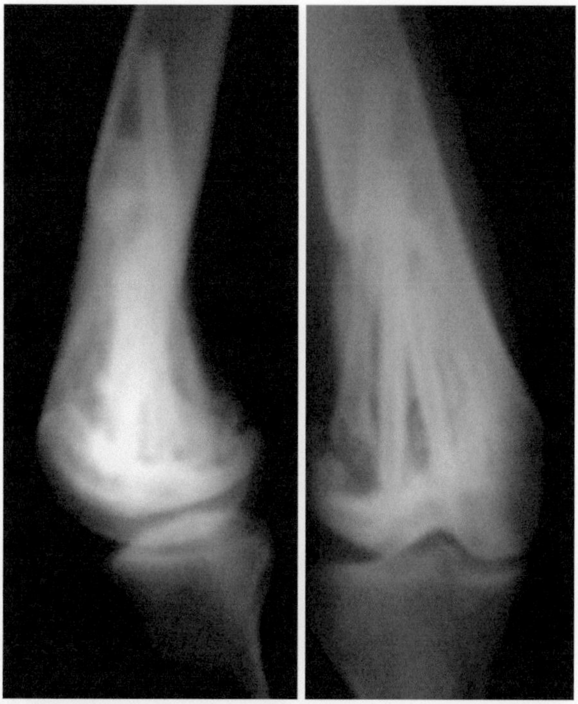

Fig. 10.2 A case of GCT of the lateral condyle of the femur with thorough curettage and fibular strut grafting. Note the healing of the struts with the parent bone

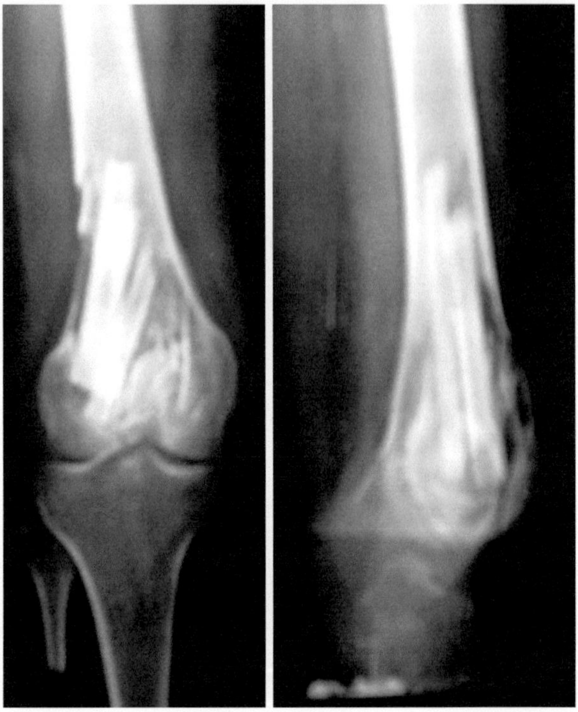

Fig. 10.3 AP and lateral radiographs of another case of GCT of the lower end of the femur. The cavity filled with fibular strut grafts after curettage revealed healing

Suggested Readings

1. Wu PK, Chen CF, Chen CM, Tsai SW, Cheng YC, Chang MC, Chen WM. Grafting for bone defects after curettage of benign bone tumor – analysis of factors influencing the bone healing. J Chin Med Assoc. 2018;81(7):643–8.
2. Hettwer WH, Petersen MM. Treatment of benign and borderline bone tumors with combined curettage and bone defect reconstruction. J Orthop Surg. 2018;
3. Enneking WF. Fibrous/cartilaginous lesions in bone. Musculoskeletal tumor surgery. 1st ed. New York: Churchill Livingstone; 1983. p. 807–939.
4. Abraham JA, Schwartz HS, Henshaw R, et al. Section 2: benign bone tumors. In: Biermann JS, editor. Orthopaedic knowledge update: musculoskeletal tumors. 3rd ed. Rosemont: American Academy of Orthopaedic Surgeons; 2013. p. 87–156.
5. Campanacci M. Bone tumors/tumor like lesions of bone. Bone and soft tissue tumors. 2nd ed. Vienna: Springer Vienna; 1999. p. 73–905.
6. Roberts TT, Rosenbaum AJ. Bone grafts, bone substitutes and orthobiologics. The bridge between basic science and clinical advancements in fracture healing. Organogenesis. 2012;8(4):114–24.
7. Fraquet N, Faizon G, Rosset P, et al. Long bones giant cells tumors: treatment by curettage and cavity filling cementation. Orthop Traum Surg Res. 2009;95(6):402–6.
8. Chen CJ, Brien EW. Early postoperative compilations of bone filling in curettage defects. J Orthop Surg Res. 2019;14:261.

Chapter 11
Twin NVFG Used for Fixation of Early Femoral Neck Fractures

11.1 Twin NVFG Used for Fixation of Early Femoral Neck Fractures

11.1.1 The Technique

The patient is fixed on a hip spica table, and the fracture is reduced. Under suitable anaesthesia, a 10-cm incision is made on the lateral aspect of the greater trochanter and a suitable window is made over the base of the greater trochanter. A Kirschner wire is passed along the calcar femorale, reaching the sub-articular level. Another Kirschner wire is passed in the same direction about 1 cm above the previous one. Twenty centimetres of the fibular shaft is retrieved subperiosteally and divided into two struts of 10 cm each. The struts are now slid over the Kirschner wires proximally up to the subchondral level (Fig. 11.1a–c). With this procedure, the fibular struts occupy the entire neck of the femur with a biological fixation of the fracture. In case the fixation is stable, the Kirschner wires can also be removed.

To achieve osteosynthesis of femoral neck fractures is a challenge to the treating surgeon. A plethora of devices and methods has been described. A new technique of achieving union of femoral neck fractures by twin fibular fixation has been reported. Twin fibular struts provide autologous bone, filling the whole of the osteopenic femoral neck and also preventing rotational forces (Fig. 11.2a–d).

The fibular shaft is tri-flanged and works on the principle of the classic Smith-Petersen nail. Twin fibular struts simulate twin Smith-Petersen nails that have a biological and osteogenic property. The added volume of bone occupies the entire neck of the femur from the calcar femorale to the top.

Another complication of femoral neck fractures, more so in an osteoporotic neck of the femur, is posterior comminution which usually does not allow a stable and sustained reduction of such fractures. Since total fixation is biologically active, the technique has proven advantageous even when stable/desirable reduction is not

S. S. Yadav, *Non-Vascularised Fibular Grafts in Orthopaedic Practice*, https://doi.org/10.1007/978-981-95-1794-7_11

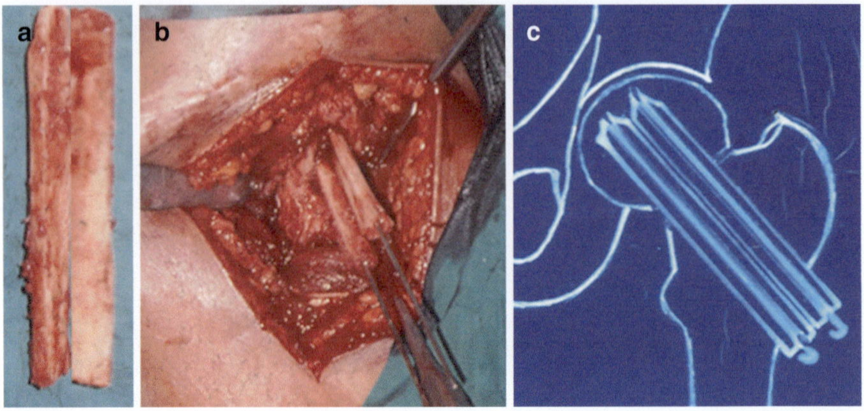

Fig. 11.1 (**a**) Twin fibular strut grafts simulate two Smith-Petersen nails. (**b**) Intraoperative demonstration of driving the fibular struts in the neck of the femur. The Kirschner wires can be seen. (**c**) The concept and diagrammatic representation of twin fibular grafts fixing the fracture. The Kirschner wires are seen inserted into the struts

possible. Being autologous bone, the twin fibular graft is advantageous even when there is 'subsequent loss of reduction' of the fracture (Fig. 11.3). It is, therefore, suggested that this simple, inexpensive and biological technique has many advantages over the existing methods of fixation of these fractures (Figs. 11.4a–c and 11.5a, b). Even in cases with difficult clinical conditions like marble bone disease, the technique can be used and has proven to be quite effective (Fig. 11.6a–c).

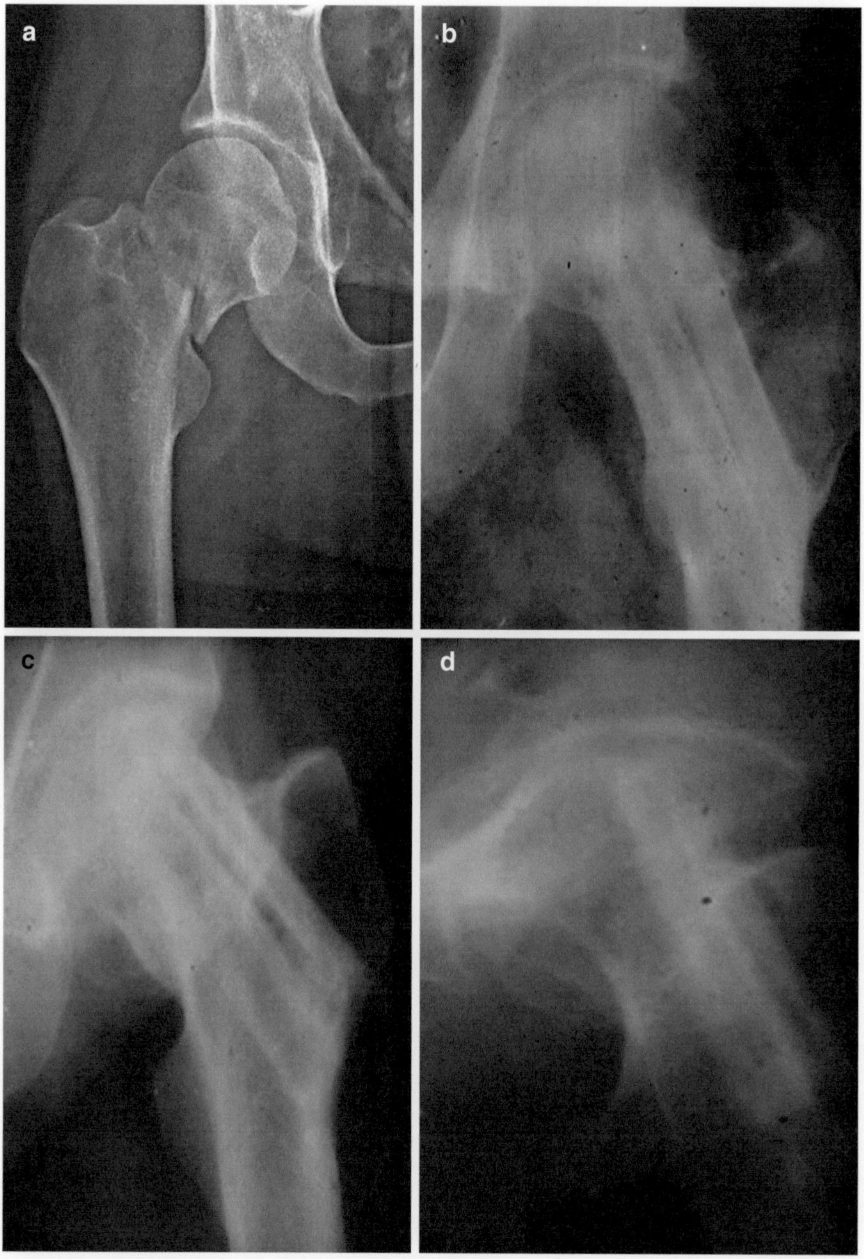

Fig. 11.2 (**a**) Roentgenogram revealing a displaced transcervical fracture of the neck of the left femur. (**b**) Postoperative roentgenogram taken after 2 months shows complete occupation of the neck of the femur by fibular struts. (**c**, **d**). AP and lateral roentgenograms of the patient after treatment. Note the total occupation of the neck by the twin fibular struts that favours the union of the fracture

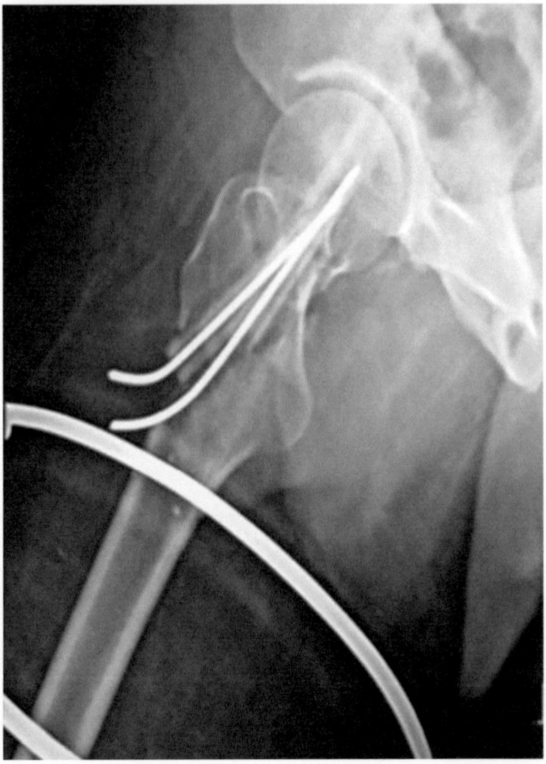

Fig. 11.3 Roentgenogram showing transcervical fracture of the neck of the right femur. Although the placement of the struts has not been in ideal position, the fracture had united

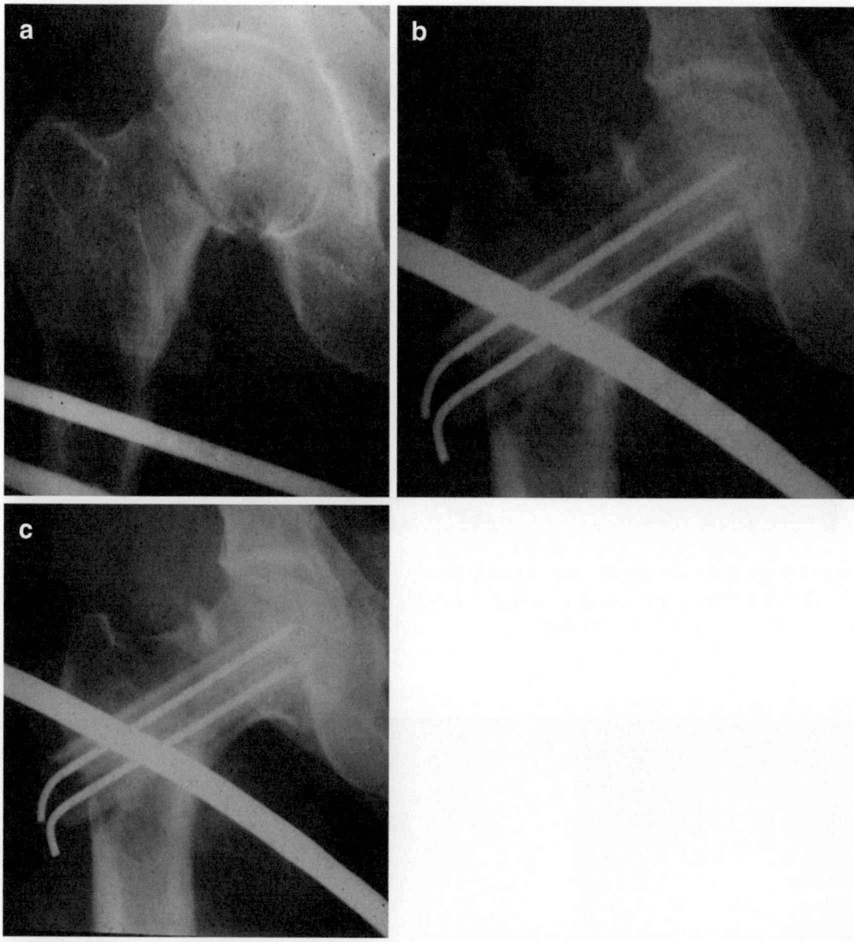

Fig. 11.4 **(a–c)** Radiograph illustrates a transcervical fracture of the neck of the right femur, fixed with twin fibular grafts which had resulted in union. Note the position of the twin grafts occupying the major part of the femoral neck along the calcar femorale

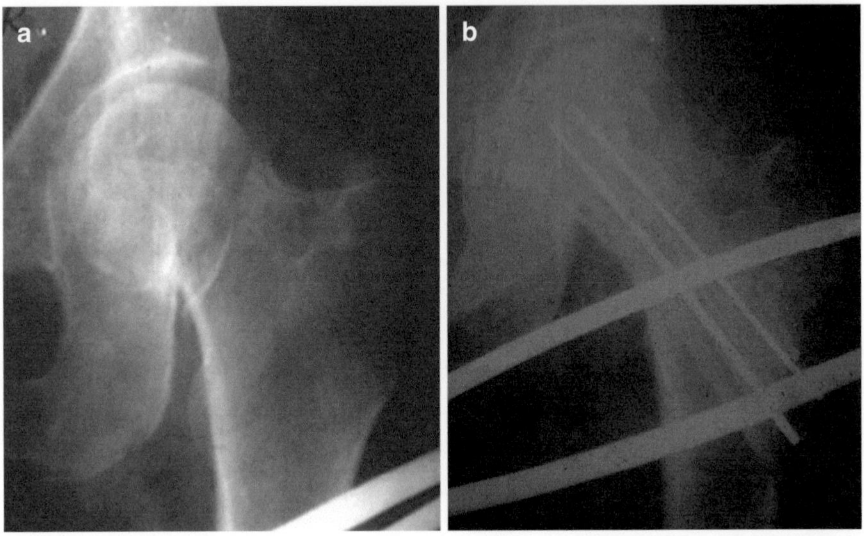

Fig. 11.5 (**a**) AP radiograph revealing undisplaced fracture of the femoral neck. (**b**) Radiograph showing twin fibular grafts with Kirschner wires. The twin grafts are seen occuping the major part of the neck. The fracture had healed

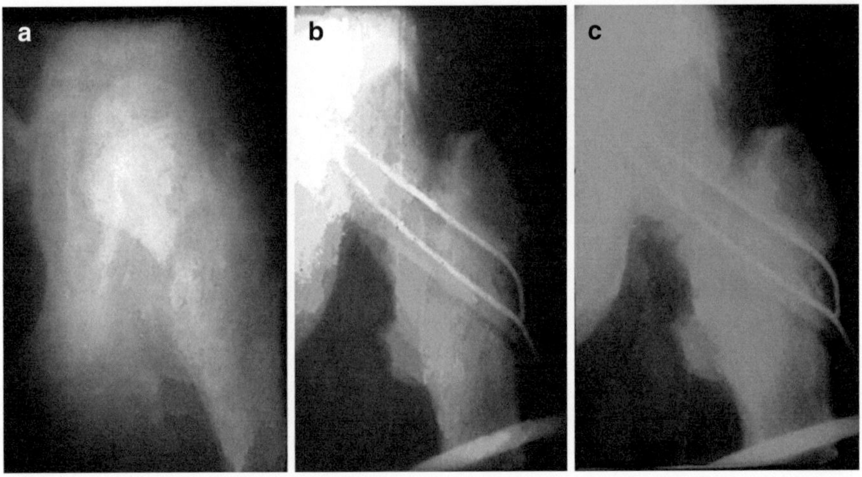

Fig. 11.6 (**a**, **b**) A transcervical fracture in a case of marble bone disease has been fixed with twin fibular grafts. (**c**) Roentgenogram revealed healing of the fracture

Suggested Readings

1. Nagi ON, Gautam VK, Marya SK. Treatment of femoral neck fractures with a cancellous screw and fibular graft. J Bone Joint Surg. 1986;68:387–91.
2. Sandhu HS, Sandhu PS, Kapoor A. Neglected fractured neck of the femur: a predictive classification and treatment by osteosynthesis. Clin Orthop Relat Res. 2005;431:14–20.
3. Chandra PP, Binod K, Karuna SD, Pulkesh S, Harish K, Goyal RK. Fixation with cancellous screws and fibular strut grafts for neglected femoral neck fractures. J Orthop Surg. 2014;22(2):181–5.
4. Wu CC, Shih CH, Chen WJ, Tai CL. Treatment of femoral neck nonunions with a sliding compression screw: comparison with and without subtrochanteric valgus osteotomy. J Trauma. 1999;46:312–7.
5. Hou SM, Hang YS, Liu TK. Ununited femoral neck fractures by open reduction and vascularized iliac bone graft. Clin Orthop Relat Res. 1993;294:176–80.
6. LeCroy CM, Rizzo M, Gunneson EE, Urbaniak JR. Free vascularized fibular bone grafting in the management of femoral neck nonunion in patients younger than fifty years. J Orthop Trauma. 2002;16:464–72.
7. Haidukewych GJ, Rothwell WS, Jacofsky DJ, Torchia ME, Berry DJ. Operative treatment of femoral neck fractures in patients between the ages of fifteen and fifty years. J Bone Joint Surg. 2004;86:1711–6.
8. Mathews V, Cabanela ME. Femoral neck nonunion treatment. Clin Orthop Relat Res. 2004;419:57–64.
9. Beris AE, Payatakes AH, Kostopoulos VK, Korompilias AV, Mavrodontidis AN, Vekris MD, et al. Non-union of femoral neck fractures with osteonecrosis of the femoral head: treatment with combined free vascularized fibular grafting and subtrochanteric valgus osteotomy. Orthop Clin North Am. 2004;35:335–43.
10. Azam MQ, Iraqi A, Sherwani M, Sabir AB, Abbas M, Asif N. Free fibular strut graft in neglected femoral neck fractures in adult. Indian J Orthop. 2009;43:62–6.
11. Yadav SS, Dual fibular grafting. A new technique of fixation of the femoral neck fractures. Indian J Orthop. 2005;39:21–5.
12. Hartford JM, Patel A, Powell J. Intertrochanteric osteotomy using a dynamic hip screw for femoral neck nonunion. J Orthop Trauma. 2005;19:329–33.

Chapter 12
'The Biological IM Nail': Bone-in-Bone Fixation with Osteogenic Advantage

12.1 Autologous Fibular Strut Used as Biological IM Nail

Challenging non-union of the long bones is difficult to manage and usually results in failures. After repeated implant failures, non-unions become resistant to treatment. In most of such cases, the bone is often osteoporotic, with a large bone gap between the bone segments, and union is usually difficult to achieve (Fig. 12.1). The selection of a viable technique for the treatment of osteoporotic bones has been a problem for the treating surgeon. As a result of repeated attempts of fixation using metallic nails or plates, the osteogenic capacity of the already osteoporotic bone is further compromised.

The advanced technology provides potential benefits related to the surgical treatment of non-union in osteoporotic long bones. The stabilization of fractures in such patients with soft bones has become a necessity. Osteopenia and severe soft tissue damage with extensive skin scars increase the possibility of repeated failure with metallic implants. The persistence of disuse osteoporosis can result in the widening of the medullary canal of long bones such as the femur, tibia, and humerus (Fig. 12.2a–d).

A metallic nail or plate of any type may not be able to provide adequate fixation in such an ailing bone with severe osteopenia with a wide medullary canal. To achieve union of osteopenic bone, an osteogenic stimulating factor in the form of an autologous bone graft may be needed to initiate healing—bone-in-bone fixation (Fig. 12.3).

As a breakthrough, the non-vascularized fibular strut graft has been used as a 'biological nail' which has proven its superiority over conventional metallic nails in strengthening osteoporotic long bones with gap non-unions. Fibular strut fixation in such a situation provides 'bone-to-bone' contact throughout the length of the strut with the host bone which in turn promotes further osteogenesis (Fig. 12.4a–c).

S. S. Yadav, *Non-Vascularised Fibular Grafts in Orthopaedic Practice*, https://doi.org/10.1007/978-981-95-1794-7_12

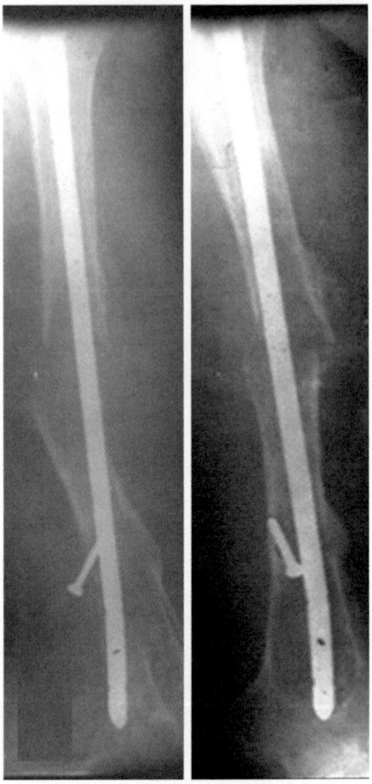

Fig. 12.1 Roentgenogram revealing gap non-union of the humeral shaft after a failed interlocking nail. Note the severe osteoporosis throughout the bone with a huge gap

This biological nail can also be inserted in long bones with a benign lesion of the shaft which may result in a pathological fracture. A fibular strut can also be inserted in any fragile long bone at risk of fracture. The use of such a biological nail in challenging clinical conditions has been published for the first time.

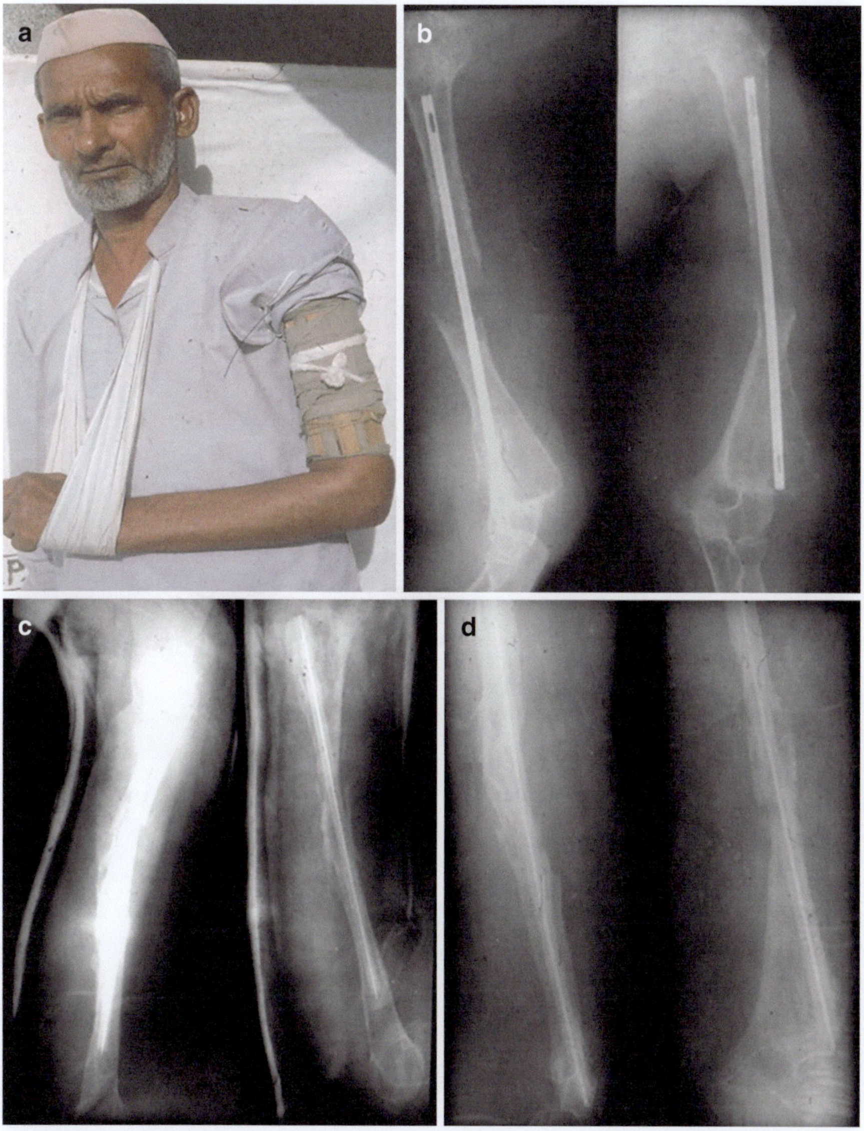

Fig. 12.2 (**a**) A 64-year-old male had fracture of the left humerus. He had local treatment and was then operated using a Kuntscher nail. (**b**) Upon arrival of the patient, the humerus revealed gross osteoporosis with a wide medullary canal throughout the length of the bone and a challenging non-union. (**c**) AP and lateral radiographs reveal a Kirschner wire inserted in the fibular strut and the fibular strut in the parent bone supported with a POP cast. (**b**) The fracture healed in 11 weeks

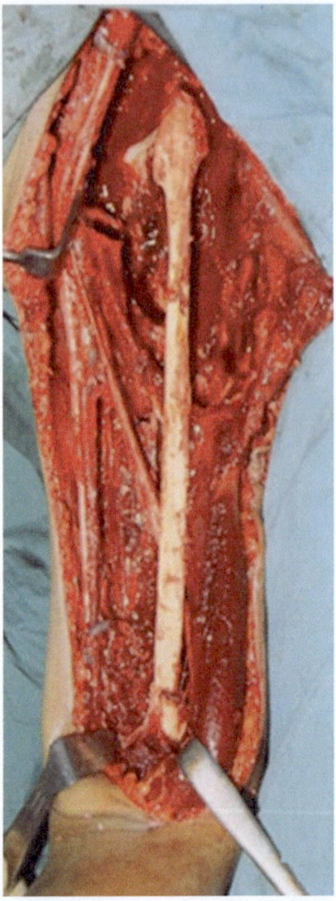

Fig. 12.3 Intraoperative picture of the fibula including its head. The long strut simulates the length and width of a metallic intramedullary nail

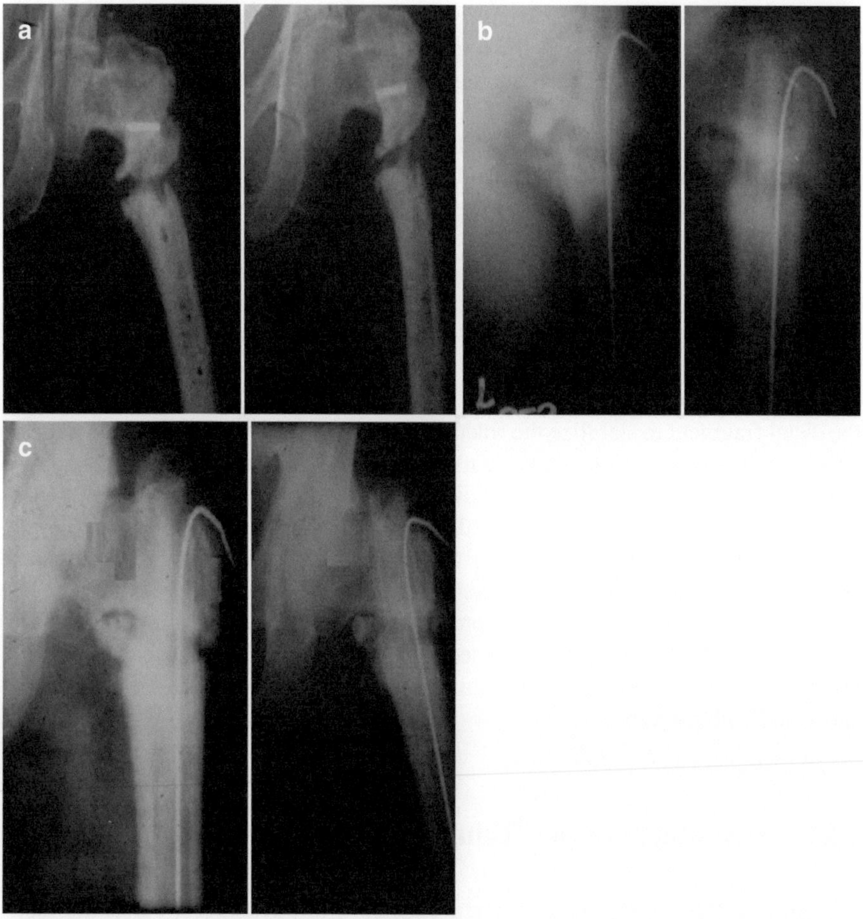

Fig. 12.4 (**a**) AP and lateral radiographs show subtrochanteric non-union after four surgeries—two attempts with nail and plate, both removed after failure at other centres. (**b**) Since the fragments were in alignment, the fibular strut graft with Kirschner wire was inserted into the proximal femur in a manner similar to closed nailing. Since the trochanteric area was wide, an additional small strut was also inserted alongside the main strut. Postoperative roentgenogram after 3 weeks revealed early healing. (**c**) AP and lateral roentgenograms after 11 weeks resulted in complete union of the fracture

12.2 Surgical Technique

The basic principles of biological nail fixation are similar to those of metallic nail fixation. In cases where the bone fragments are aligned, closed fibular fixation is recommended.

The host site is prepared using either a closed or open technique, similar to that for a metallic nail. The required autologous fibular strut is retrieved, with the distal 8–10 cm of the fibula left in place for ankle stability. In cases where a long strut is required, the head of the fibula can also be taken after carefully protecting the peroneal nerve. The fibular strut, or 'biological nail', is fashioned to fit the host medullary canal. The biological strut should be inserted into the host bone as early as possible to maximize its viability. If the surgeon thinks that the fibular strut should be strengthened, a Kirschner wire can be passed through the medullary canal of the strut graft. Following a procedure involving the femur or tibia, the extremity is supported with a Thomas splint. Following a procedure involving the humerus, the arm is initially supported with a U-cast.

In non-unions that are aligned, a small incision is made over the greater tuberosity or the greater trochanter as the case may be, similar to the approach used for a closed metallic nail. The fibular strut is now inserted into the host long bone. If required, the medullary canal is reamed. An appropriately sized fibular strut removed subperiosteally is shaped to be driven first into the proximal fragment and then into the distal fragment to stabilize the fracture. In cases with a relatively narrow medullary canal, the edges of the fibular graft are shaved before insertion of the graft into the medullary canal of the host. In a displaced fracture, the fracture site is opened. The full length of the graft is inserted into the proximal fragment in a retrograde fashion and then advanced into the distal fragment like a metallic nail to the extent that half of the strut is placed on either side of the fracture.

In the tibia, fixation can be attempted with an open method, with the non-union site exposed. The strut graft is passed on the proximal side and can be slowly inserted into the distal fragment after the non-union is reduced. The limb is initially supported with a splint.

12.3 Advantages of the Technique

The proposed technique is associated with several advantages. First, the technique is simple and based on the principles of Kuntscher nail fixation. Second, the technique involves 'bone-in-bone fixation' and is biological. As a result, the large contact area between the strut and the endosteal surface of the host bone results in early union and strengthens the osteopenic host bone. Third, the autogenous fibular strut also provides the much-needed osteogenesis and stability at the site of the non-union that takes place throughout the length of the graft in the parent bone. Fourth, usually no reaming is required. The tri-flanged fibula engages both the non-union fragments. If considered necessary by the surgeon to strengthen the strut, a Kirschner wire can be inserted into the graft before it is inserted into the parent bone. No additional fixation is necessary. Fifth, once united, the fibular strut does not require removal. Sixth, the periosteum of the host bone is minimally displaced.

The success of 'the biological fixation' is an important development in the surgical treatment of difficult fractures and non-unions. Ordinarily, a metallic nail or plate acts as an internal splint and does not abolish motion completely in osteoporotic cases, and the fracture heals with peripheral callus formation. Even the best of metallic implants may not prove adequate in severely osteoporotic fractured bone with wide medullary canal with a thin cortex (Figs. 12.5 and 12.6).

Because the fibula has three surfaces and three boarders, the graft functions as a tri-flanged nail and engages the host bone firmly. In bones with a wide medullary canal, reaming is not necessary for fixing the non-union. Another major advantage is that the periosteum of the host bone is undisturbed, similar to closed nailing. If required, reaming may also be helpful in establishing contact between the reamed endosteum of the host bone and the fresh autologous nail graft. The three borders of the fibula fix firmly to the inner cortices of the fractured fragments. In this technique, union can also be achieved even when the surrounding soft tissues around the non-union were grossly damaged and there was potential need for an amputation. Evidently, the intramedullary graft also sufficiently reduces rotational and other undesirable forces acting on the construct.

The technique has some of the advantages of both closed and open fixation. In cases in which the non-union had occurred after the failure of a metallic nail, the fragments are in alignment and the fibular strut could be easily inserted through the same track in the parent bone. With this technique, there is no need to use additional screws or a plate because the strong fibular strut can be hammered into the parent bone (Figs. 12.7, 12.8, and 12.9).

The large contact area between the fibular strut graft and the host bone promotes dependable union. With a firmly fixed autologous graft, compression may not be required. However, in rare cases involving a very wide medullary canal and a thin cortex, screws can be used to achieve a four-cortex fixation (Fig. 12.6a–d). These minor changes to the basic technique can be employed, when necessary. The insertion of a free autologous intramedullary fibular strut graft also provides mechanical stability (Fig. 12.5a–i).

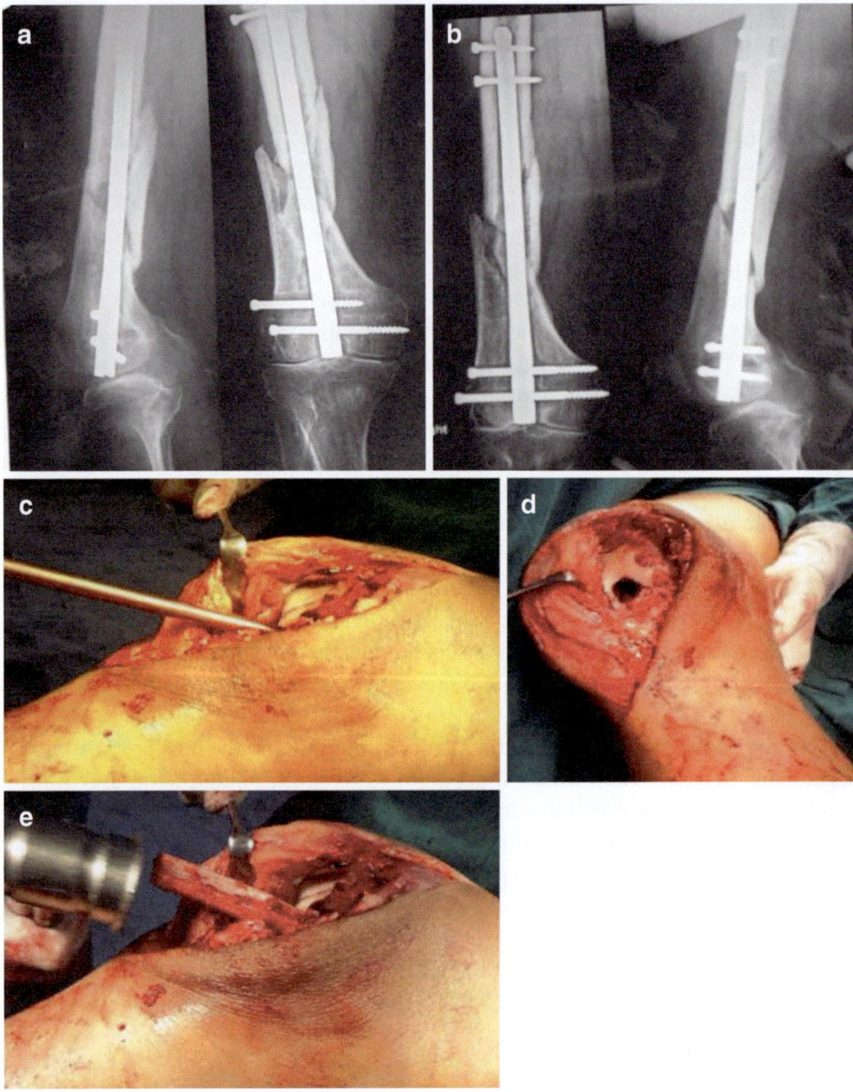

Fig. 12.5 **(a, b)** AP and lateral roentgenograms revealed bilateral symmetrical fractures of the distal third of the femur treated with interlocking nails. Upon arrival of the patient, the fractures had not yet united and the nails were protruding into the joints, causing severe pain in both the knees. (**c**) Intraoperative picture showing removal of the inter-condylar nail. (**d**) The passage after removal of the nail. (**e**) An autologous fibular strut was introduced through the same hole and stabilized at the fracture site on both sides. (**f, g**) AP and lateral postoperative rontgenograms of both sides. The inlay fibular grafts are seen at the fracture site on either side showing early healing. (**h, i**) Bilateral roentgenograms taken after 6 months revealed union of the fracture on either side

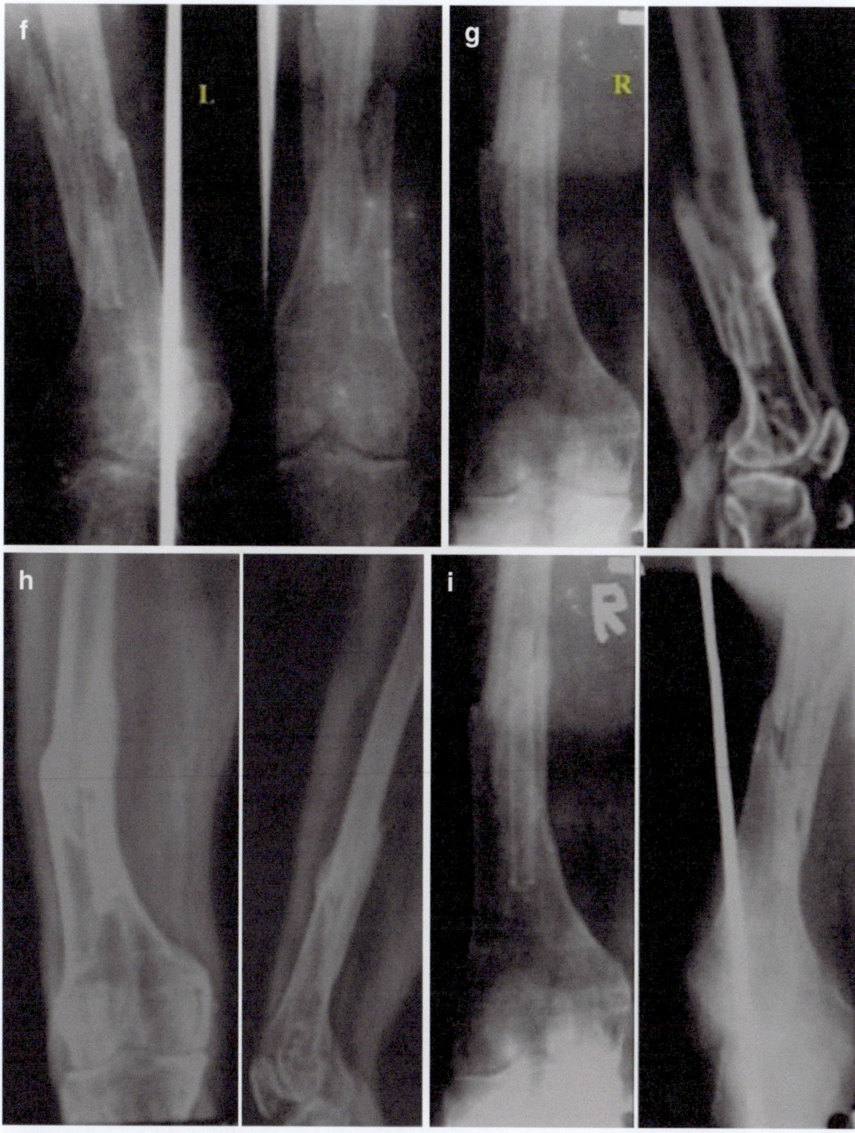

Fig. 12.5 (continued)

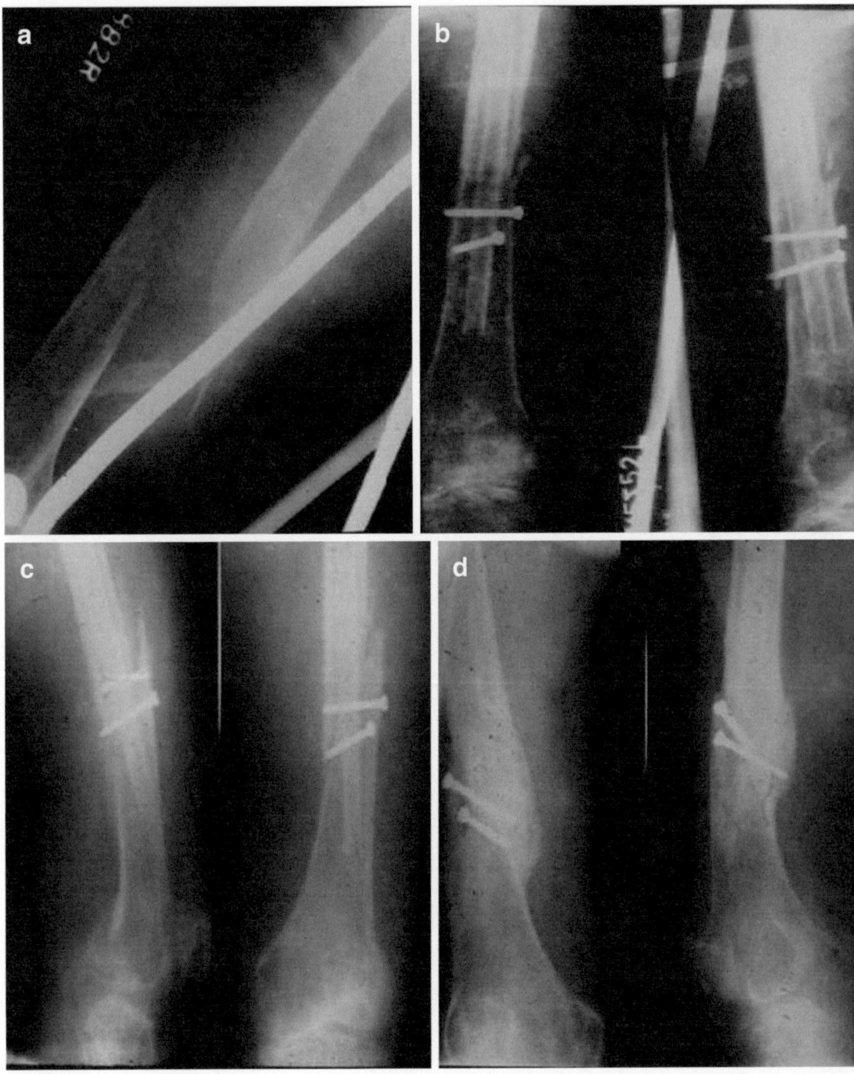

Fig. 12.6 (**a**) Roentgenogram of oblique fracture of the distal third of the femur with severe osteoporosis. (**b**) Autologous fibular graft was inserted at the fracture site. Since the medullary canal was very wide, the fibular strut also was a loose fit. The site was fixed with two cortical screws to achieve a 'four-cortex' fixation. (**c**) The roentgenogram taken after 10 weeks revealed early healing. (**d**) Roentgenogram revealed complete healing and remodelling after 24 weeks

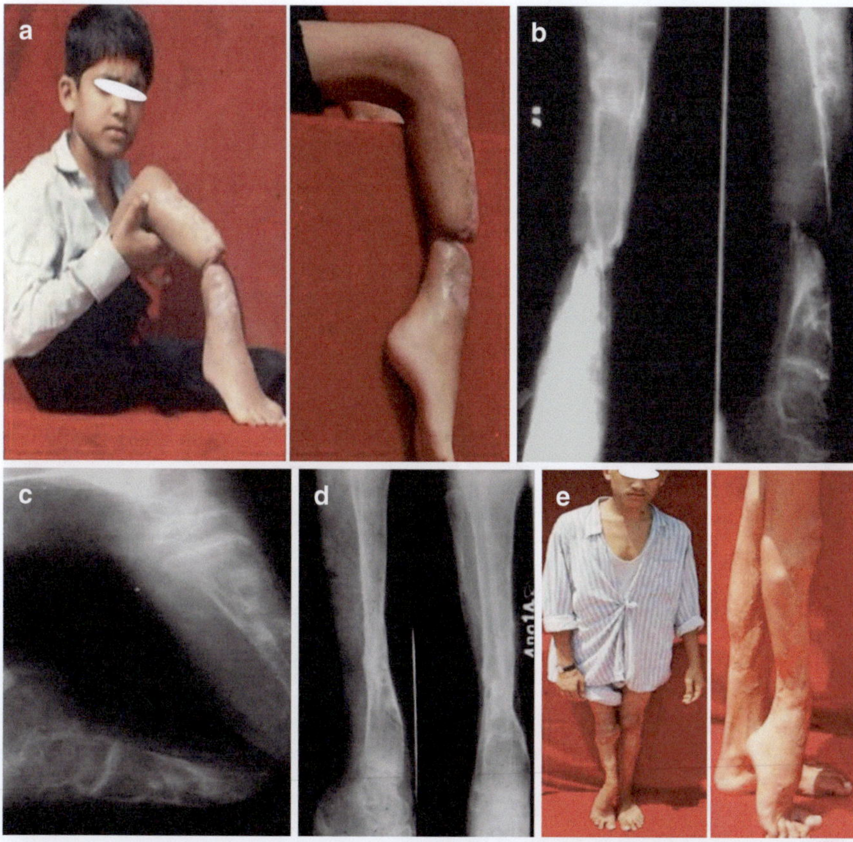

Fig. 12.7 (**a**) A 12-year-old boy with complete circumferential injury of the right distal leg. There was a narrow isthmus through which the vessels and the nerve were connecting the proximal and distal extremity. A very rare presentation indeed. (**b**, **c**) AP and lateral roentgenograms revealed a challenging gap non-union with very severe osteoporosis. An amputation was suggested at other centres, which he refused. (**d**) A full-thickness cross-leg skin graft was performed. After healing, a long autologous fibular graft was inserted into the tibia. AP and lateral radiographs taken after 18 months revealed complete diaphyseal healing. Note the fibular graft in the tibial diaphysis showing massive bone formation. (**e**) Clinical picture 18 months after the insertion of the biological fibular nail. The patient had developed equinus deformity which compensated the shortening. The patient was so happy and satisfied that he refused any further treatment for the equinus deformity

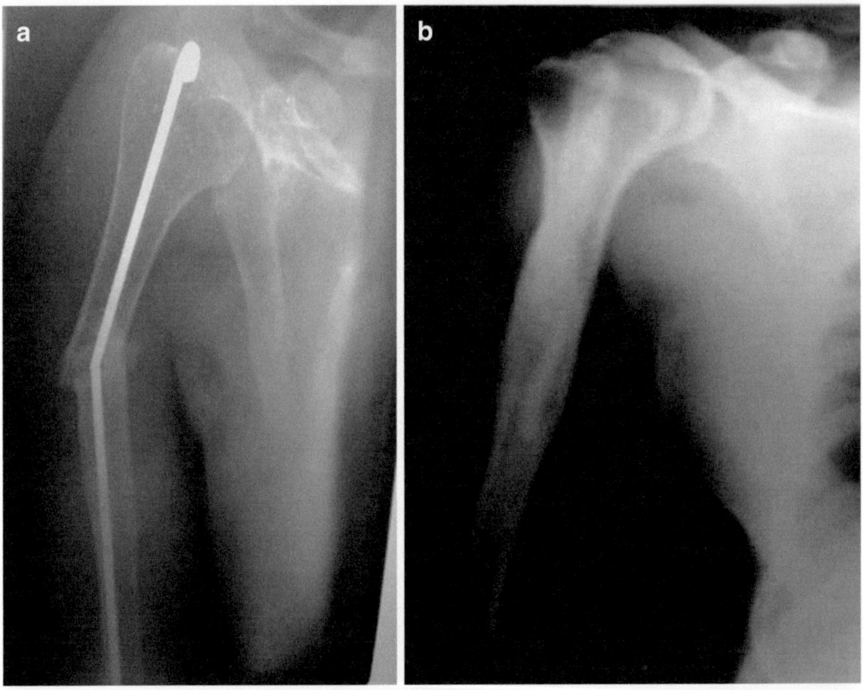

Fig. 12.8 (**a**) Roentgenogram of the right humerus shows non-union with a broken Rush pin. (**b**) Roentgenogram 2 months after insertion of the fibular strut reveals complete healing

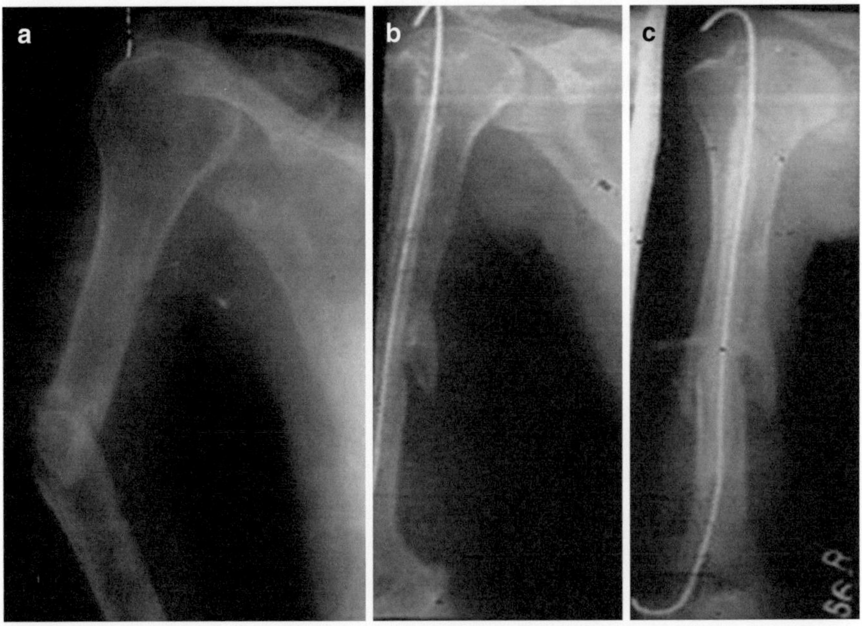

Fig. 12.9 (**a**) Roentgenogram shows non-union of the humeral shaft. (**b**) An inlay fibular graft was attempted with a Kirschner wire in the fibular strut. (**c**) The graft acted as a biological nail and helped in healing of the fracture in 8 weeks

Suggested Reading

1. Trotter DH, Dobozi W. Nonunion of the humerus: rigid fixation, bone grafting, and adjunctive bone cement. Clin Orthop Relat Res. 1986;204:162–8.
2. Rosen H. The treatment of nonunions and pseudarthroses of the humeral shaft. Orthop Clin North Am. 1990;21(4):725–42.
3. Wright TW, Miller GJ, Vander Griend RA, Wheeler D, Dell PC. Reconstruction of thehumerus with an intramedullary fibular graft. A clinical and biomechanical study. J Bone Joint Surg Br. 1993;75(5):804–7.
4. Lynch JR, Taitsman LA, Barei DP, Nork SE. Femoral nonunion: risk factors and treatment options. J Am Acad Orthop Surg. 2008 Feb;16(2):88–97.
5. Somford MP, van den Bekerom MPJ, Kloen P. Operative treatment for femoral shaft nonunions, a systematic review of the literature. Strategies Trauma Limb Reconstr. 2013;8(2):77–88.
6. Jupiter JB. Complex non-union of the humeral diaphysis. Treatment with a medial approach, an anterior plate, and a vascularized fibular graft. J Bone Joint Surg Am. 1990;72(5):701–7.
7. Cannada LK. Viable bone and circulatory factors required for survival of bone grafts [table of contents.]. Orthop Clin North Am. 2010;41(1):5–13.
8. Maheshwari P, Maheshwari P. Non-union distal femur fracture: causes and management options. Trauma Int. 2016;2(1):28–33.
9. Cameron HU, Jacob R, Macnab I, Pilliar RM. Use of polymethylmethacrylate to enhance screw fixation in bone. J Bone Joint Surg Am. 1975;57(5):655–6.
10. Epps CH Jr, Grant RE. Fractures of the shaft of the humerus. In: Rockwood Jr CA, Green DP, Bucholz RW, editors. Rockwood and Green's fractures in adults. 3rd ed. Philadelphia: J.B. Lippincott; 1991. p. 843–69.
11. Li XK, Wang HQ, Wei YY, Wu ZX, LiXK. Treatment of nonunions of humeral fractures with interlocking intramedullary nailing. Chin J Traumatol. 2008;11(6):335–40.
12. Ring D, Jupiter JB, Sanders RA, Quintero J, Santoro VM, Ganz R, Marti RK. Complex non-union of fractures of the femoral shaft treated by wave-plate osteosynthesis. J Bone Joint Surg Br. 1997;79(2):289–94.
13. Mukhopadhaya J, Shivapuri S. Functional outcome after open reduction and internal fixation for symptomatic delayed union and nonunion after fracture clavicle: a series of 31 cases. Indian J Orthop. 2007;41(3):209–13.
14. Vidyadhara S, Vamsi K, Rao SK, Gnanadoss JJ, Pandian S. Use of intramedullary fibular strut graft: a novel adjunct to plating in the treatment of osteoporotic humeral shaft nonunion. Int Orthop. 2009;33(4):1009–14.
15. Tarr RR, Wiss DA. The mechanics and biology of intramedullary fracture fixation. Clin Orthop Relat Res. 1986;212:10–7.
16. Esterhai JL Jr, Brighton CT, Heppenstall RB, Thrower A. Nonunion of the humerus. Clinical, roentgenographic, scintigraphic, and response characteristics to treatment with constant direct current stimulation of osteogenesis. Clin Orthop Relat Res. 1986;211:228–34.
17. Healy WL, White GM, Mick CA, Brooker AF Jr, Weiland AJ. Nonunion of the humeral shaft. Clin Orthop Relat Res. 1987;219:206–13.
18. Ray RD. Vascularization of bone grafts and implants. Clin Orthop Relat Res. 1972;87(87):43–8.
19. Schuh R, Panotopoulos J, Puchner SE, Willegger M, Hobusch GM, Windhager R, Funovics PT. Vascularised or non-vascularised autologous fibular grafting for the reconstruction of a diaphyseal bone defect after resection of a musculoskeletal tumour. Bone Joint J. 2014;96(9):1258–63.
20. Yadav SS. Radical resection of bone tumours and reconstruction by autologous bone grafting. Indian J Orthop. 1980;14(2):150–4.
21. Yadav SS. Observations on enbloc resection and reconstruction of malignant bone tumours. Indian J Cancer. 1981;18(3):206–10.
22. Yadav SS. Dual-fibular grafting for massive bone gaps in the lower extremity. J Bone Joint Surg Am. 1990;72(4):486–94.

23. Marino JT, Ziran BH. Use of solid and cancellous autologous bone graft for fractures and nonunions. Orthop Clin North Am. 2010;41(1):15–26.
24. Livani B, Belangero W, Medina G, Pimenta C, Zogaib R, Mongon M. Anterior plating as a surgical alternative in the treatment of humeral shaft non-union. Int Orthop. 2010;34(7):1025–31.
25. Trader JE, Johnson RP, Kalbfleisch JH. Bone-mineral content, surface hardness, and mechanical fixation in the human radius. A correlative study. J Bone Joint Surg Am. 1979;61(8):1217–20.
26. Brown CR, Boden SD. Fracture repair and bone grafting. In: Fischgrund JS, editor. Orthopaedic knowledge update 9. Rosemont: AAOS; 2008. p. 13–22.
27. Khan SN, Cammisa FP Jr, Sandhu HS, Diwan AD, Girardi FP, Lane JM. The biology of bone grafting. J Am Acad Orthop Surg. 2005;13(1):77–86.
28. Yadav SS. Bridging of large skeletal defects by twin fibular grafts supported by Lplatefixation. Orthopaedics (Int Ed). 1995;3(3):213–21.

Chapter 13
Biological Nail for Strengthening the Long Bones with Benign Diaphyseal Lesions

13.1 Biological Nail for Strengthening the Long Bones with Benign Diaphyseal Lesions

This biological nail can also be inserted into long bones with a benign lesion of the shaft, which may otherwise result in a pathological fracture (Fig. 13.1a–d). A fibular strut can also be inserted into any fragile long bone with severe osteoporosis and diaphyseal lesions threatening a fracture (Fig. 13.2a–d). The insertion of a free autologous intramedullary fibular strut graft provided mechanical stability, and osteogenesis occurred inside the medullary canal of the host bone.

S. S. Yadav, *Non-Vascularised Fibular Grafts in Orthopaedic Practice*, https://doi.org/10.1007/978-981-95-1794-7_13

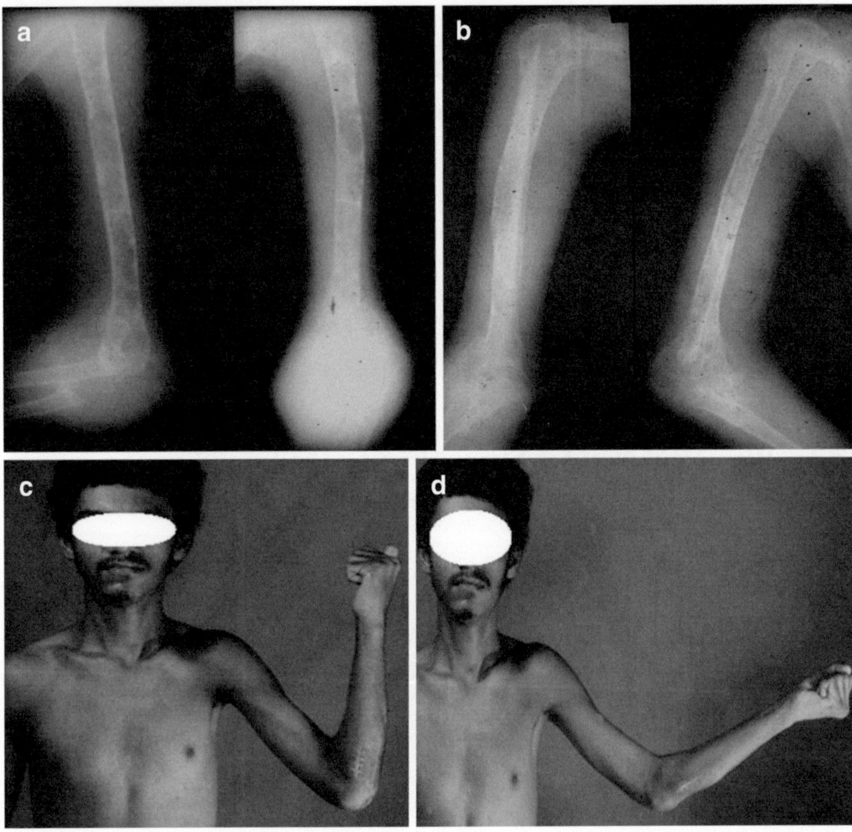

Fig. 13.1 (**a**) AP and lateral roentgenograms revealing fibrous dysplasia involving the whole shaft of the left humerus. (**b**) Roentgenogram 3 months after curettage and insertion of the biological nail strengthening the entire length of the bone. (**c**, **d**) The clinical picture of the patient showing flexion and extension at the elbow

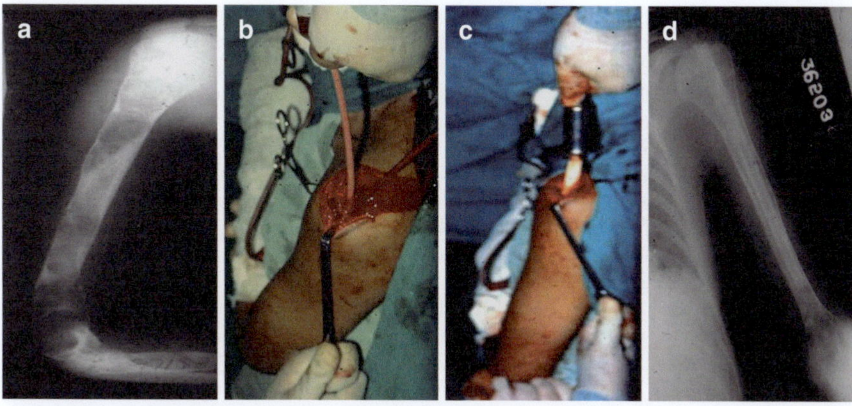

Fig. 13.2 (**a**) Radiograph of a patient from Bangladesh with ABC involving the whole diaphysis of the humerus, threatening a pathological fracture. (**b**) Intraoperative picture showing a catheter washing the medullary canal after curettage. (**c**) Intraoperative picture revealing insertion of the fibular strut into the humerus. (**d**) Roentgenogram of the humerus after insertion of the fibular nail filling the medullary cavity and strengthening the entire humeral shaft

Suggested Readings

1. Trotter DH, Dobozi W. Nonunion of the humerus: rigid fixation, bone grafting, and adjunctive bone cement. Clin Orthop Relat Res. 1986;204:162–8.
2. Rosen H. The treatment of nonunions and pseudarthroses of the humeral shaft. Orthop Clin North Am. 1990;21(4):725–42.
3. Wright TW, Miller GJ, Vander Griend RA, Wheeler D, Dell PC. Reconstruction of the humerus with an intramedullary fibular graft. A clinical and biomechanical study. J Bone Joint Surg (Br). 1993;75(5):804–7.
4. Lynch JR, Taitsman LA, Barei DP, Nork SE. Femoral nonunion: risk factors and treatment options. J Am Acad Orthop Surg. 2008;16(2):88–97.
5. Somford MP, van den Bekerom MPJ, Kloen P. Operative treatment for femoral shaft nonunions, a systematic review of the literature. Strategies Trauma Limb Reconstr. 2013;8(2):77–88. Epub 2013 Jul 27
6. Jupiter JB. Complex non-union of the humeral diaphysis. Treatment with a medial approach, an anterior plate, and a vascularized fibular graft. J Bone Joint Surg Am. 1990;72(5):701–7.
7. Cannada LK. Viable bone and circulatory factors required for survival of bone grafts [table of contents.]. Orthop Clin North Am. 2010;41(1):5–13.
8. Maheshwari P, Maheshwari P. Non-union distal femur fracture: causes and management options. Trauma Int. 2016;2(1):28–33.
9. Cameron HU, Jacob R, Macnab I, Pilliar RM. Use of polymethylmethacrylate to enhance screw fixation in bone. J Bone Joint Surg Am. 1975;57(5):655–6.
10. Epps CH Jr, Grant RE. Fractures of the shaft of the humerus. In: Rockwood Jr CA, Green DP, Bucholz RW, editors. Rockwood and Green's fractures in adults. 3rd ed. Philadelphia: J.B. Lippincott; 1991. p. 843–69.
11. Li XK, Wang HQ, Wei YY, Wu ZX, Li XK. Treatment of nonunions of humeral fractures with interlocking intramedullary nailing. Chin J Traumatol. 2008;11(6):335–40.

12. Ring D, Jupiter JB, Sanders RA, Quintero J, Santoro VM, Ganz R, Marti RK. Complex nonunion of fractures of the femoral shaft treated by wave-plate osteosynthesis. J Bone Joint Surg (Br). 1997;79(2):289–94.
13. Mukhopadhaya J, Shivapuri S. Functional outcome after open reduction and internal fixation for symptomatic delayed union and nonunion after fracture clavicle: a series of 31 cases. Indian J Orthop. 2007;41(3):209–13.
14. Vidyadhara S, Vamsi K, Rao SK, Gnanadoss JJ, Pandian S. Use of intramedullary fibular strut graft: a novel adjunct to plating in the treatment of osteosteoporotic humeral shaft nonunion. Int Orthop. 2009;33(4):1009–14. Epub 2008 Jun 18
15. Tarr RR, Wiss DA. The mechanics and biology of intramedullary fracture fixation. Clin Orthop Relat Res. 1986;212:10–7.
16. Esterhai JL Jr, Brighton CT, Heppenstall RB, Thrower A, Esterhai JL Jr. Nonunion of the humerus. Clinical, roentgenographic, scintigraphic, and response characteristics to treatment with constant direct current stimulation of osteogenesis. Clin Orthop Relat Res. 1986;211:228–34.
17. Healy WL, White GM, Mick CA, Brooker AF Jr, Weiland AJ. Nonunion of the humeral shaft. Clin Orthop Relat Res. 1987;219:206–13.
18. Ray RD. Vascularization of bone grafts and implants. Clin Orthop Relat Res. 1972;87(87):43–8.
19. Schuh R, Panotopoulos J, Puchner SE, Willegger M, Hobusch GM, Windhager R, Funovics PT. Vascularised or non-vascularised autologous fibular grafting for the reconstruction of a diaphyseal bone defect after resection of a musculoskeletal tumour. Bone Joint J. 2014;96-B(9):1258–63.
20. Yadav SS. Radical resection of bone tumours and reconstruction by autologous bone grafting. Indian J Orthop. 1980;14(2):150–4.
21. Yadav SS. Observations on enbloc resection and reconstruction of malignant bone tumours. Indian J Cancer. 1981;18(3):206–10.
22. Yadav SS. Dual-fibular grafting for massive bone gaps in the lower extremity. J Bone Joint Surg Am. 1990;72(4):486–94.
23. Marino JT, Ziran BH. Use of solid and cancellous autologous bone graft for fractures and nonunions. Orthop Clin North Am. 2010;41(1):15–26.
24. Livani B, Belangero W, Medina G, Pimenta C, Zogaib R, Mongon M. Anterior plating as a surgical alternative in the treatment of humeral shaft non-union. Int Orthop. 2010;34(7):1025–31.
25. Trader JE, Johnson RP, Kalbfleisch JH. Bone-mineral content, surface hardness, and mechanical fixation in the human radius. A correlative study. J Bone Joint Surg Am. 1979;61(8):1217–20.
26. Brown CR, Boden SD. Fracture repair and bone grafting. In: Fischgrund JS, editor. Orthopaedic knowledge update 9. Rosemont: AAOS; 2008. p. 13–22.
27. Khan SN, Cammisa FP Jr, Sandhu HS, Diwan AD, Girardi FP, Lane JM. The biology of bone grafting. J Am Acad Orthop Surg. 2005;13(1):77–86.
28. Yadav SS. Bridging of large skeletal defects by twin fibular grafts supported by L-plate fixation. Orthopaedics (Int Ed). 1995;3(3):213–21.
29. Yadav SS. The use of a free fibular strut as a "biological intramedullary nail" for the treatment of complex nonunion of long bones. J Bone Joint Surg; Open Access. 2018:e0050. https://doi.org/10.2016/JBJS.OA.17.00050.

Chapter 14
NVFG Used to Achieve Arthrodesis in Challenging Cases

14.1 NVFG Used to Achieve Arthrodesis in Challenging Cases

Arthrodesis continues to be a dependable procedure in stabilizing the diseased joints where movements are persistently painful. The procedure is more useful in the lower extremity where stability is preferred to mobility. Arthrodeses are usually performed for salvage, except in the foot, where sub-talar, triple and pan-talar arthrodeses are used with great advantage in stabilizing the foot after realignment. A painful joint with fibrous ankylosis can also be managed by achieving arthodesis in a weight-bearing joint (Fig. 14.1a, b). Arthrodesis is a useful and dependable method in patients with repeatedly failed arthroplasty, such as TKR (total knee replacement) with severe osteoporosis and infection.

Arthrodesis has also proved advantageous for stabilizing joints in certain selected cases of cerebral palsy and poliomyelitis. It is also indicated in neuropathic joints. In a paralytic shoulder, an arthrodesis in a functional position is of a great advantage. The scapulo-thoracic articulation provides functional abduction of the shoulder. However, strong trapezius and serratus anterior muscles are necessary for this outcome.

Non-vascularized and vascularized fibular grafts have been used earlier for tibio-talo-calcaneal arthrodesis. Tibio-talo-calcaneal arthrodesis with an intramedullary nail has been the procedure of choice for patients with involvement of the ankle and sub-talar joints. However, complications include non-union, mal-union, delayed-union and infection. Moreover, the techniques described earlier are expensive, extensive and time-consuming.

The author has used non-vascularized autologous fibular struts in achieving arthrodesis of various joints in difficult cases. The fibular strut has been used as an inlay graft to achieve tibio-talo-calcaneal arthrodesis without an implant. It is a simple, biological, dependable and cost-effective technique (Fig. 14.2a–g). For unicondylar involvement of the femur and tibia, the author has also suggested a

S. S. Yadav, *Non-Vascularised Fibular Grafts in Orthopaedic Practice*,
https://doi.org/10.1007/978-981-95-1794-7_14

technique for arthrodesis of the knee with a single fibular strut (Figs. 14.3 and 14.4a, b).

Another technique for achieving arthrodesis at the knee with a fibular strut is used in unicondylar lesions of the tibia and femur. The proposed technique is indicated for unicondylar lesions of the distal femur and proximal tibia. After the diseased condyle is excised, the large gap is bridged by a fibular strut and the remaining normal condyle, resulting in arthrodesis.

The Technique

After the diseased condyle of the femur or tibia is excised (as shown in the diagram), the articular cartilage of the remaining condyle and the corresponding areas

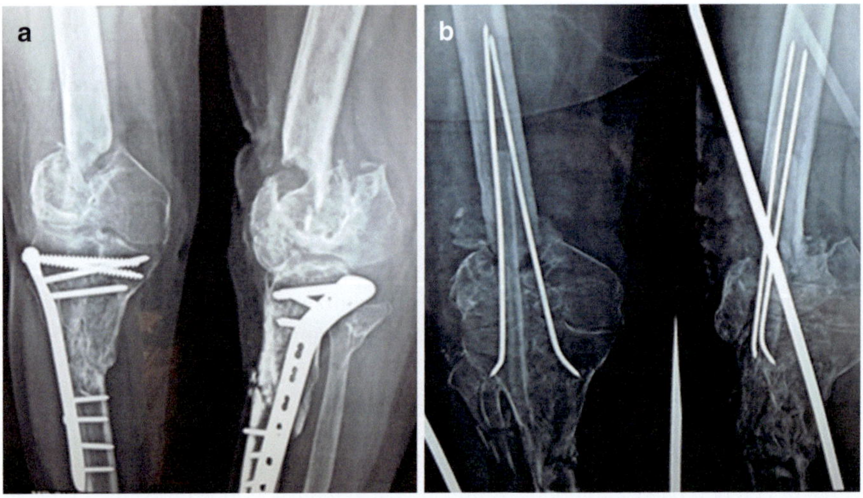

Fig. 14.1 (**a**) The radiograph reveals non-union of a supra-condylar fracture of the femur, and the proximal tibia was plated in another centre. (**b**) Postoperative radiograph reveals a long fibular strut passing through the fracture and knee joint. Twin Kirschner wires are visible on either side of the fibular nail to provide support to the strut graft. This finally resulted in healing of the supra-condylar fracture and arthrodesis of the knee joint

Fig. 14.2 (**a**) A 45-year-old male had a trophic ulcer under the left heel. He has been an old case of spina bifida cystica with foot drop. (**b**) The radiograph illustrates involvement of the under-surface of the calcaneum corresponding to the trophic ulcer track under the heel (arrow). (**c**) The ulcer was excised, and a reamer is passed through the straight track crossing the calcaneum and talus to the lower end of the tibia. The fibular strut is passed through the reamed track up to the lower end of the tibia. (**d**) AP and lateral postoperative radiographs illustrate the placement of the fibular strut to achieve a tibio-talo-calcaneal arthrodesis. (**e**) AP and lateral radiographs reveal complete healing of the ulcer. Note the final position of the fibular strut filling the calcaneal defect, resulting in tibio-talo-calcaneal arthodesis 6 months after surgery. The ulcer had healed and the tibio-talo-calcaneal arthrodesis had helped him for his foot drop also. (**f**) Clinical picture of the heel. (**g**) The patient after treatment

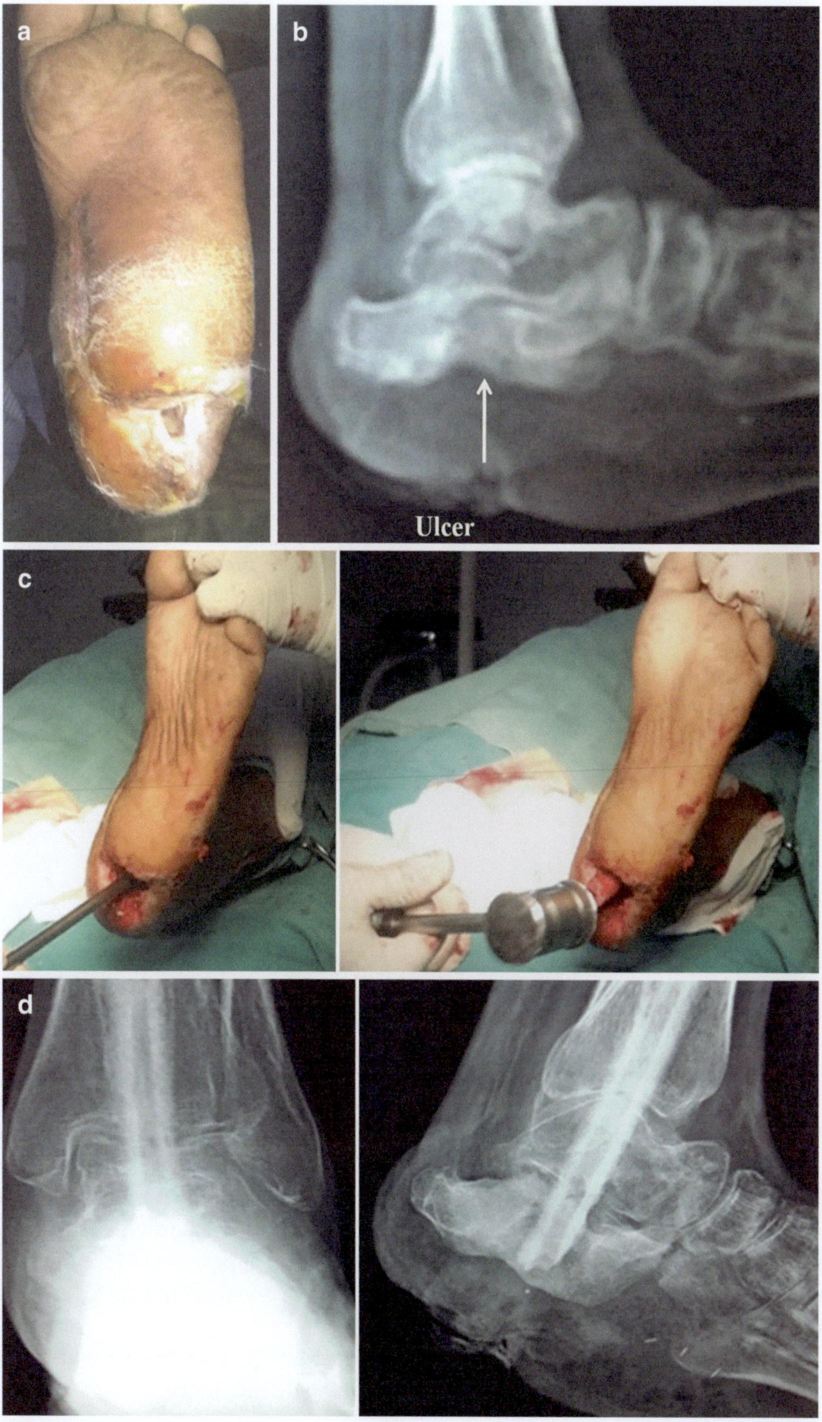

(continued)

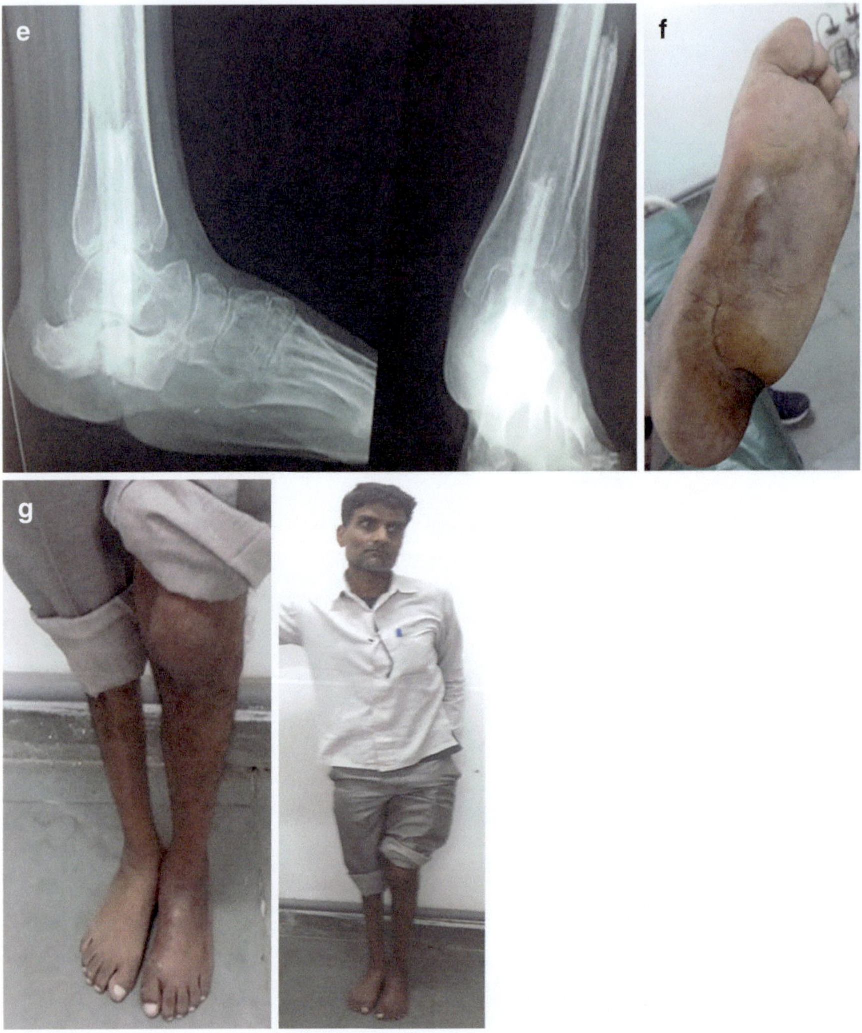

Fig. 14.2 (continued)

of the normal bone are shaved. A long fibular strut is placed with the remaining normal condyle, stabilized by insertion into the medulla of the femur above and the tibia below (as shown in the diagram). The projecting ends of the normal condyle of the normal bone (femur and tibia) are nibbled. This not only provides additional cancellous bone graft but also gives a smooth, cosmetic appearance to the knee/leg. Further stability to the construct is provided by an above-knee POP cast for 2 weeks, followed by a brace.

It is a simple, biological, dependable and cost-effective technique and can be practised by most orthopaedic surgeons, even at the district level.

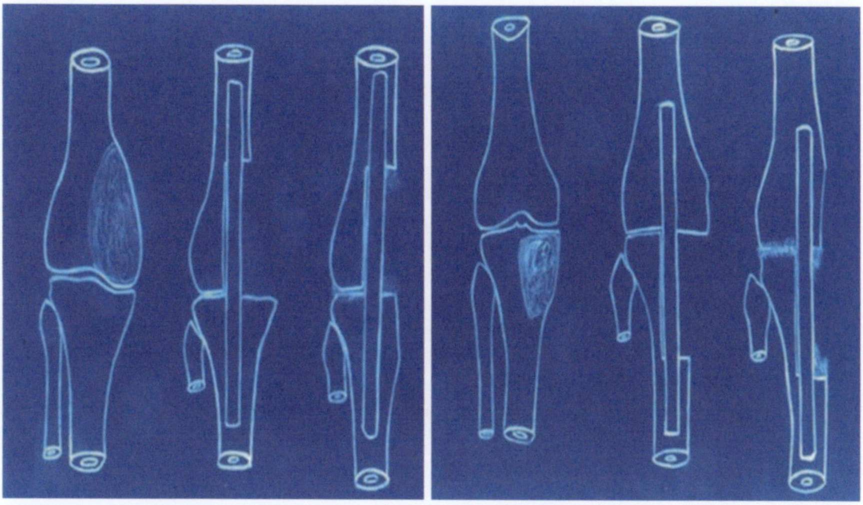

Fig. 14.3 Diagrammatic representation of the proposed technique. After excision of the diseased condyle, the knee is further stabilized with a single fibular graft along with the normal condyle in the femur and tibia

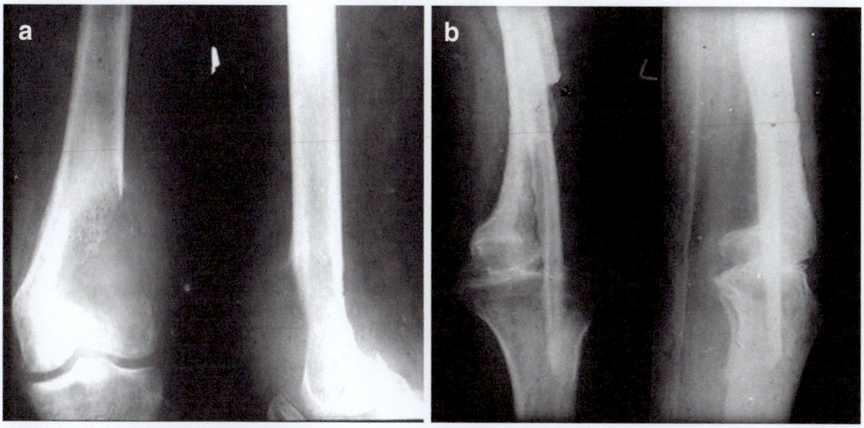

Fig. 14.4 (**a**) AP and lateral radiographs reveal a giant cell tumour involving the lateral condyle of the left femur which was excised. (**b**). AP and lateral postoperative radiographs illustrate arthrodesis achieved using the normal condyle and a single fibular strut graft stabilized at both ends. Note the healing of the construct after 6 months

Suggested Reading

1. Jeong ST, Bin PH, Hwang SC, Kim DH, Nam DC. Use of intramedullary nonvascularized fibular graft with external fixation for revisional charcot ankle fusion: a case report. J Foot Ankle Surg. 2012;51(2):249–53. [PubMed] [Google Scholar].
2. Shah AB, Araoye I, Elattar O. Fibular nail/strut graft for hindfoot fusion plantar exposure and fibular graft placement. Tech Orthop 2017;00: 000–000) 2017.
3. Monaco SJ, Lowery N, Crim B. Fibular strut graft for revisional tibiotalocalcaneal arthrodesis. Foot Ankle Spec. 2016;9(6):560–2. [PubMed] [Google Scholar].
4. Ebraheim NA, Elgafy H, Stefancin JJ. Intramedullary fibular graft for. Clin Orthop Relat Res. 2001;385:165–9. [PubMed] [Google Scholar].
5. Shah AB, Jones C, Elattar O, Naranje SM. Tibiotalocalcaneal arthrodesis with intramedullary fibular strut graft with adjuvant hardware fixation. J Foot Ankle Surg. 2017;56(3):692–6. [PubMed] [Google Scholar].
6. Woods JB, Burns PR. Advances in intramedullary nail fixation in foot and ankle surgery. Clin Podiatr Med Surg. 2011;28:633–48.
7. Ebraheim NA, Elgafy H, Stefancin JJ. Intramedullary fibular graft for tibiotalocalcaneal arthrodesis. Clin Orthop Relat Res. 2001;385:165–9.
8. DiDomenico LA, Wargo-Dorsey M. Tibiotalocalcaneal arthrodesis using a femoral locking plate. J Foot Ankle Surg. 2012;51:128–32.
9. Kile TA, Donnelly RE, Gehrke JC, Werner ME, Johnson KA. Tibiotalocalcaneal arthrodesis with an intramedullary device. Foot Ankle Int. 2002;23:704–10.
10. Mudgal CS, Wilson MG. Revision tibiotalocalcaneal arthrodesis after a failed intramedullary rod: a technique tip. Foot Ankle Int. 1999;20:210–1.
11. Patzakis MJ, Zalavras CG. Chronic posttraumatic osteomyelitis and infected nonunion of the tibia: current management concepts. J Am Acad Orthop Surg. 2005;13:417–42.

Chapter 15
Twin NVFG Used for Achieving Stabilization of a Spinal Segment

15.1 Twin NVFG Used for Achieving Stabilization of a Spinal Segment

Spinal fusion with either non-vascularized or vascularized bone grafts has been well documented for inflammatory, degenerative, post-oncological and post-traumatic reconstruction. In such cases, the said fusion is usually achieved with instrumentation and bone grafting.

A few reports have indicated that free vascularized fibular grafts have been used for reconstruction and stabilization of the thoracolumbar spine with good clinical results. However, all vascularized bone grafting is supported by instrumentation with rods and plates. The existing techniques used are technically challenging, complicated, extensive and expensive. Moreover, their availability and cost are an issue that needs consideration.

15.2 GCT of the Spine

GCT of the spine is a rare disease. Any osteolytic lesion in the spine is diagnosed as GCT or ABC, pending a biopsy report. Smaller lesions need only curettage. However, the large ones do require stabilization after thorough curettage. There are many ways for fixation of the spine. We have used autologous twin fibular grafts after wedging the grafts between the healthy vertebra above and below with success (Fig. 15.1a–h).

In some cases, we have also used twin grafts fixed posteriorly to the raw laminae like any other implant. The strong struts provide biological fixation in stabilizing the spine even in other diseases requring spinal stability.

S. S. Yadav, *Non-Vascularised Fibular Grafts in Orthopaedic Practice*,
https://doi.org/10.1007/978-981-95-1794-7_15

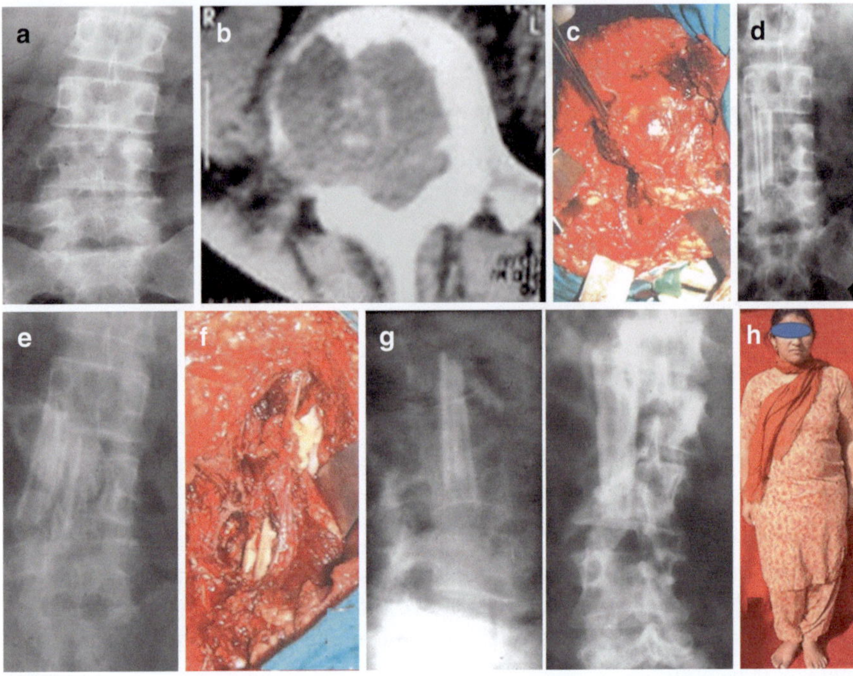

Fig. 15.1 (**a**) A 34-year-old lady was diagnosed with a GCT involving the L-4 vertebra. (**b**) A CT scan revealing the extent of the diseased vertebra. (**c**) Intraoperative picture showing excision of the lesion. (**d**) Radiograph reveals twin fibular grafts in situ after excision of the lesion and the soft tissue extension with thorough curettage. The resultant gap was bridged by dual fibular struts fixed between the healthy vertebrae on either side. (**e**) Radiograph illustrates evidence of recurrence of the lesion. (**f**) Intraoperative picture reveals recurrence eroding the twin graft. The lesion was excised and a fresh twin fibular graft was stabilized in the vertebra above and below. (**g**) Radiograph reveals twin fibular grafts in situ. Healing took place in 10 months. (**h**) Clinical picture of the patient who is now symptom free after 3 years

The autologous fibula is strong and straight, making it an ideal choice for stabilization of the spine. NVFG is effective and makes it an option for obtaining a bony fusion in patients who need stability of the spine (Fig. 15.2a–e). Moreover, fibular graft fixation can help address pseudarthrosis, implant breakage and screw pullout secondary to osteoporosis.

In a few cases, we have attempted twin NVFG for achieving spinal fusion of the dorso-lumbar spine in diseases that needed fusion. The principle of the technique is similar to that of metallic spinal instrumentation/fixation. The advantage of the technique is that it provides autologous bone with osteogenic effect between the laminae and the fibular struts (Fig. 15.3a–g).

This technique may be considered as one of the methods for achieving spinal fusion in various spinal diseases needing fusion.

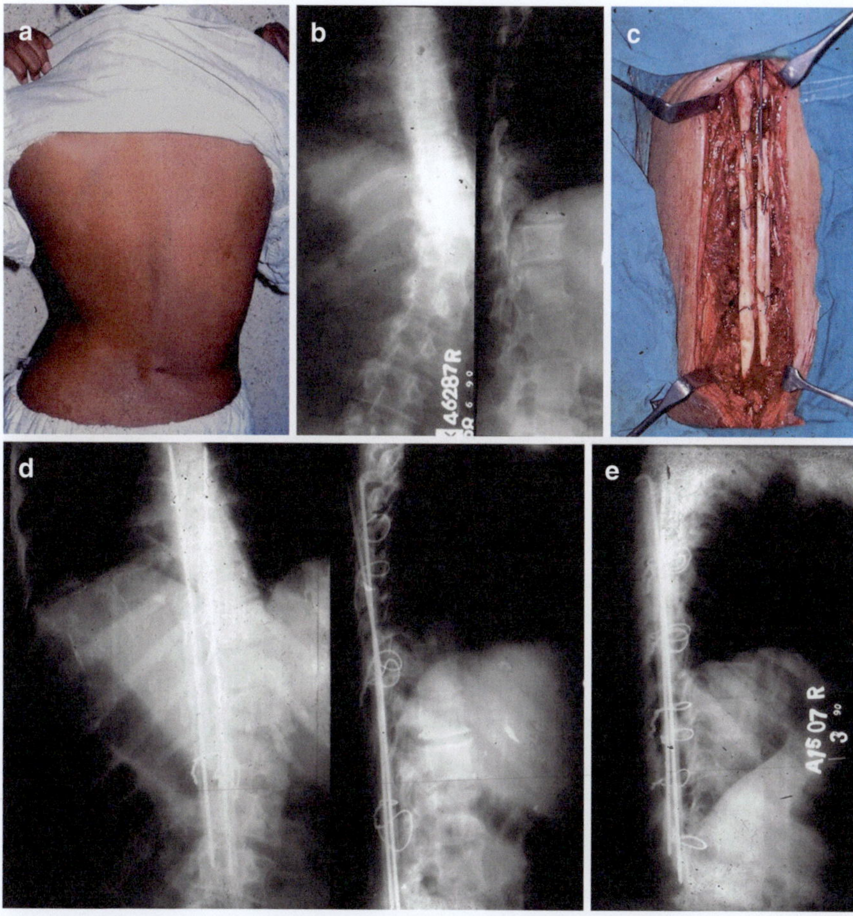

Fig. 15.2 (**a**) A 25-year-old patient of post-polio residual paralysis with mild but painful scoliosis. (**b**) Radiograph revealing the dorsal-lumbar scoliotic curve. (**c**) Intraoperative picture of twin fibular grafts over the laminae. Note the interlaminar wiring fixing the fibular struts to the laminae like a metallic rod. (**d**) Postoperative radiographs revealing the fibular struts fixed to the spine. (**e**) Radiograph taken 9 months after surgery revealing union of the host and the graft. The wires were removed

Surgical Technique

- After a thorough clinical examination and radiological assessment, the surgery is carefully planned.
- The patient is put in a prone position under suitable anaesthesia. An incision is made over the spine, keeping the primary disease in its centre. The laminae are exposed and cleaned.
- The spinus processes of the vertebrae required to be fused are removed.
- The laminae are made raw with a burr machine.

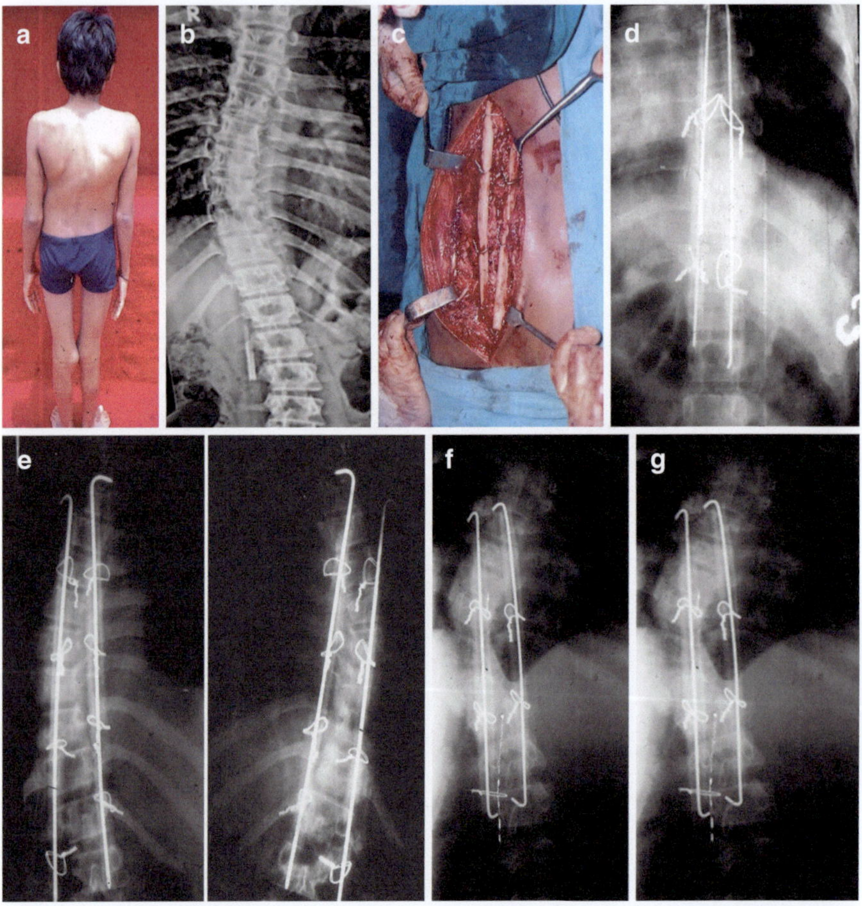

Fig. 15.3 (**a**) A 16-year-old girl with PPRP (post polio residual paralysis) and mild kyphoscoliosis. (**b**) Radiograph of the patient. (**c**) Intraoperative picture with fibular grafts fixed to the laminae with interlaminar wiring. (**d**) Postoperative roentgenogram showing a straight spine with the fibular grafts fixed to the laminae. (**e**) Radiographs 6 months after surgery revealing new bone formation in between the two fibular struts. (**f**) In another case, a radiograph taken 8 months after surgery shows enough bone formation at the proximal and distal ends and hypertrophy in one of the fibular struts. The wires were removed. (**g**) Postoperative radiograph of a different patient revealing healing after 8 months

- The required length of fibular struts can be harvested subperiosteally and placed over the raw laminae on either side of the spine.
- To provide strength to the graft in the initial stages, suitably sized Kirschner wires are inserted into the fibular struts.
- Inter-laminar wiring is attempted for fixing the fibular struts to the laminae, similar to metallic rods.
- The removed spinus processes are placed over and in between the two fibular struts.

- The wound is closed in layers.
- Postoperatively, the patient is kept in bed for 2–3 weeks. Depending on a particular case, a suitable brace is applied to provide further stability to the spine.

The ischemic time of the fibular strut outside the body should be minimal. The fibular strut should be removed only after the host site is prepared to receive the graft. An early fixation of the graft to the vertebrae makes it more viable as the surface osteoblasts and osteocytes survive and add to the quality of the graft to be more osteogenic and viable for achieving union with the laminae.

The advantage of the technique is that it is simple, biological and cost-effective. Moreover, the structural viability, osteogenesis and strength are maintained throughout the healing process. Once the healing process is achieved, the Kirschner wires are removed through small incisions which will allow the graft to get remodelled. After removal of the Kirschner wires, the struts get contoured according to the curvature of the spine. However, depending on a particular case, a suitable brace may be used. The technique can also be attempted in mild but painful cases of dorsolumbar scoliosis where only a spinal fusion is required. Ultimately, indications and techniques of spinal fusion should be individualized to the patient and based on surgeon preference and experience.

Suggested Readings

1. Chen ZC, Fan KF, Wu WC, Chen HC. Fusion of the lumbar spine with a free vascularized fibular bone grafts: case report. Changgeng Yi Xue Za Zhi. 1998;21(4):463–8.
2. Moran SL, Bakri K, Mardini S, Shin AY, Bishop AT. The use of vascularized fibular grafts for the reconstruction of spinal and sacral defects. Microsurgery. 2009;29(5):393–400.
3. Shen FH, Mason JR, Shimer AL, Arlet VM. Pelvic fixation for adult scoliosis. Eur Spine J. 2013;22(2):S265–75.
4. Agarwal A, Chauhan V, Singh D, Shailendra R, Maheshwari R, Juyal A. A comparative study of pedicle screw fixation in dorsolumbar spine by freehand versus image-assisted techniques: a cadaveric study. Indian J Orthop. 2016;50(3):243–9.
5. Maruyama T, Takeshita K. Surgical treatment of scoliosis: a review of techniques currently applied scoliosis and spinal disorders. Scoliosis. 2008 Apr 18:3:6. doi: 10.1186/1748-7161-3-6.

Chapter 16
Maternal Fibular Graft Used in Children with Congenital Pseudarthrosis of Long Bones

16.1 Congenital Pseudarthrosis of Long Bones

Congenital pseudarthrosis of long bones occurs commonly in the tibia and also in the radius, ulna and clavicle. Neurofibromatosis or skin manifestations occur in up to 50% of patients with pseudarthrosis. The defect may be noted at birth but is usually observed later in early childhood. In most cases, there is a pathological fracture, bone pain and deformity. The cortex is thin and the medulla wide. An area of radiolucency is seen at the site of pseudarthrosis. There is progressive tapering of the bone ends towards the site of pseudarthrosis.

Fibrous dysplasia and congenital ring syndrome also have been described in association with congenital tibial pseudarthrosis. Neurofibromas are rarely seen at the site of pseudarthrosis. MR imaging of congenital pseudarthrosis provides valuable information regarding the extent of the disease and an accurate evaluation.

16.2 Congenital Pseudarthrosis of the Radius

Congenital pseudarthrosis of the radius is a rare condition (Fig. 16.1a, b). It is reported to be associated with neurofibromatosis (von Recklinghausen's disease) or fibrous dysplasia. Various treatment options have been described with varying degrees of success, and the reports have revealed successful healing. The literature discloses the difficulties in treating this condition. It has been reported that vascularized fibular grafts have been used successfully. The author reports a case of congenital pseudarthrosis of the radius managed successfully with a maternal graft (Fig. 16.2a–d).

S. S. Yadav, *Non-Vascularised Fibular Grafts in Orthopaedic Practice*,
https://doi.org/10.1007/978-981-95-1794-7_16

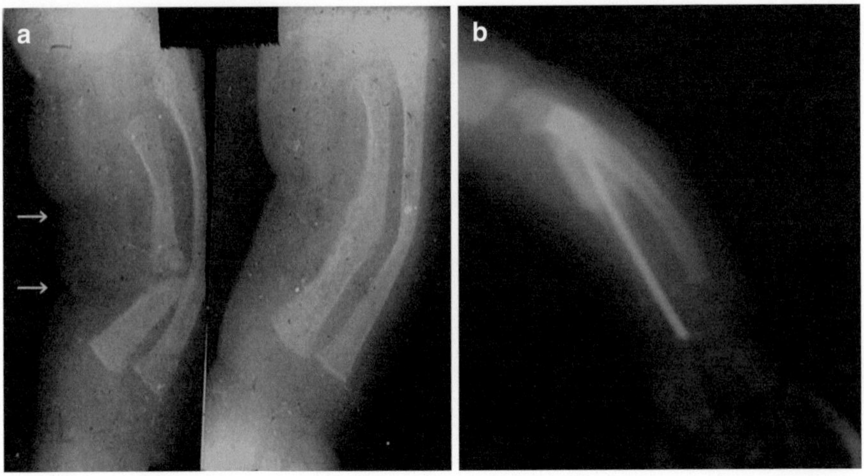

Fig. 16.1 (**a**) Roentgenogram shows congenital pseudarthrosis of the radial shaft. Note the congenital furrows in the soft tissues of the forearm which are diagnostic in such cases (arrows). (**b**) Postoperative roentgenogram after excision of the pseudarthrosis and reconstruction with a maternal fibular graft stabilized by a Kirschner wire

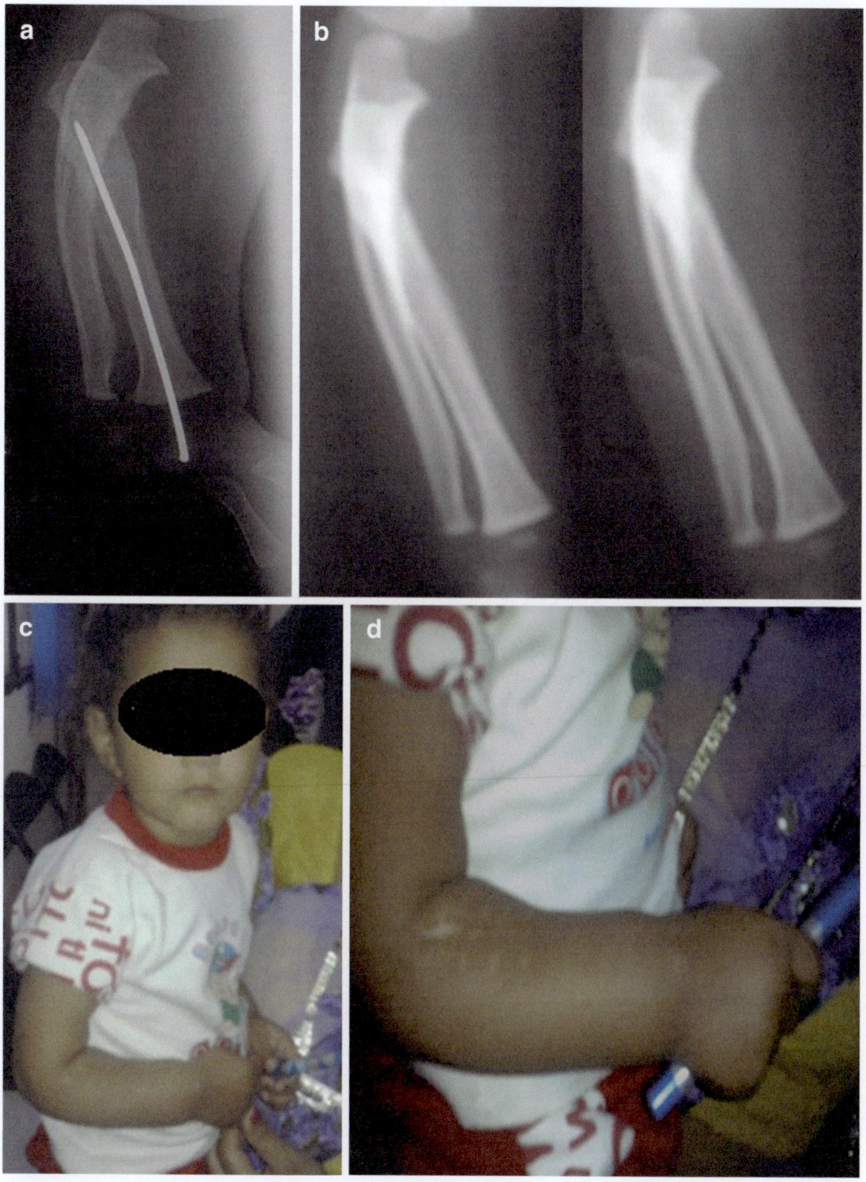

Fig. 16.2 (**a**) A follow-up roentgenogram reveals union of the graft with early remodelling. (**b**) The Kirschner wire has been removed. The graft has completely merged with the radius. There is no deformity, and the forearm shows signs of normal growth. (**c**, **d**) Postoperative clinical pictures of the patient after 24 weeks with straight right forearm which shows normal growth, no deformity and a fully functional hand. Note the postoperative scar

Suggested Reading

1. Sprague BL, Brown GA. Congential pseudarthrosis of the radius. JBJS. 1974;56-A(1):191–4.
2. Mukhopadaya S, Shivapuri. Congential pseudarthrosis of the radius. A case report. Strat Traum Limb Recon. 2006;1:51–4. https://doi.org/10.1007/s11751-006-0006-0.
3. Ali MS, Hopper G. Congenital pseudarthrosis of the ulna due to neurofibromatosis 1982 British Editorial Society of Bone and Joint Surgery 0301-620X/82/5120–0600.
4. Witoonchart K, Uerpairojkit C, Leechavengvongs S, Thuvasethakul P. Congenital pseudarthrosis of the forearm treated by free vascularised fibular graft: a report of three cases and a review of the literature. J Hand Surg Am. 1990;24:1045–55.
5. Talab YA. Congenital pseudarthrosis of the radius, a case report and the review of the literature. Clin Orthop Relat Res. 1993;291:246–50.
6. Kameyama O, Ogawa R. Pseudarthrosis of the radius associated with neurofibromatosis: report of a case and review of the literature. J Pediatr Orthop. 1990;10:128.
7. Gregg PJ, Price BA, Ellis HA, Strvens J. Pseudarthrosis of the radius associated with neurofibromatosis. A case report. Clin Orthop Relat Res. 1982;171:175–9.
8. Less KS, Lee SH, Ha KH, Lee SJ. Congenital pseudarthrosis of ulna treated by free vascularised fibular graft – a case report. Hand Surg. 2000;5:61–7.
9. Cleneland RH, Gilsanz V, Wilkinson RH. Congenital Pseudarthrosis of the radius. Am J Roentgenol. 1978;130:955–7.
10. Ansari MT, Gautam D, Kotwal PP. Mother's fibula in son's forearm: use of maternal bone grafting for aneurysmal bone cyst not amenable to curettage – a case report with review of literature. SICOT J. 2016;2:18.
11. Brown GA, Osebold WR, Ponseti IV. Congenital pseudarthrosis of long bones: a clinical, radiographic, histologic and ultrastructural study. Clin Orthop Relat Res. 1977;128:228–42.

Chapter 17
Maternal Fibular Grafting in Congenital Pseudarthrosis of the Tibia

17.1 Congenital Pseudarthrosis of the Tibia (CPT)

Although rare, CPT continues to be one of the most challenging diseases in orthopaedics. The disease has a variable history and usually occurs during the first decade of life. It is characterized by gradual anterolateral angulation of the distal third of the leg and is associated with fracture non-union. Its incidence is reported to be from 1:140,000 to 1:250,000 live births. CPT is known to be associated with neurofibromatosis type I. Its skin manifestations are known as 'café au lait spots' that occur in up to 50% of patients with CPT. CPT may also involve other tubular bones including the radius, ulna and clavicle.

Paget (1891) was the first to describe a case of congenital pseudarthrosis of the tibia. The tibia is the most frequently affected site associated with congenital anterolateral tibial deformity. Spontaneous fracture at the distal third of the tibia progresses to non-union (Fig. 17.1). Recurrence after treatment is well known, but the incidence diminishes with age and is rarely reported after puberty. There have been sporadic reports of bilateral and familial involvement.

Morphologically, three classifications have been proposed by Andersen, Boyd and Crawford. Radiologically, all the three classifications include sclerotic, cystic and dysplastic types. These changes included cortical tapering, sclerosis and formation of cysts in the region of the involved medullary canal. Because the appearance changes during the course of the disease, all the classifications have limited value. The main determining factor is the stage of the disease at which it has been classified. With the classical deformity, diagnosis can easily be made on a radiograph (Fig. 17.2a, b). However, MRI may provide valuable information on the extent of the disease, and the soft tissue changes may be accurately defined.

The site of pseudarthrosis is usually surrounded by thickened periosteum and massive fibrous tissue (Fig. 17.3). It has been reported that periosteal cells in the hamartoma of CPT have decreased osteoblastic responses. Emphasis has been laid

S. S. Yadav, *Non-Vascularised Fibular Grafts in Orthopaedic Practice*,
https://doi.org/10.1007/978-981-95-1794-7_17

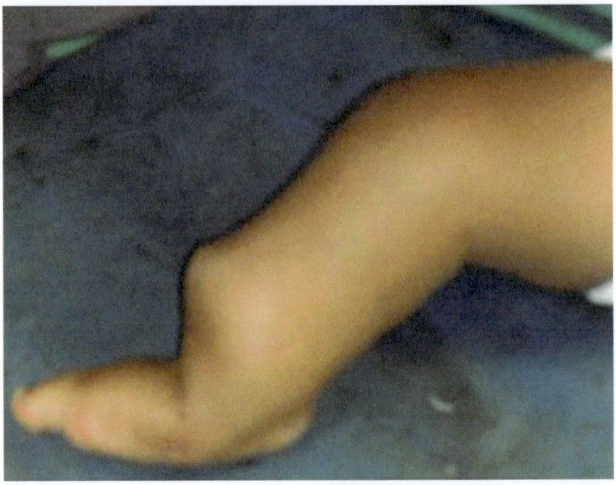

Fig. 17.1 Clinical picture of a 2-year-old patient with congenital pseudarthrosis of the tibia with a kyphotic deformity

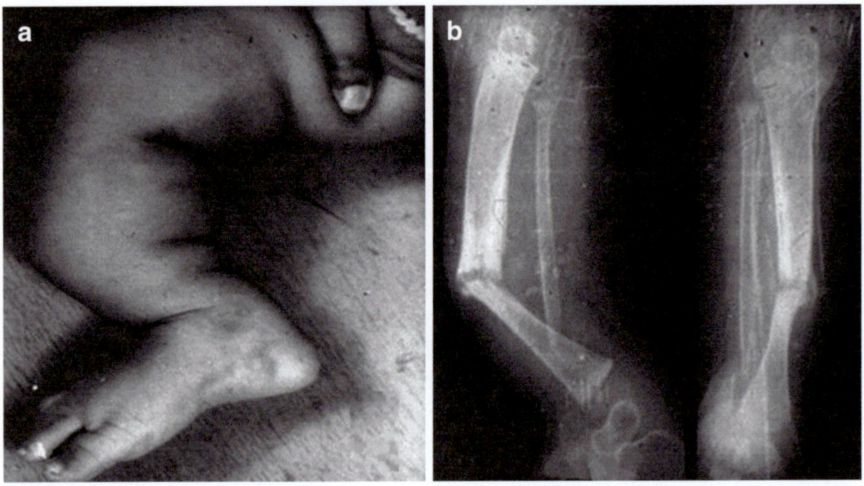

Fig. 17.2 (**a**, **b**) Clinical picture and radiograph of a classical case of congenital pseudarthrosis of the tibia and fibula

on the importance of the periosteum to treat CPT. Fibrous hamartoma is known to replace the healthy periosteum and leads to osteolysis. A report of managing CPT with bone and periosteal grafting from the child's mother has been mentioned [36].

Fracture of the fibula, when present, leads to proximal migration of its distal end and results in valgus deformity of the ankle joint. A cross-union between the tibia and fibula has also been created as part of the treatment of CPT.

Management of CPT remains difficult, controversial and uncertain. Various methods have been described to manage CPT. Intramedullary rodding, the Ilizarov treatment and vascularized fibular grafting have been reported with

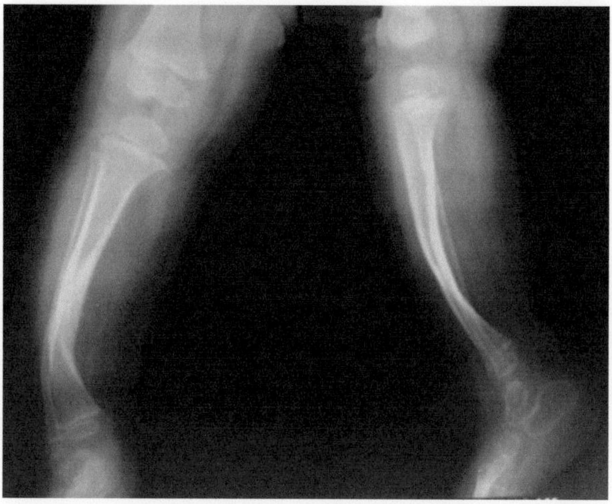

Fig. 17.3 Roentgenogram revealing a pre-pseudarthrotic tibia

almost similar results. The problems in the management include persistent non-union, re-fracture and leg and ankle deformities along with limb length inequality. Generally, in older children, the prognosis is better after surgical treatment and recurrences are rare after skeletal maturity. However, there is currently no standard accepted technique.

Bone grafting in congenital tibial pseudarthrosis may follow certain guidelines: (1) The hamartoma and the fibrous tissue should be widely excised along with the tibial ends. (2) The bone and soft tissues at the CPT site should be viable. (3) Solid fixation with the proposed strut bone graft is achieved between the tibial ends, further stabilized with a Kirschner wire or plate and screws, and supported with plaster cast. (4) Autogenous iliac bone grafting may be performed around the construct. (5) The needed length of the proposed strut graft is calculated on the basis of the expected length of the leg after the affected bone and fibrous tissues have been excised and the angular deformity has been corrected. (6) The Kirschner wire maybe removed after solid clinical and radiographic union has taken place. (7) Prolonged orthotic protection of the leg is required.

Amputation is known to be the final option in a child with CPT. Foot deformities, the number of operations and other severe problems such as repeated non-union have been described as factors that determine the need for amputation. The author is of the opinion that, in a viable limb with sensate foot, amputation should be the last resort and avoided as far as possible. Access to appropriate prosthetic care has been a matter of consideration in developing countries.

We have used maternal fibular grafts in all but one patient, within the age group of 4–14 years. In one patient, a maternal fibular graft was not available as the fibulae were already used by previous surgeons in this bilateral case with prior failure. In this patient, on one side, we had used a paternal fibular strut as an onlay graft after wide excision of the pseudarthrosis. The construct had healed, and a 55-year follow-up for this rare case is available.

The Author's Concept About CPT

Congenital pseudarthrosis of the tibia is a disease affecting the tibia, particularly in its distal third. However, its exact cause is not fully understood. Since it is not possible to judge the exact extent of the diseased tibia, it is considered necessary that enough tibial shaft is excised on either side of the pseudarthrosis to achieve a disease-free site. It is also proposed that the pseudarthrosis may be excised with the bone ends without disturbing its pseudocapsule. A wide excision of the tibial shaft may also result in preventing recurrent non-union.

Pseudarthrosis of the tibia is usually noted at the distal third or fourth of the tibia. The distal end is usually small and tapering. After adequate excision of the distal end along with the pseudarthrosis, a very little part of it is left or it may even need complete excision. In such cases, the required fixation at the distal end is not possible. To achieve a stable fixation, the maternal strut graft is fixed to the remaining distal end of the tibia, talus and calcaneus. A tibio-talo-calcaneal arthrodesis has been recommended to fix the distal end of the maternal fibular graft. Arthrodesis at these joints is a small price to pay for achieving good fixation in such a challenging disease. This may be taken as a necessary step rather than a disadvantage.

Emphasis has been laid on the importance of the periosteum to treat CPT. A report on the management of CPT using bone and periosteal grafting from the child's mother has been mentioned by Paley [36].

The Technique of Fixing Maternal Fibular Strut Graft in CPT

The pseudarthrotic site is exposed, and a wide excision of the fibrous hamartoma is attempted including a part of the normal-looking tibia. Since it is not possible to judge the length of the diseased tibia with the naked eye, it is considered necessary that enough tibial shaft is excised on either side of the pseudarthrosis to achieve a disease-free site. The wide excision of the tibial shaft may also result in preventing recurrent non-union.

Another team retrieved an appropriate size of the maternal fibular graft and transplanted it at the host site as early as possible, stabilizing it between the tibial ends. A delay may affect the osteogenic cells on and within the graft.

At the proximal end of the tibia, a window is made anteriorly by gently lifting the cortex. This is possible as the child's tibia is not brittle. The proximal end of the appropriately sized maternal fibular graft is wedged or fitted into the medullary canal of this tibial fragment. The lifted portion of the cortex is placed back over the graft and stabilized circumferentially by a wire or even a chromic cat-gut (Fig. 17.4). A transcalcaneal long Kirschner wire of appropriate size may be inserted into the strut graft, stabilizing it further on the principle of three-point fixation between the tibial ends. To support the extremity further, an above-knee POP cast is applied for a period of 12 weeks. Periodic roentgenograms are taken to assess the progress of the healing process (Fig. 17.5a–d).

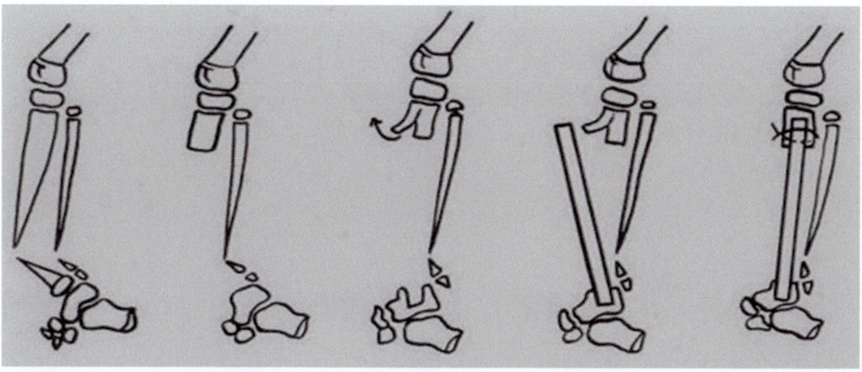

Fig. 17.4 Steps of the surgical technique described in the text. The diseased tibia has been excised. The maternal fibular strut has been used to bridge the gap, as described

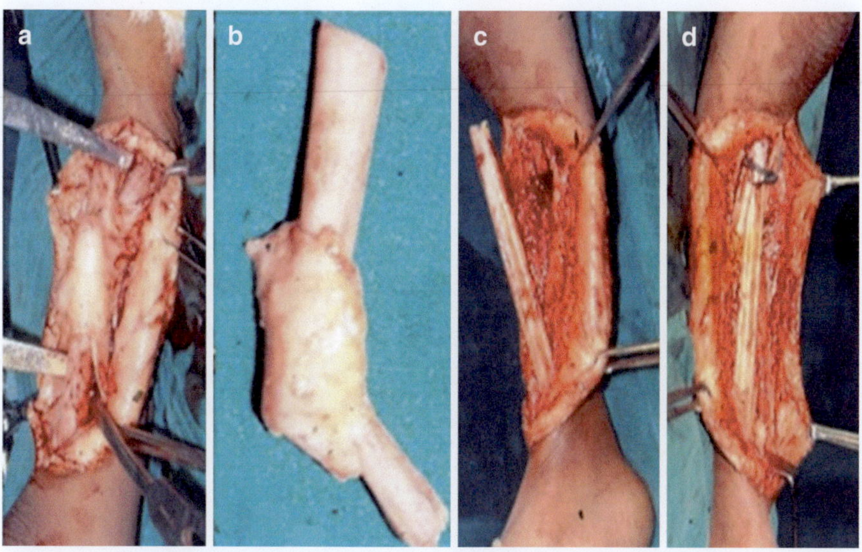

Fig. 17.5 Intraoperative steps of the surgical procedure. (**a**) Exposure. (**b**) The liberally excised diseased segment. (**c**) The distal and of the fibular strut is fixed, arthrodesing the distal joints. (**d**) The maternal fibular strut is shown bridging the tibial gap as suggested

17.2 Some of the Patients with Congenital Pseudoarthrosis of the Tibia Managed Using the Above Technique with Maternal Fibular Grafting

(Figs. 17.6a–f, 17.7a–e, 17.8a–g, 17.9a–i, 17.10a–d, 17.11a–c, 17.12a, b, and 17.13)

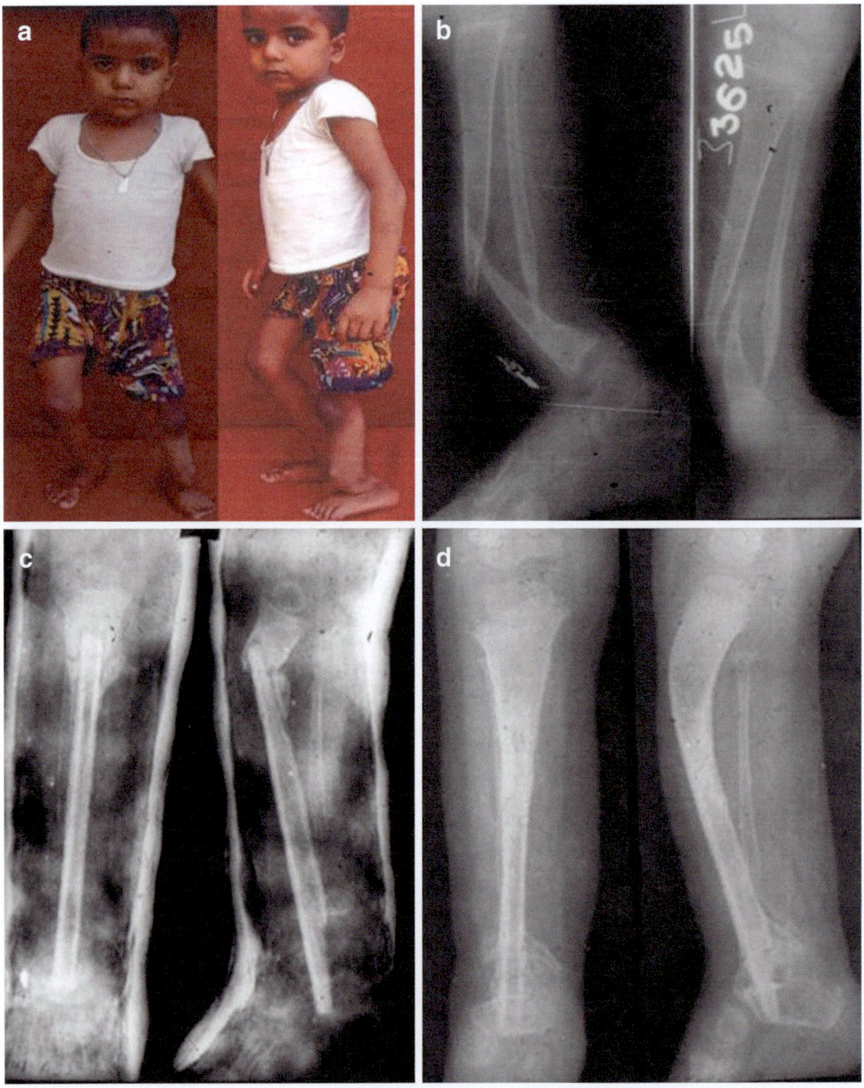

Fig. 17.6 (**a**) Congenital pseudarthrosis of the left tibia. (**b**) Roentgenogram showing the tapering ends at the site of pseudarthrosis. (**c**) Postoperative radiograph reveals slight anterior angulation at the proximal end. (**d**) However, union has taken place. Note the hypertrophy of the fibular strut. (**e**) Roentgenogram reveals complete healing and hypertrophy of the maternal fibular graft at both its ends. (**f**) An angiogram taken after healing reveals near-normal vasculature

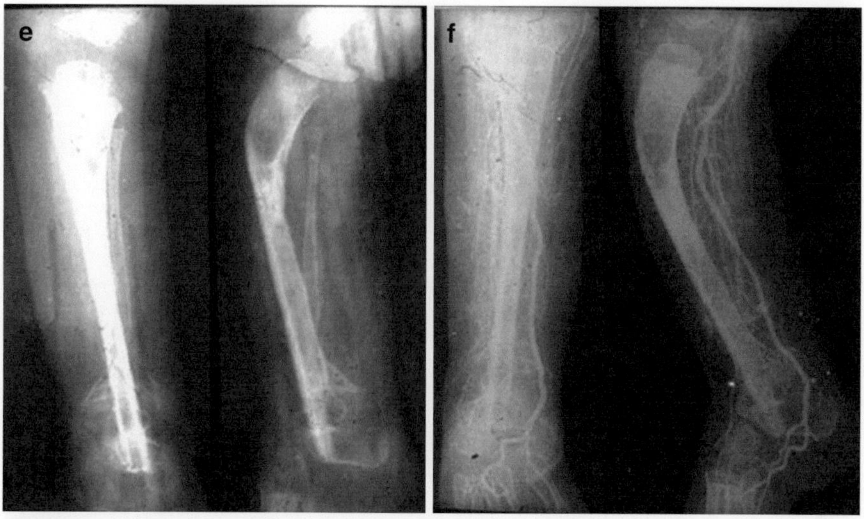

Fig. 17.6 (continued)

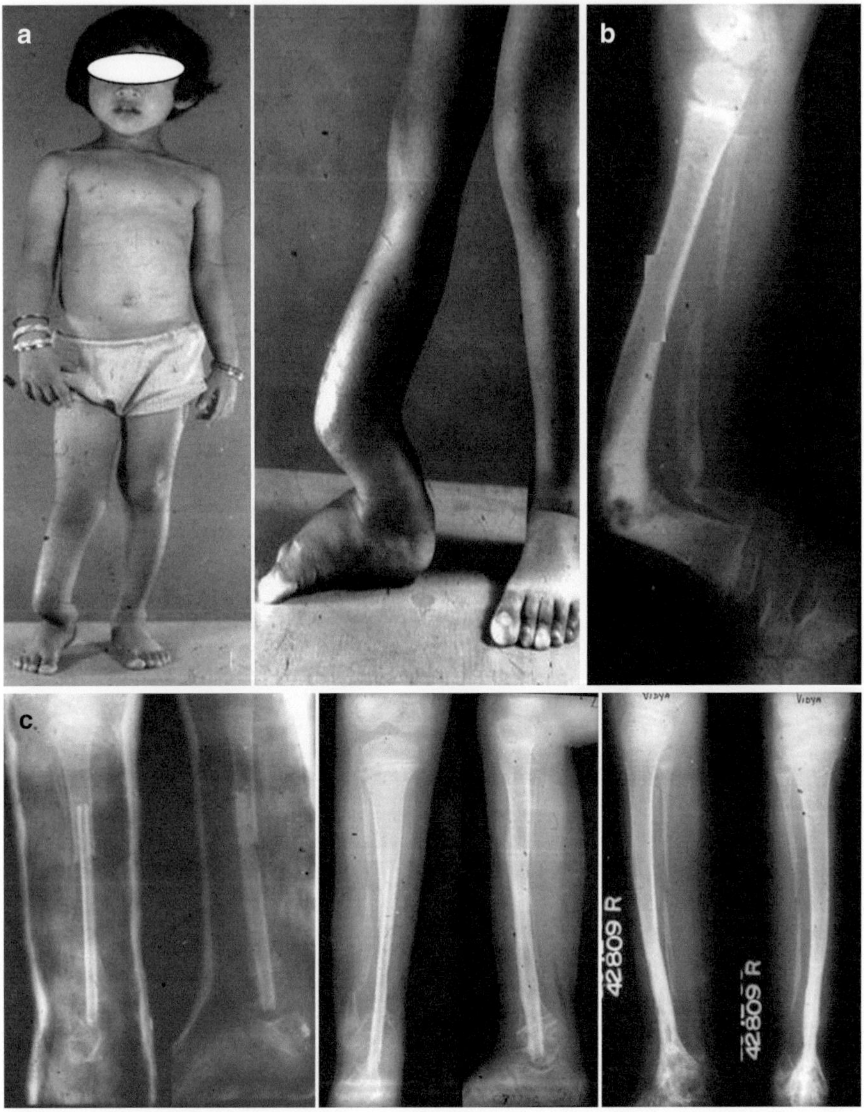

Fig. 17.7 (**a**, **b**) Clinical picture and roentgenogram of a girl with congenital pseudarthrosis of the right tibia. (**c**) AP and lateral postoperative roentgenograms taken at various stages of management reveal healing and remodelling of the graft with ankle arthrodesis. (**d**, **e**) The roentgenogram reveals complete healing, and the patient stands in a protective boot

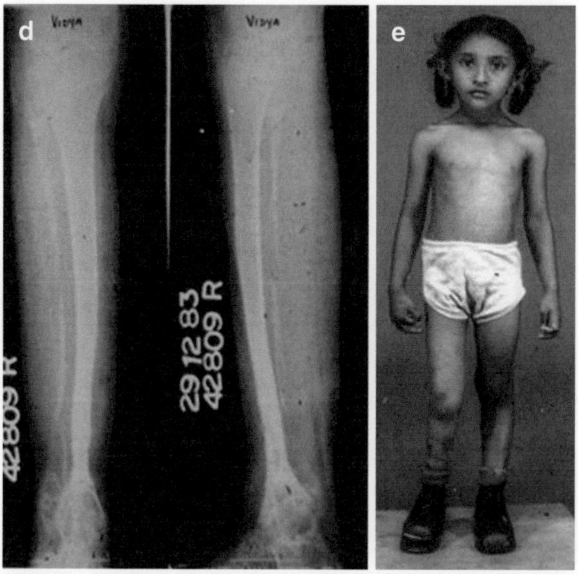

Fig. 17.7 (continued)

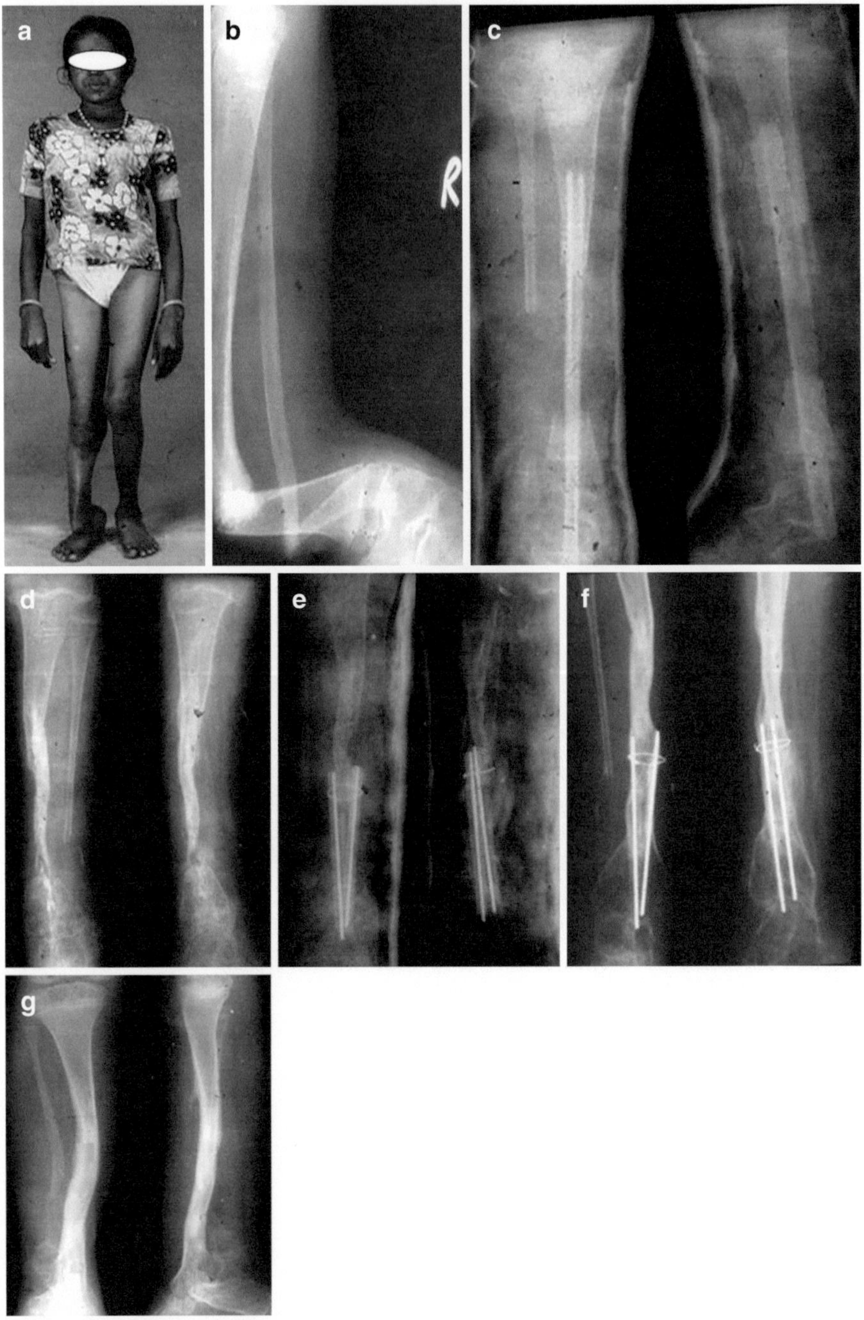

Fig. 17.8 (**a**, **b**) Clinical picture and roentgenogram of a 14-year-old girl revealing congenital pseudarthrosis of the right tibia. (**c**) Postoperative AP and lateral roentgenogram after maternal fibular graft. (**d**) The patient had a fracture at the site of pseudarthrosis after 10 months. (**e**, **f**) Two onlay fibular struts from the contralateral fibula with Kirschner wires were fixed with circumferential wiring. The limb was further supported by a POP cast. The fracture revealed union after 1 year. (**g**) The final radiograph showing complete healing and hypertrophy of the construct

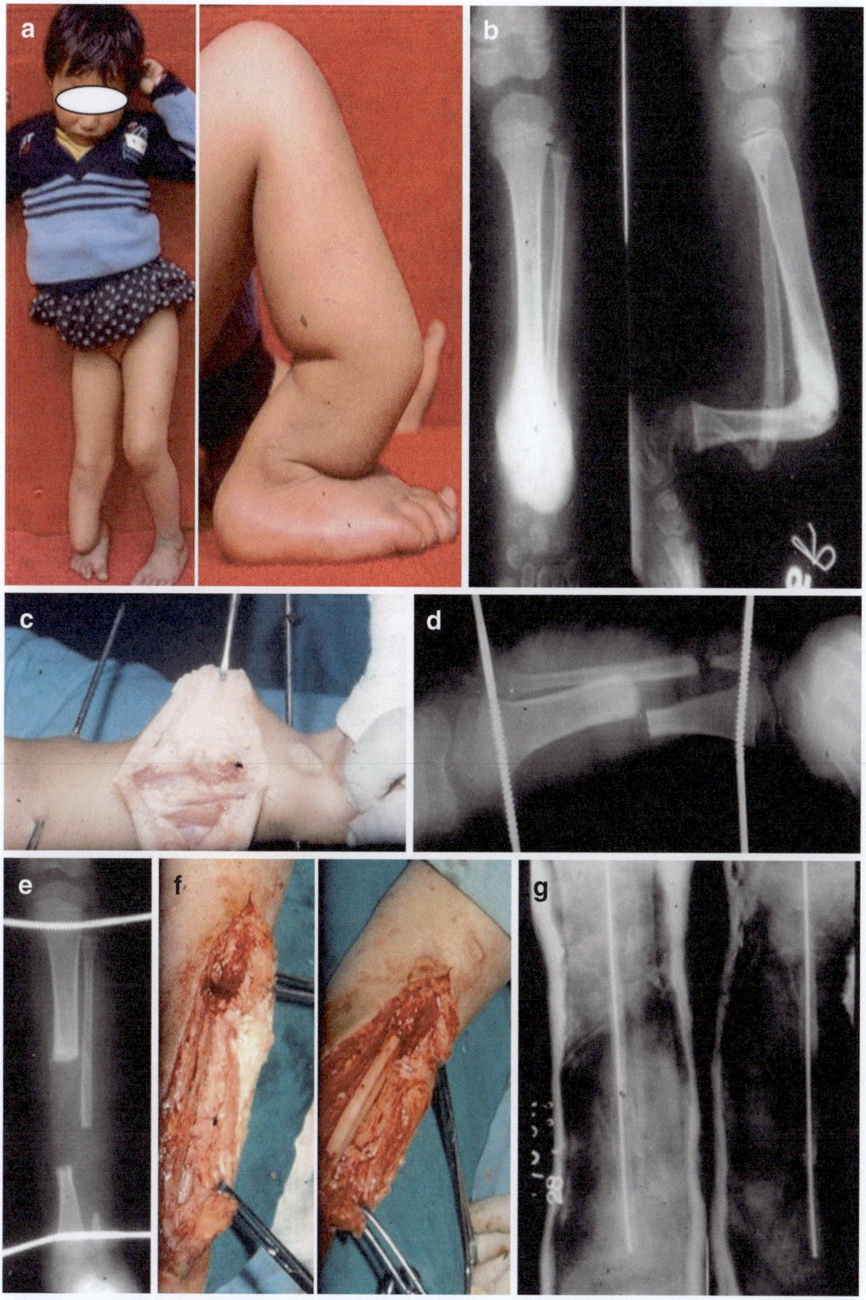

Fig. 17.9 (**a**) Clinical picture of a 3-year-old girl with classical deformity of pseudarthrosis of the tibia. (**b**) Roentgenogram shows pseudarthrosis of the right tibia. (**c**) Intraoperative picture shown after excision of the lesion. (**d**) AP roentgenogram reveals the excision after which the leg had become very short. (**e–g**) Tibial traction on either end subsequently led to the lengthening of the leg. Note the increased gap. Radiograph after the second surgery reveals bridging of the gap with a maternal fibula with inlay Kirschner wires, further supported by a POP cast. (**h**) Roentgenograms reveal healing. (**i**) Note the complete healing at the site of pseudarthrosis. However, the wires were not removed for next 2 years as a support to the graft

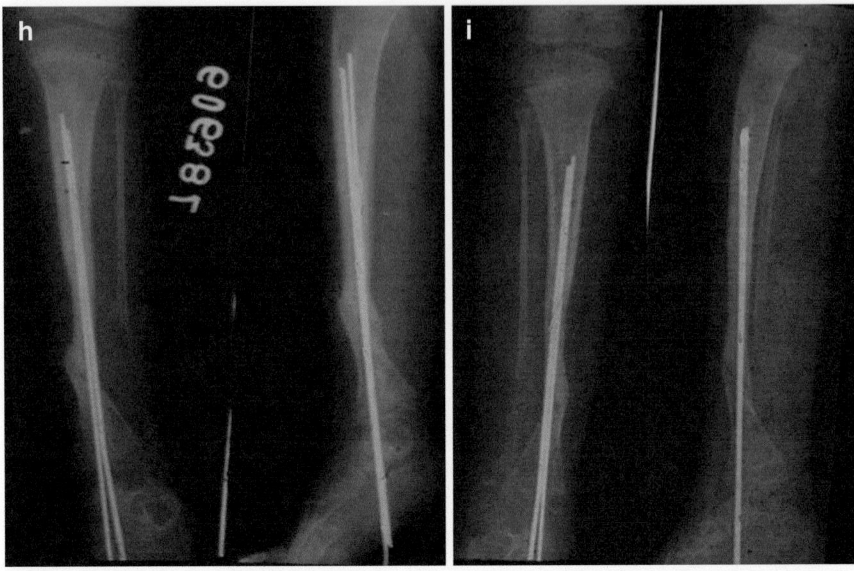

Fig. 17.9 (continued)

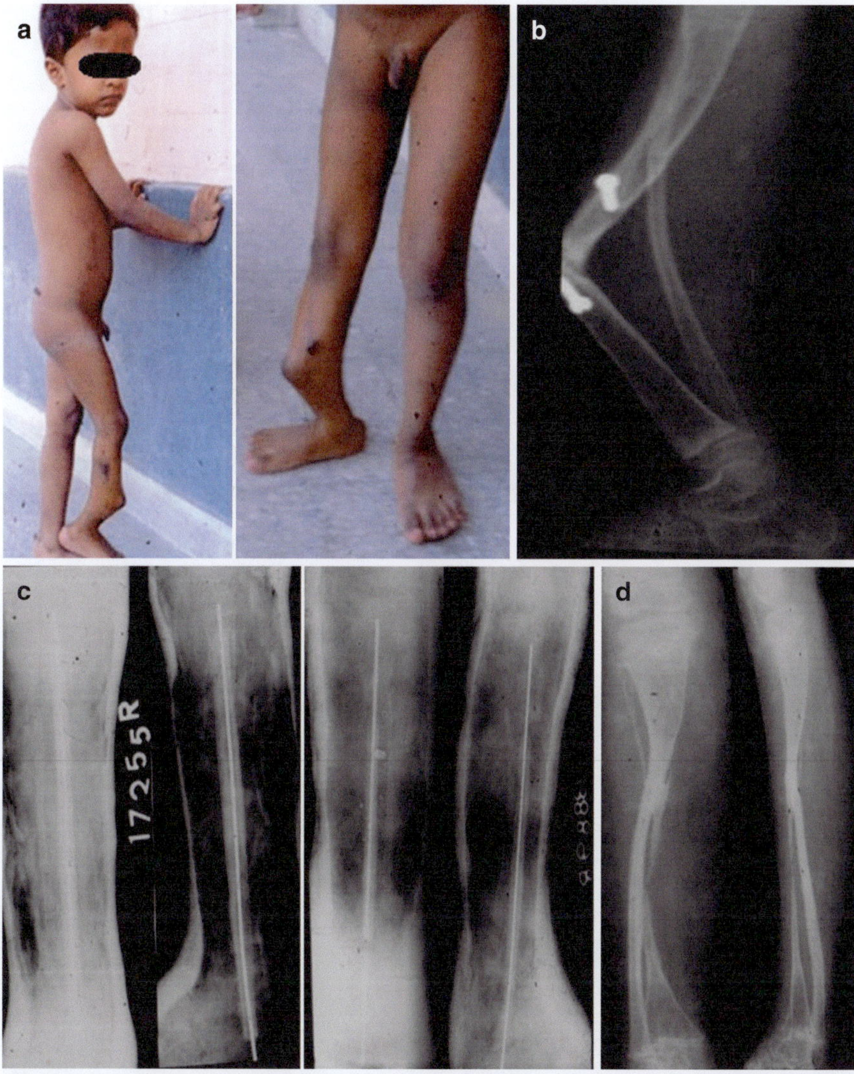

Fig. 17.10 (**a**) A 6-year-old boy with congenital pseudarthrosis of the tibia on the right side. (**b**) Roentgenogram shows failed surgery which was done in an earlier centre. (**c**) Roentgenograms revealing excision of the lesion and bridging of the gap with the mother's fibula, stabilized by a long Kirschner wire. (**d**) The final picture revealed tibio-fibular union which was supported by a brace for 2 years

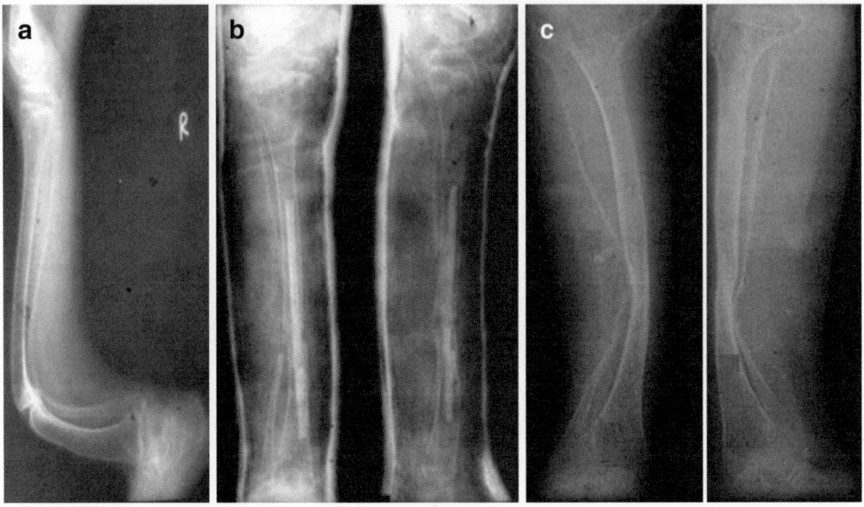

Fig. 17.11 (**a**) Roentgenogram reveals congenital pseudarthrosis of the right tibia. (**b**) Managed using the mother's fibula. (**c**) The final roentgenogram shows healing and remodelling. Since the distal tibial end was long enough, an ankle arthrodesis was not attempted in this case

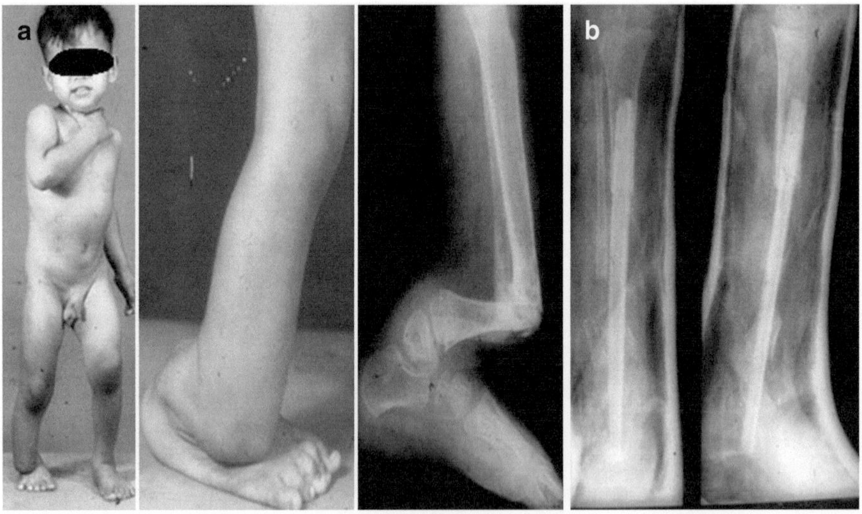

Fig. 17.12 (**a**) Congenital pseudarthrosis of the right tibia with severe angulation. (**b**) Wide excision of the lesion bridged by the mother's fibula which revealed union after 10 months

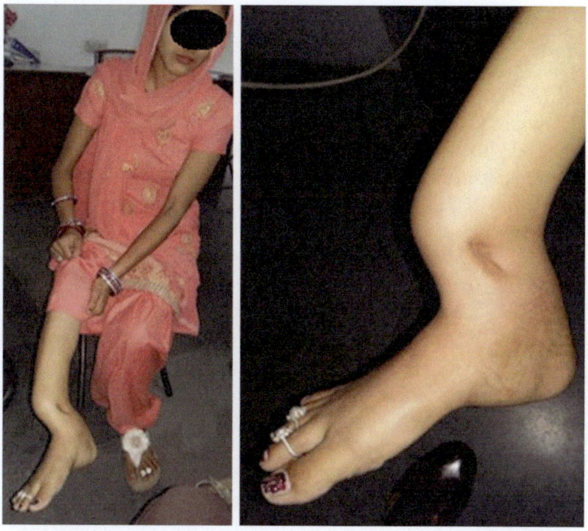

Fig. 17.13 A 35-year-old lady had typical deformity of congenital pseudarthrosis of the tibia. She did not agree for radiograph and treatment. She had been managing with the leg

Suggested Readings

1. Pannier S. Congenital pseudarthrosis of the tibia. Orthop Traumatol Surg Res. 2011;97(7):750–61.
2. El-Rosasy MA. Congenital pseudarthrosis of the tibia: the outcome of a pathology-oriented classification system and treatment protocol. J Pediatr Orthop B. 2020;29(4):337–47.
3. Ohnishi I, Sato W, Matsuyama J, Yajima H, Haga N, Kamegaya M, Minami A, Sato M, Yoshino S, Oki T, Nakamura K. Treatment of congenital pseudarthrosis of the tibia: a multicenter study in Japan. J Pediatr Orthop. 2005;25(2):219–24.
4. Khan T, Joseph B. Controversies in the management of congenital pseudarthrosis of the tibia and fibula. Bone Joint J. 2013;95-B(8):1027–34.
5. Dobbs MB, Rich MM, Gordon JE, Szymanski DA, Schoenecker PL. Use of an intramedullary rod for treatment of congenital pseudarthrosis of the tibia. A long-term follow-up study. J Bone Joint Surg Am. 2004;86(6):1186–97.
6. Paley D, Catagni M, Argnani F, Prevot J, Bell D, Armstrong P. Treatment of congenital pseudoarthrosis of the tibia using the Ilizarov technique. Clin Orthop Relat Res. 1992;280:81–93.
7. Mathieu L, Vialle R, Thevenin-Lemoine C, Mary P, Damsin JP. Association of Ilizarov's technique and intramedullary rodding in the treatment of congenital pseudarthrosis of the tibia. J Child Orthop. 2008;2(6):449–55.
8. Sakamoto A, Yoshida T, Uchida Y, Kojima T, Kubota H, Iwamoto Y. Long-term follow-up on the use of vascularized fibular graft for the treatment of congenital pseudarthrosis of the tibia. J Orthop Surg Res. 2008;3:13.
9. Balci Hİ, Bayram S, Pehlivanoglu T, Anarat FB, Eralp L, Şen C, Kocaoğlu M. Effect of lengthening speed on the quality of callus and complications in patients with congenital pseudarthrosis of tibia. Int Orthop. 2021;45(6):1517–22.
10. Boyd HB. Pathology and natural history of congenital pseudarthrosis of the tibia. Clin Orthop Relat Res. 1982;166:5–13.

11. Crawford AH. Neurofibromatosis in children. Acta Orthop Scand Suppl. 1986;218:1–60.
12. Roach JW, Shindell R, Green NE. Late-onset pseudarthrosis of the dysplastic tibia. J Bone Joint Surg Am. 1993;75(11):1593–601.
13. McCarthy RE. Amputation for congenital pseudarthrosis of the tibia. Indications and techniques. Clin Orthop Relat Res. 1982;4:58–61. [PubMed] [Google Scholar].
14. Codivilla A. On the cure of the congenital pseudoarthrosis of the tibia by means of periosteal transplantation. J Bone Joint Surg Am. 1906;S2-4-A:163–9. [Google Scholar].
15. Boyd HB. Pathology and natural history of congenital pseudarthrosis of the tibia. Clin Orthop Relat Res. 1982;166:5–13. [PubMed] [Google Scholar].
16. El-Rosasy M, Paley D, Herzenberg J. Ilizarov techniques for the management of congenital pseudarthrosis of the tibia. Tanta: Tanta University; 2001. [Google Scholar].
17. Thabet AM, Paley D, Kocaoglu M, et al. Periosteal grafting for congenital pseudarthrosis of the tibia: a preliminary report. Clin Orthop Relat Res. 2008;466:2981–94. doi: 10.1007/s11999-008-0556-1 [DOI] [PMC free article] [PubMed] [Google Scholar]..
18. Hermanns-Sachweh B, Senderek J, Alfer J, et al. Vascular changes in the periosteum of congenital pseudarthrosis of the tibia. Pathol Res Pract. 2005;201:305–12. [DOI] [PubMed] [Google Scholar].
19. Cho T-J, Seo J-B, Lee HR, et al. Biologic characteristics of fibrous hamartoma from congenital pseudarthrosis of the tibia associated with neurofibromatosis type 1. J Bone Joint Surg Am. 2008;90-A:2735–44. [DOI] [PubMed] [Google Scholar].
20. Madhuri V, Mathew SE, Rajagopal K, Ramesh S, Antonisamy B. Does pamidronate enhance the osteogenesis in mesenchymal stem cells derived from fibrous hamartoma in congenital pseudarthrosis of the tibia? Bone Rep. 2016;5:292–8. [DOI] [PMC free article] [PubMed] [Google Scholar].
21. Dobbs MB, Rich MM, Gordon JE, Szymanski DA, Schoenecker PL. Use of an intramedullary rod for treatment of congenital pseudarthrosis of the tibia. A long-term follow-up study. J Bone Joint Surg Am. 2004;86-A:1186–97. [DOI] [PubMed] [Google Scholar].
22. Keret D, Bollini G, Dungl P, et al. The fibula in congenital pseudoarthrosis of the tibia: the EPOS multicenter study. European Paediatric Orthopaedic Society (EPOS). J Pediatr Orthop B. 2000;9:69–74. [DOI] [PubMed] [Google Scholar].
23. Joseph B, Mathew G. Management of congenital pseudarthrosis of the tibia by excision of the pseudarthrosis, onlay grafting, and intramedullary nailing. J Pediatr Orthop B. 2000;9:16–23. [DOI] [PubMed] [Google Scholar].
24. Joseph B, Somaraju VVJ, Shetty SK. Management of congenital pseudarthrosis of the tibia in children under 3 years of age: effect of early surgery on union of the pseudarthrosis and growth of the limb. J Pediatr Orthop. 2003;23:740–6. [DOI] [PubMed] [Google Scholar].
25. Kim HW, Weinstein SL. Intramedullary fixation and bone grafting for congenital pseudarthrosis of the tibia. Clin Orthop Relat Res. 2002;405:250–7. [DOI] [PubMed] [Google Scholar].
26. Liu Y, Mei H, Zhu G, et al. Congenital pseudarthrosis of the tibia in children: should we defer surgery until 3 years old? J Pediatr Orthop B. 2018;27:17–25. [DOI] [PubMed] [Google Scholar].
27. Vigouroux F, Mezzadri G, Parot R, et al. Vascularised fibula or induced membrane to treat congenital pseudarthrosis of the tibia: a multicentre study of 18 patients with a mean 9.5-year follow-up. Orthop Traumatol Surg Res. 2017;103:747–53. [DOI] [PubMed] [Google Scholar].
28. Ohnishi I, Sato W, Matsuyama J, et al. Treatment of congenital pseudarthrosis of the tibia: a multicenter study in Japan. J Pediatr Orthop. 2005;25:219–24. [DOI] [PubMed] [Google Scholar].

29. Shabtai L, Ezra E, Wientroub S, Segev E. Congenital tibial pseudarthrosis, changes in treatment protocol. J Pediatr Orthop B. 2015;24:444–9. [DOI] [PubMed] [Google Scholar].
30. Westberry DE, Carpenter AM, Tisch J, Wack LI. Amputation outcomes in congenital pseudarthrosis of the tibia. J Pediatr Orthop. 2018;38:e475–81. [DOI] [PubMed] [Google Scholar].
31. Zhu GH, Mei HB, He RG, et al. Combination of intramedullary rod, wrapping bone grafting and Ilizarov's fixator for the treatment of Crawford type IV congenital pseudarthrosis of the tibia: mid-term follow up of 56 cases. BMC Musculoskelet Disord. 2016;17:443. [DOI] [PMC free article] [PubMed] [Google Scholar].
32. Kesireddy N, Kheireldin RK, Lu A, et al. Current treatment of congenital pseudarthrosis of the tibia. J Pediatr Orthop B. 2018;27:541–50. [DOI] [PubMed] [Google Scholar].
33. Seo SG, Lee DY, Kim YS, et al. Foot and ankle function at maturity after Ilizarov treatment for atrophic-type congenital pseudarthrosis of the tibia a comprehensive outcome comparison with normal controls. J Bone Joint Surg Am. 2016;98:490–8. [DOI] [PubMed] [Google Scholar].
34. Andersen KS. Radiological classification of congenital pseudarthrosis of the tibia. Acta Orthop Scand. 1973;44:719–27. [DOI] [PubMed] [Google Scholar].
35. Crawford AH, Bagamery N. Osseous manifestations of neurofibromatosis in childhood. J Pediatr Orthop. 1986;6:72–88. [DOI] [PubMed] [Google Scholar].
36. Paley D. Congenital pseudarthrosis of the tibia: biological and biomechanical considerations to achieve union and prevent refracture. J Child Orthop. 2019;13(2):120–33. https://doi.org/10.1302/1863-2548.13.180147.

Chapter 18
Bilateral Congenital Pseudarthroses of the Tibiae

18.1 Bilateral Congenital Pseudarthroses of the Tibiae

Congenital pseudarthrosis of the tibia is a rare and challenging condition. It occurs in 1 in 150,000 children. The aetiology of congenital pseudarthrosis of the tibia is controversial. Its association with neurofibromatosis type I has been well described. There is anterolateral bowing of the tibia at its distal third with non-union. Usually, the disease is unilateral. Bilateral occurrence is very rare. The author has successfully managed a case of bilateral congenital pseudarthroses of the tibiae treated with onlay paternal fibular graft and a long follow-up of 55 years.

Case History
An 8-year-old girl was brought in with congenital deformities of both legs. The available radiographs with the parents revealed bilateral congenital pseudarthroses of the tibiae. She had been operated three times on each leg in other centres, with no success. The patient had no clinical evidence of neurofibromatosis type I (Figs. 18.1 and 18.2).

Left Side
On the left side, the radiograph revealed evidence of pseudarthrosis with failed plating. The plate was removed and the pseudarthrosis was excised. The fibulae from the mother were not available as they were already used by the earlier surgeons. The resultant gap was bridged using a paternal onlay fibular graft, fixed on either side with screws and further supported by a POP cast.

The radiograph after 2 years revealed union at both ends. The leg was straight and stable. Gradually, the graft showed hypertrophy and underwent remodelling (Fig. 18.3).

S. S. Yadav, *Non-Vascularised Fibular Grafts in Orthopaedic Practice*,
https://doi.org/10.1007/978-981-95-1794-7_18

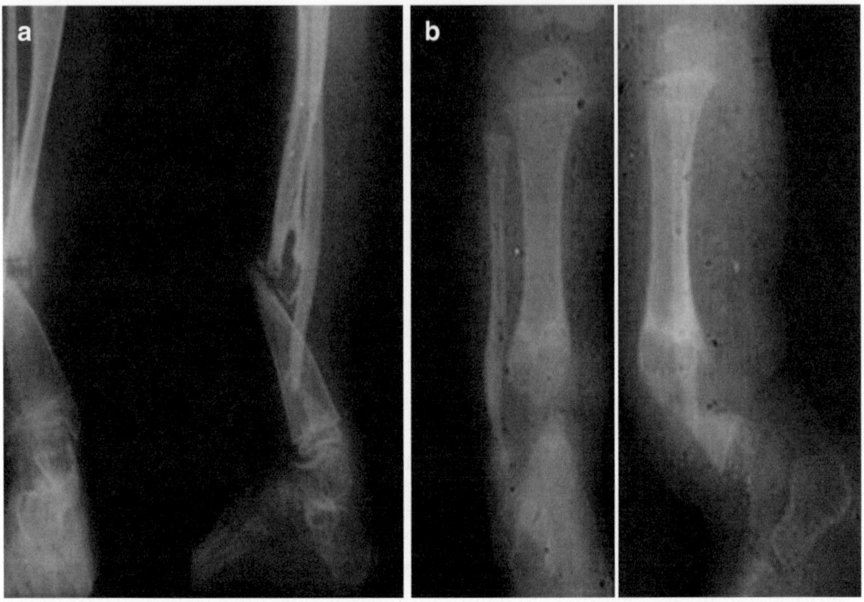

Fig. 18.1 (**a**, **b**) The only available roentgenograms of the patient with the parents revealed bilateral congenital pseudarthrosis of the tibiae

Right Side

Clinically, she had severe anterior angulation at the distal third of the right leg with valgus deformity of the foot. The radiograph revealed severe anteromedial angulation of the distal tibia. Although the tibia had united, the severe deformity was not acceptable and needed correction. The parents also wanted the deformity to be corrected. Though risky, a corrective osteotomy had to be performed and was supported with a POP cast. The osteotomy united within 6 months. The deformity was fully corrected, and the leg was straight and stable. The valgus of the foot was also gradually corrected with the now straight leg (Fig. 18.4).

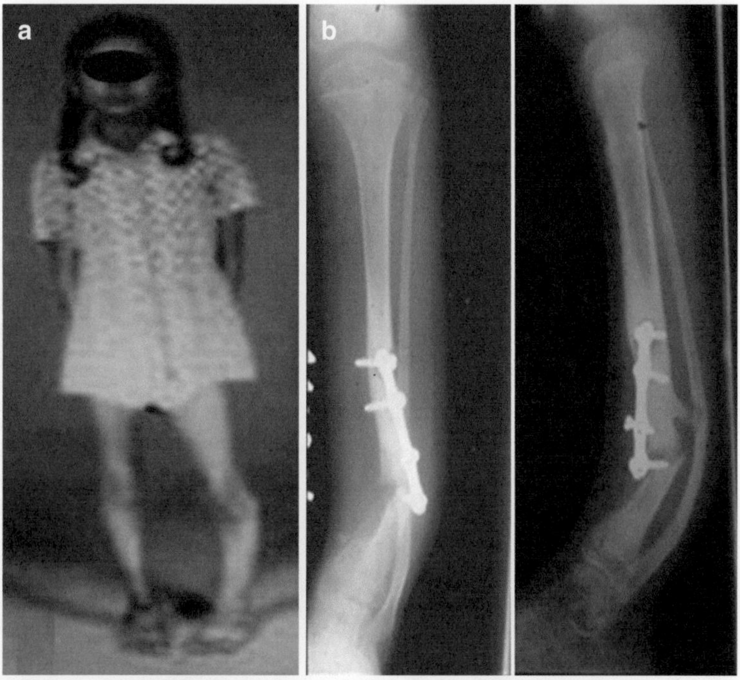

Fig. 18.2 (**a**) The patient upon arrival at our centre stands on pseudarthrosis of the left tibia with recurvatum at the knee. (**b**) The roentgenogram revealed a failed plating. The patient had three operations on either side at other centres, which resulted in failure

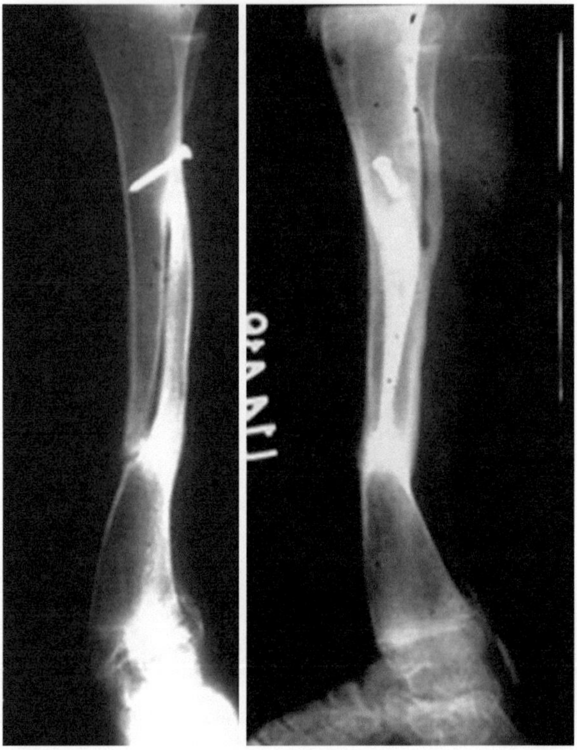

Fig. 18.3 Radiographs reveal a healed paternal onlay fibular graft on the left side. Note the hypertrophy of the paternal fibular graft after 2 years

Fig. 18.4 (**a**) On the right side, the patient had severe anteromedial angulation at the distal right leg with valgus deformity of the foot. (**b**) Although the radiograph revealed healed pseudarthrosis, the deformity was unacceptable. Though risky, a corrective osteotomy was performed which had healed in 6 months. (**c, d**) AP and lateral roentgenograms taken after the healed corrective osteotomy on the right side. Note the early remodelling that has taken place. (**e**) The patient stands on her corrected legs. The valgus deformity of the foot on the right side was gradually corrected with the now straight leg. (**f**) Clinical photographs of the patient at the age of 15 years with straight and equal size of the legs. (**g, h**) AP and lateral roentgenograms of both the legs showing complete healing and remodelling on both sides at the age of 44 years. (**i**) The final radiograph of both the legs at the age of 55 years. (**j**) The patient stands on her legs at the age of 55 years and had been gainfully employed as a teacher

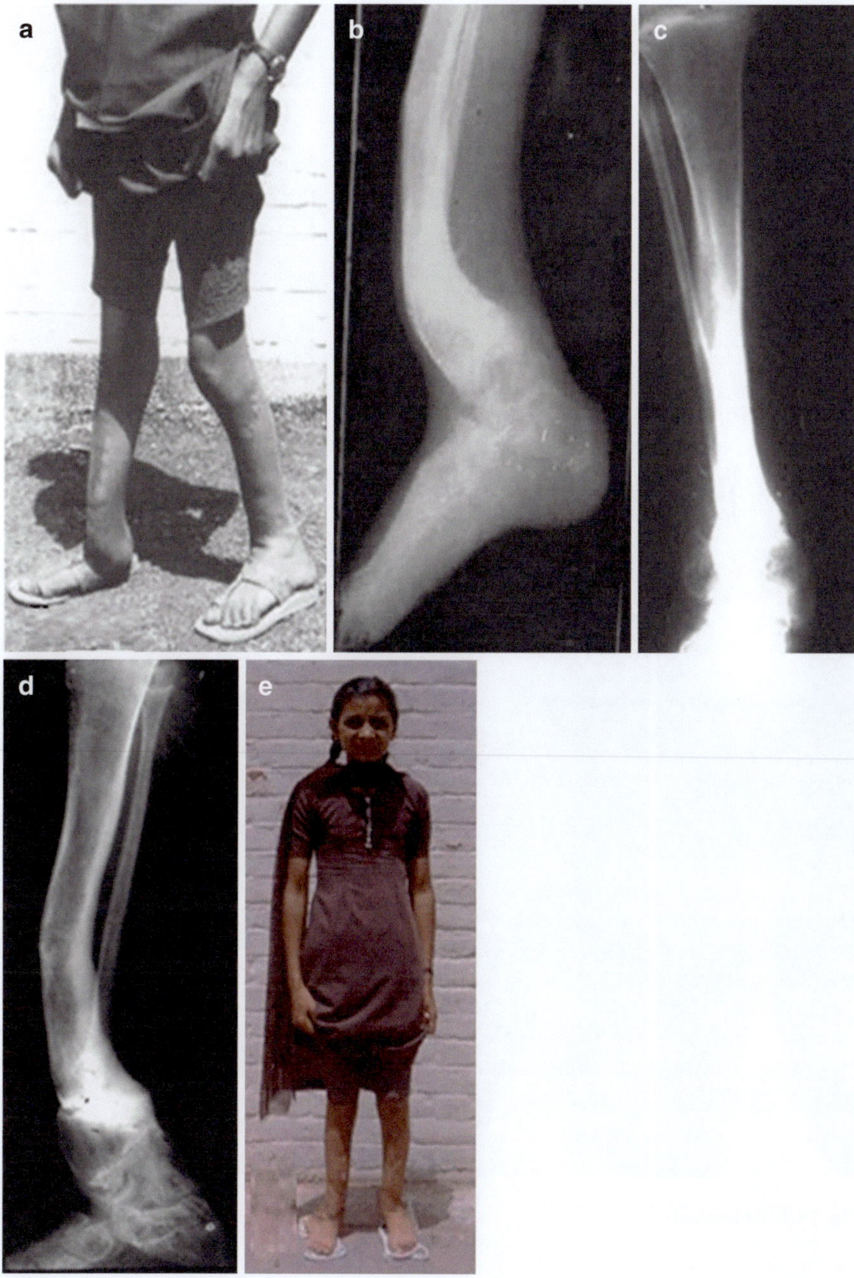

(continued)

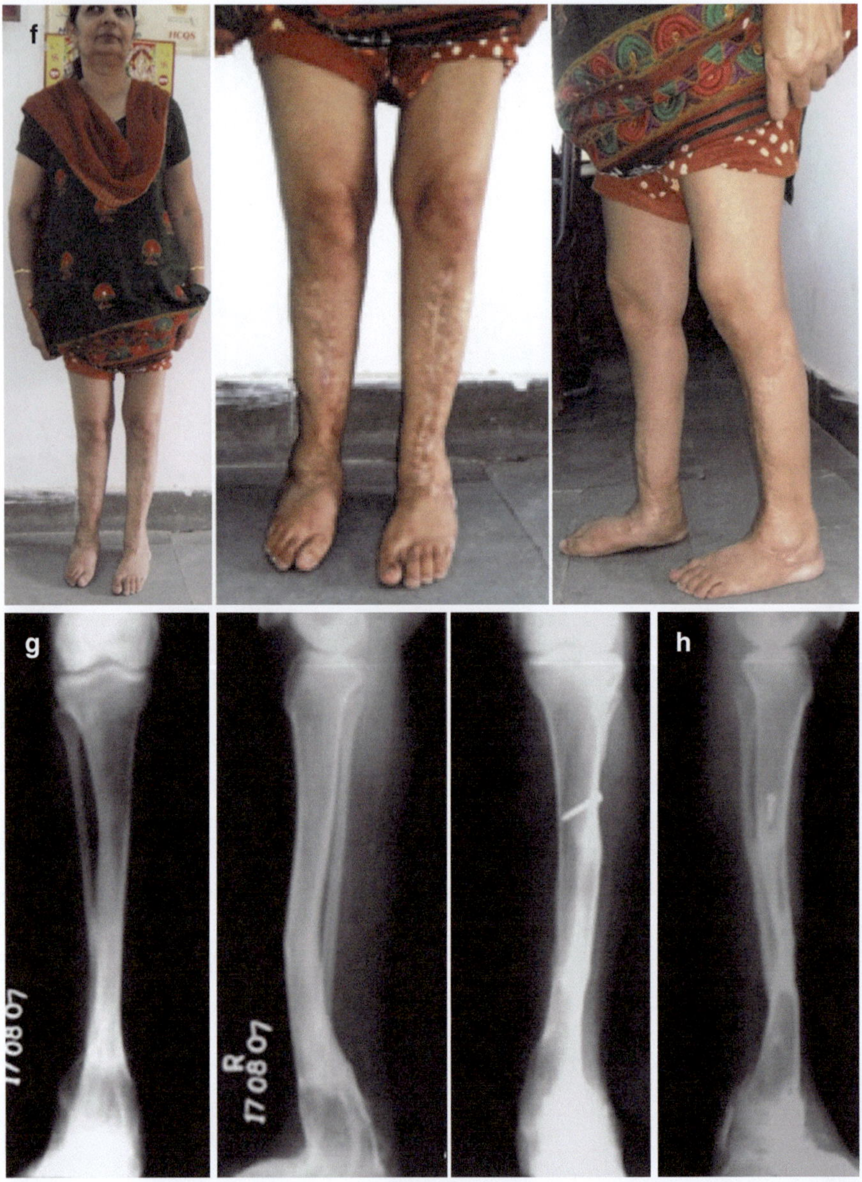

Fig. 18.4 (continued)

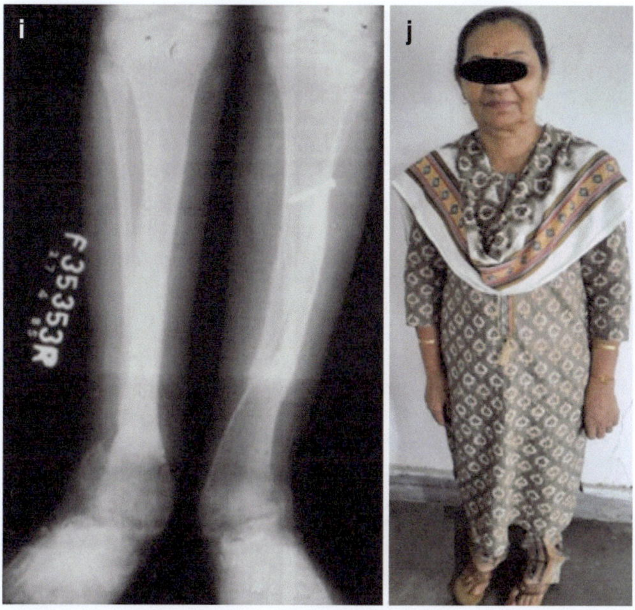

Fig. 18.4 (continued)

18.2 Conclusion

It is recommended that a maternal fibular graft has a place in the treatment of congenital pseudarthrosis of the tibia. In case a maternal graft is not available, the father's fibula can also be used with success. The onlay paternal graft had healed, revealed hypertrophy and finally got remodelled with the patient's tibia. It is also suggested that in case of unacceptable mal-union at the pseudarthrotic site, a corrective osteotomy may also be attempted.

In this bilateral case, the length of both legs has been equal and near normal. She has been married and has grown-up children. Since the patient lives in a nearby area, a 55-year follow-up of this rare success could be possible.

Suggested Readings

1. Berkshire SB Jr, Maxwell EN, Sams BF. Bilateral symmetrical pseudarthrosis in a newborn. Radiology. 1970. https://doi.org/10.1148/97.2.389.
2. Hefti F, Bollini G, Dungl P, Fixsen J, Grill F, Ippolito E, Romanus B, Tudisco C, Wientroub S. Congenital pseudarthrosis of the tibia: history, etiology, classification, and epidemiologic data. J Pediatr Orthop Part B. 2000. https://doi.org/10.1097/01202412-200001000-00003.

3. Ari B, Kuyubasi SN. Bilateral congenital pseudarthrosis of the tibia with neurofibromatosis type 1. J Pak Med Assoc. 2021;71(5). https://doi.org/10.47391/JPMA.504.
4. Van Royen K, Brems H, Legius E, Lammens J, Laumen A. Prevalence of neurofibromatosis type 1 in congenitalpseudarthrosis of the tibia. Eur J Pediatr. 2016;175:1193–8. https://doi.org/10.1007/s00431-016-2757-z.
5. Vitale MG, Guha A, Skaggs DL. Orthopaedic manifestations of neurofibromatosis in children: an update. Clin Orthop Relat Res. 2002;2002:107–18. https://doi.org/10.1097/00003086-200208000-00013.
6. Chand S, Afaque SF, Singh RK. Bilateral congenital pseudoarthrosis of the tibia: a case report and literature review. J Clin Orthop Trauma. 2024;58:102769.
7. Dobbs MB, Rich MM, Gordon JE, Szymanski DA, Schoenecker PL. Use of an intramedullary rod for treatment of congenital pseudarthrosis of the tibia. A long-term follow-up study. J Bone Joint Surg Am. 2004;86(6):1186–97.
8. Paley D, Catagni M, Argnani F, Prevot J, Bell D, Armstrong P. Treatment of congenital pseudoarthrosis of the tibia using the Ilizarov technique. Clin Orthop Relat Res. 1992;280:81–93.
9. Sakamoto A, Yoshida T, Uchida Y, Kojima T, Kubota H, Iwamoto Y. Long-term follow-up on the use of vascularized fibular graft for the treatment of congenital pseudarthrosis of the tibia. J Orthop Surg Res. 2008;3:13.
10. Borzunov DY, Chevardin AY, Mitrofanov AI. Management ofcongenital pseudarthrosis of the tibia with the Ilizarov method ina paediatric population: influence of aetiological factors. Int Orthop. 2016;40:331–9. https://doi.org/10.1007/s00264-015-3029-7.
11. Bobotas K, Lallos SN, Nikolaou VS, Korres DS, Efstathopoulos NE. Successful treatment of congenital pseudarthrosis of the tibia: stilla challenge. Eur J Orthop Surg Traumatol. 2013;23(Suppl 2):s303–10. https://doi.org/10.1007/s00590-012-1072-2.
12. Heikkinen ES, Poyhonen MH, Kinnunen PK, Seppanen UI. Congenital pseudarthrosis of the tibia. Treatment and outcome atskeletal maturity in 10 children. Acta Orthop Scand. 1999;70:275–82. https://doi.org/10.3109/17453679908997807.
13. Olumuyiwa Ifedayo Ajayi. Bilateral congenital pseudarthrosis of the tibia case contributed Radiologist based in Nigeria.
14. Udit A, Vivek T. Congenital tibial pseudarthrosis statpearls internet. Treasure Island I: StatPearls Publishing; 2024.

Chapter 19
Tibialization of the Fibula

19.1 Tibialization of the Fibula

In challenging gap non-union of the tibial shaft, tibialization of the fibula (medialization of the fibula) is a useful limb salvage procedure and an alternative to amputation. High-velocity injuries may lead to massive damage to the bones and soft tissues of the leg. Persistent gap non-unions of the tibia after repeated surgeries and prolonged sepsis also result in a difficult clinical situation for the treating surgeons. Huntington (1905) conceived the concept of tibialization of the fibula which was later popularized as an alternative reconstruction to salvage such extremities. The main requirement is the availability of the required fibular segment and a vascular limb with a sensate sole.

Various methods have been described to manage such patients. The options available for management include non-vascularized and vascularized fibular grafts and the Ilizarov procedure. All these techniques have their specific advantages and disadvantages. However, there is no consensus in the literature about which technique is optimal in a given situation. Microvascular free fibular grafting has been considered as one of the successful methods for reconstruction of the tibia. However, it is a time-consuming procedure and requires meticulous intraoperatve microsurgical technique and strict postoperative rehabilitation protocols. Moreover, there are many complications such as arterial thrombosis, deep infection, stress fractures and donor-site problems. Bone transport using the Ilizarov frame has been a known procedure to bridge such gaps. However, if the tibial ends are short or not available, distraction osteogenesis may not be indicated. Moreover, it is a highly specialized technique and has its own complications. In such patients, tibialization of the fibula is a dependable alternative to amputation (Fig. 19.1a–c).

S. S. Yadav, *Non-Vascularised Fibular Grafts in Orthopaedic Practice*,
https://doi.org/10.1007/978-981-95-1794-7_19

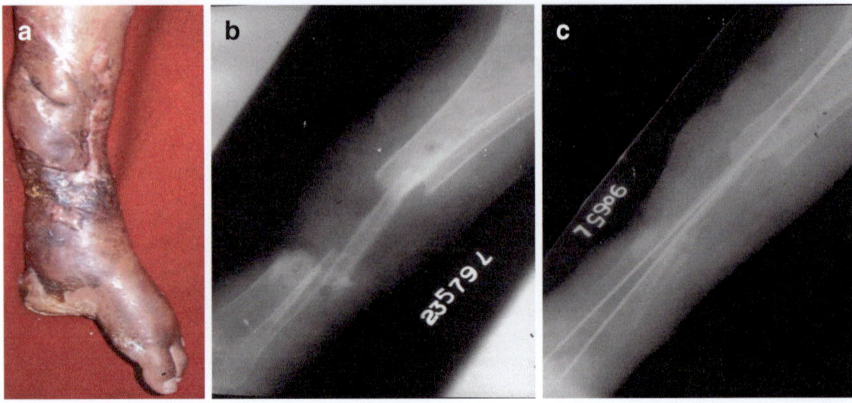

Fig. 19.1 (**a**) Extensively scarified left leg after an accident 3 years ago. (**b**) The roentgenogram revealed segmental fracture of both bones of the leg at the same level. The tibial fragment was already extruded at the arrival of the patient. (**c**) The fibular fragment was released and gently rotated medially, then wedged into the tibial ends, and further stabilized with twin long Kirschner wires. The roentgenogram after 4 months revealed union at both ends

The Technique

The main objective is to achieve a sound synostosis between the tibial ends and the osteotomized fibular ends, both proximally and distally. Thus, the level of fibular osteotomy at either end depends on the size of the gap between the tibial ends in a particular case. After performing fibular osteotomy at either end, the whole fibular segment is medialized beneath the anterior soft tissues. With the lateral soft tissue release, the fibular ends come closer to the tibial ends. The fibular ends are exposed sub-periosteally and fixed with the tibial ends with a pair of screws at both the ends (Figs. 19.2 and 19.3a, b). If possible, the fibular ends can also be wedged into the tibial ends through a trap door. In case the distal tibial end is too small or not available, the fibular end can be wedged into the body of the talus (Fig. 19.4a–e). Minimal traction correcting the angulation of the leg may be needed to achieve the required fixation. In cases where a screw fixation is not possible, a transcalcaneal Kirschner wire or a pin has also been recommended for fixation. The procedure results in a stable construct without disturbing the anteromedial surface of the leg where the skin is usually scarred and ischemic (Fig. 19.5a–f). When present, an equinus deformity can also be suitably corrected. To provide further stability to the construct, an above-knee plaster cast is applied in 10° flexion at the knee and 5–10° valgus at the ankle. Assisted walking is permitted in the POP cast.

The union at the tibiofibular ends usually takes place in 10–12 weeks. However, periodic roentgenograms should be obtained to record the progress regarding the union at the synostosis. Gradual weight-bearing without a cast is allowed only after sound radiological union has taken place which takes about 24 weeks. Once weight-bearing is allowed, the fibular segment gradually hypertrophies and attains the circumference of the original tibial shaft (Fig. 19.1a–c).

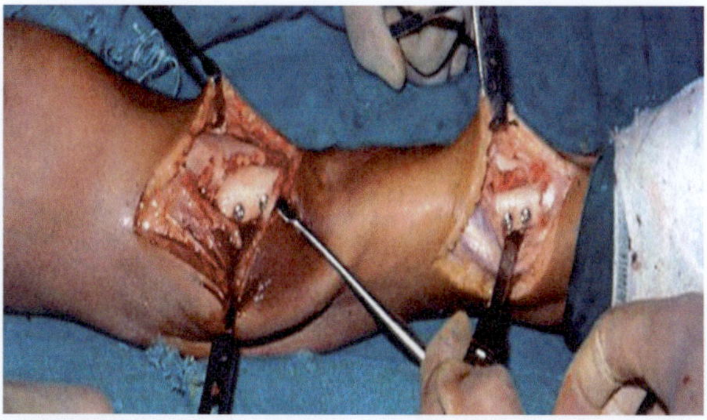

Fig. 19.2 A demonstrative intraoperative picture of stage 1 tibialization of the fibula. A pair of screws fixing the tibial segment at either end is visible

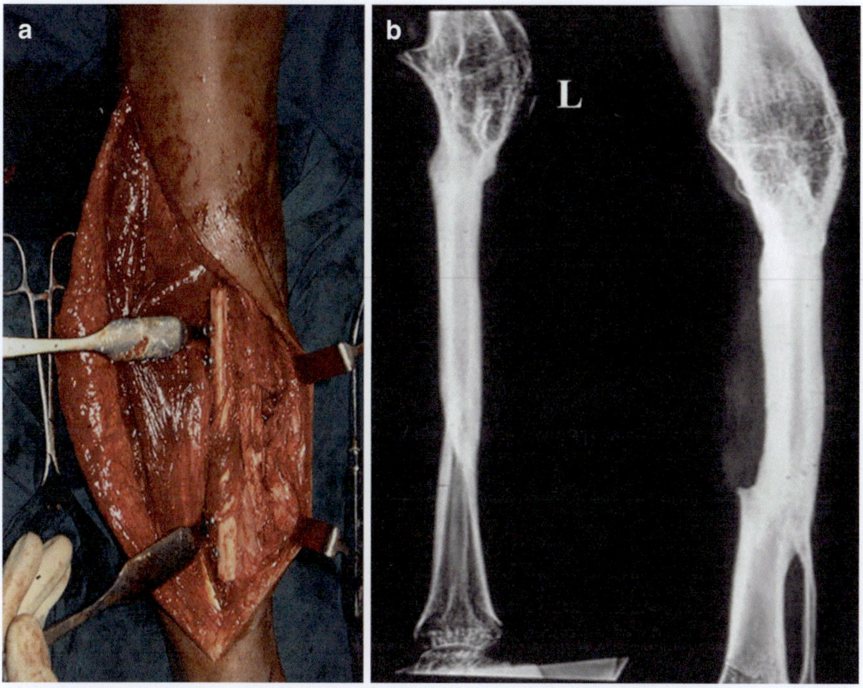

Fig. 19.3 (**a**) Intraoperative illustration of the medialized shaft of the fibula along with its muscles and intact vascularity. A pair of screws at the proximal and distal ends is visible. (**b**) The roentgenogram taken after 20 years reveals massive hypertrophy of the fibular segment. The knee was already fused in this post-infective case

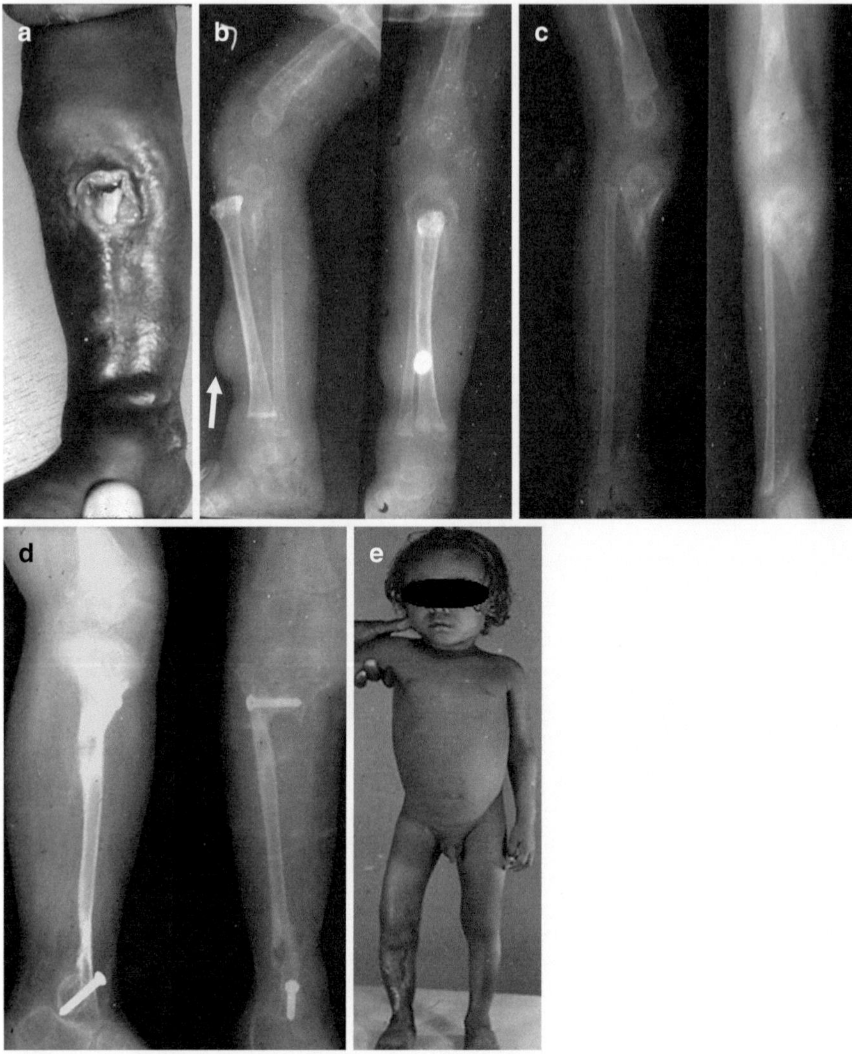

Fig. 19.4 (**a**) A 3-year-old child with acute osteomyelitis of the tibial shaft on the right side. The leg was swollen and drained pus. (**b**) The roentgenogram revealed separated diaphyseal ends at the metaphyseal level. Note the abscess on the leg (arrow). (**c**) While dressing, the whole of the separated diaphysis came out, leaving behind a small tibial end proximally, and the distal end of the tibia was missing. (**d**) After the wounds healed, almost total fibular shaft was medialized fixing it with proximal tibial end with a screw. Since the distal end of the tibia was not available, the fibular end was wedged into the body of the talus and fixed with a screw. The roentgenogram taken 6 months after fixation revealed complete union at both the ends and hypertrophy of the fibular shaft. (**e**) The patient could bear weight. Note the scarification on the anterior aspect of the entire right leg

A mind that understands the principle will work out the method.

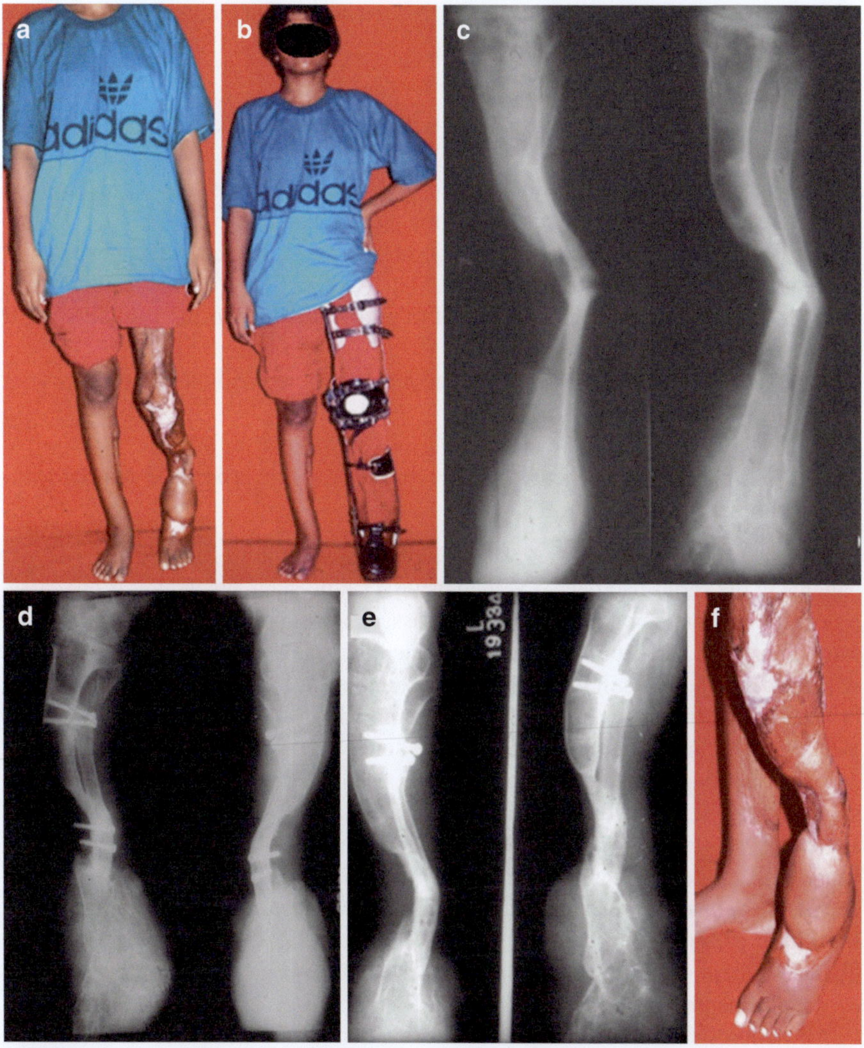

Fig. 19.5 (**a**) A 15-year-old girl came with severe post-burn scarification of the left lower extremity, especially the leg. She had a full-thickness skin graft at the ankle done elsewhere. (**b**) The tibia and fibula revealed posterolateral angulation with tapering ends. Non-union was observed at the tibial shaft for which she had been using an above-knee orthotic support. (**c**) The fibular shaft showed union. She refused amputation. Since the tibia and fibula were angulated in the same plain, the fibula was medialized as it is and fitted to the tibial ends with screws. (**d**) A roentgenogram taken after 1 year revealed that the tibial ends had not only united with its companion fibula but also revealed hypertrophy of the involved tapering ends. (**e**) The patient could bear weight without any support. (**f**) Although cosmetically the leg did not appear acceptable, the patient was happy for getting her own sensate limb to bear weight without orthosis

Finally, it results in a straight, stable and functional leg. The resultant shortening of the extremity can be compensated by a shoe raise. The patient is able to carry out the activities of daily living.

Advantages of the Technique

1. The fibular segment is medialized with its total vascularity along with the muscles.
2. The vascular ends of the fibula unite with the tibial ends like a fracture and restore tibial continuity in a shorter time than any other procedure.
3. Screw fixation at both ends provides good fixation. A transcalcaneal pin can also be used for fixing the fibular segment.
4. It does not disturb the often scarred or ischemic skin on the middle side of the leg.
5. After healing, the fibular segment gets hypertrophied and attains the diameter similar to that of the tibial shaft.
6. An amputation can well be avoided.
7. It is a simple, biological, cost-effective and dependable procedure in a challenging clinical situation.

Tibialization of the fibula can be attempted in a single stage or two stages. All patients in the series had been operated using a single-stage procedure. A one-stage procedure is more suitable when the soft tissues are supple (Fig. 19.6a–e). A two-stage procedure has been recommended when there is extensive peri-fibular fibrosis, and it may be difficult to mobilize or medialize the fibular segment at one stage. In such cases, the second stage can be attempted 3–6 weeks after the first stage. When present, an equinus deformity can be suitably corrected.

Long-standing cases with large tibial loss usually reveal varus angulation at the ankle and leg. It is suggested that while applying a POP cast after tibialization, the ankle may be kept in 5–10° of valgus position. This keeps the leg straight and prevents varus at the leg, needing a subsequent corrective osteotomy.

Hypertrophy of the medalized fibular segment takes place in all such patients and starts after partial weight-bearing is permitted in the POP cast. It continues until the fibular segment simulates the diameter of the tibia. We are in agreement with the earlier reports that it takes place in about 3–4 years (Fig. 19.7a–f).

All patients with a stable leg after tibialization are able to perform quadriceps and ankle exercises in a much better way. Shortening of the leg is observed in all patients and could be compensated by a shoe raise. Tibialization of the fibula is a simple, safe and dependable salvage procedure for managing difficult gap nonunions of the tibial shaft with scarification of the leg. Moreover, this procedure can be attempted by most orthopaedic surgeons, even at the district-level hospitals (Fig. 19.8).

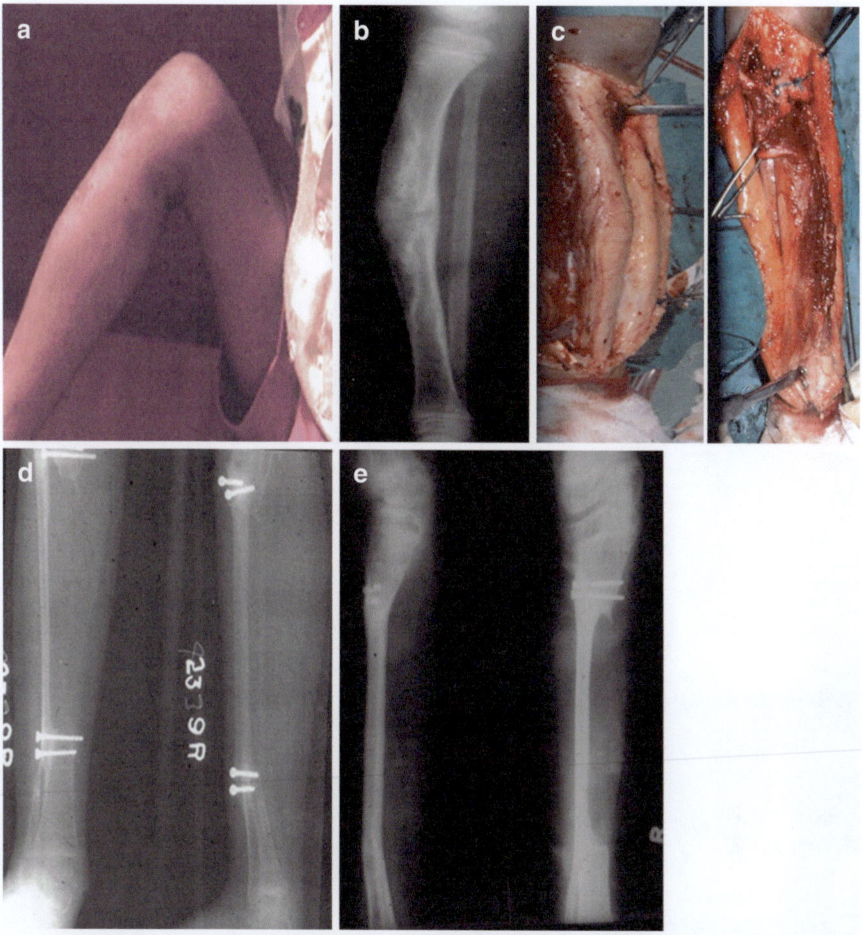

Fig. 19.6 (**a**) Photograph of a boy with tibial swelling of the right leg. Biopsy revealed adamantinoma of the right tibia. (**b**) Radiograph revealing the lesion at mid-diaphysis with anterior bowing of the tibia. (**c**) Intraoperative picture of the tibia and after excision of the tibial shaft. (**d**) Radiograph showing bridging of the gap with tibialization of the fibula. (**e**) Radiograph showing healing 1 year after tibialization of the fibula. Note the hypertrophy of the transferred fibula

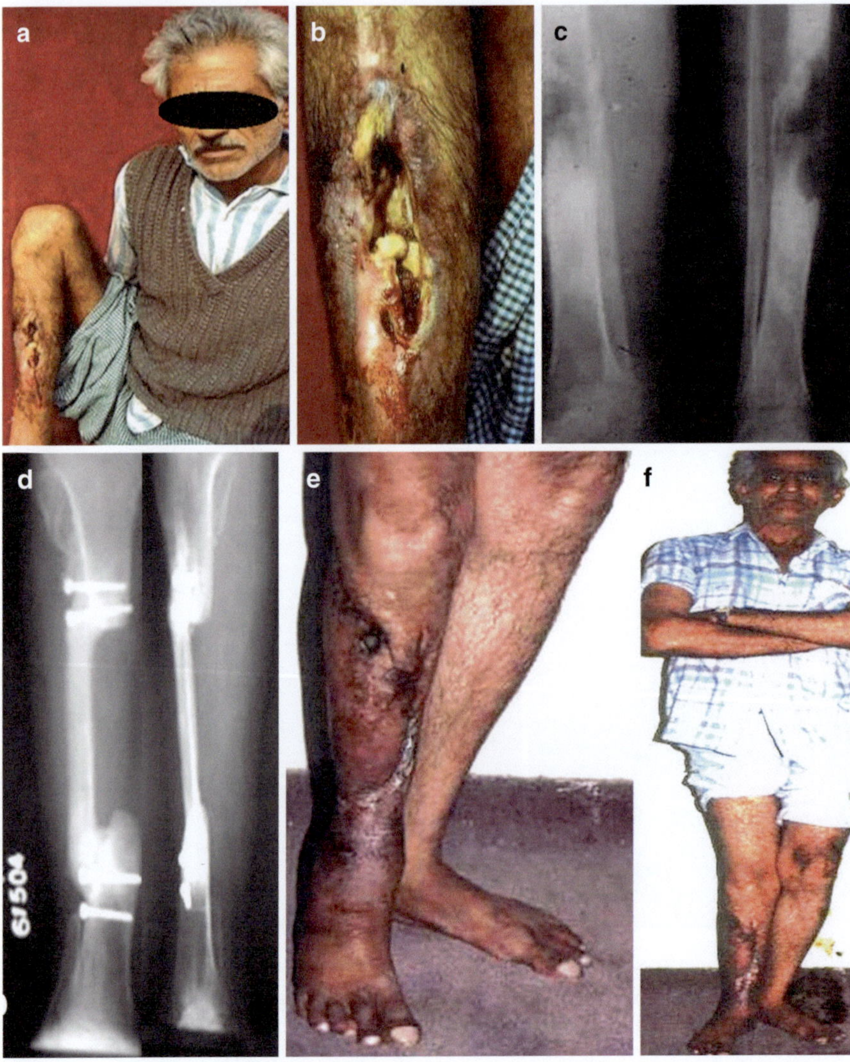

Fig. 19.7 (**a**, **b**) Clinical picture of a 50-year-old male with fungal-bacterial osteomyelitis of the right tibial shaft with unusual ulcerations. (**c**) The roentgenogram revealed extensive lytic appearance at the mid shaft of the tibia. (**d**) The necrotic skin, soft tissues and the involved area of tibial diaphysis were excised. After a thorough surgical toilet, the corresponding shaft of the fibula was medialized and fixed to the tibial ends with a pair of screws on both sides. A posterolateral skin release incision was made which permitted the wound closure anteriorly. A roentgenogram taken 15 months after fixation revealed sound union at both ends and hypertrophy of the transplanted fibular shaft—a bypass operation. (**e**, **f**) The clinical picture of the leg and the patient bearing weight

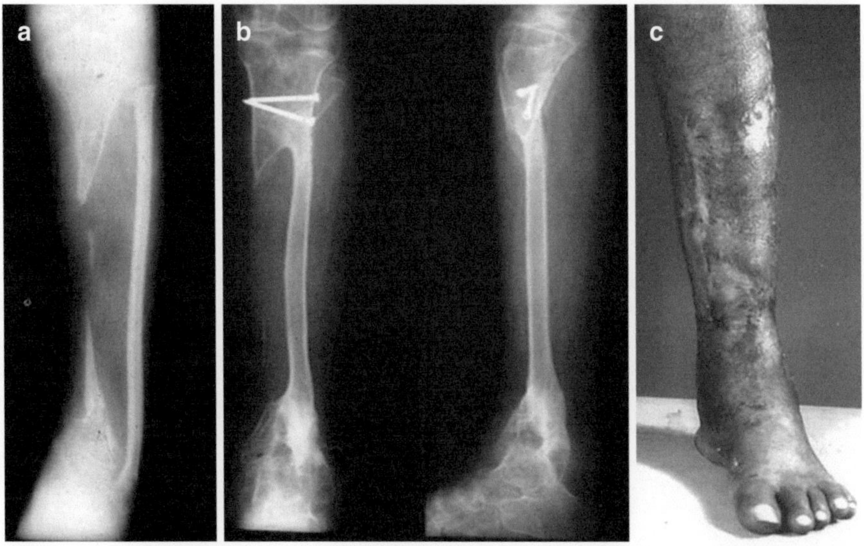

Fig. 19.8 (**a**) A post-infective bone loss of the left tibial shaft. A one-stage tibialization of the fibula was attempted. (**b**) Roentgenogram taken 1 year after tibialization revealed sound healing and hypertrophy of the fibular shaft. (**c**) The clinical picture revealed a straight and stable leg. Note the extensive scarification on the anterior aspect of the left leg

Suggested Readings

1. Huntington TW. Case of bone transference: use of segment of fibula to supply a defect in the tibia. Ann Surg. 1905;41:249–51.
2. Tuli SM. Tibialization of the fibula a viable option 230 to salvage limbs with extensive scarring and gap nonunions of the tibia. Clin Orthop Relt Res. 2005;431:80–4.
3. Kundu ZS, Gupta V, Sangwan SS, Kamboj P. Gap nonunion of tibia treated by Huntington's procedure. Indian J Orthop. 2012;46(6):653–8.
4. Meulemeester CD, Verdonk R, Bongaerts W. The fibula pro tibia procedure in the treatment of nonunion of the tibia. Acta Orthop Belg. 1992;58(Suppl1):187–9.
5. Khan AQ, Siddiqui YS, Julfiqar AM, Sabir AB. Role of Huntington procedure asa limb salvage surgery for complex gap nonunion of tibia in children. J Clin Orthop Trauma. 2021;18:20–4.
6. Agarwal P, Savant R, Sharma D. Huntington's procedure revisited. J Clin Orthop Trauma. 2019;10(6):1128–31.
7. Rahimnia A, Fitoussi F, Penneçot G, Mazda K. Treatment of segmental loss of the tibiaby tibialisation of the fibula: a review of the literature. Trauma Mon. 2012;16(4):154–9.
8. Kassab M, Samaha C, Saillant G. Ipsilateral fibular transposition in tibial nonunion using Huntington procedure: a 12-year follow-up study. Injury. 2003;34(10):770–5.
9. Nwokike OC, Esezobor EE, Olomu DO, Edomwonyi EO, Onuminya JE. Tibialization of fibula in treatment of major bone gap defect of the tibia: a case report. Open Journal of Orthopedics. 2015;05(08):Article ID:58628, 4 pages.
10. Yadav SS. Dual fibular grafting for massive bone gaps in the lower extremity. J Bone Joint Surg Am. 1990;72(4):486–94.
11. Morsi E. Tibial reconstruction using a non-vascularised fibular transfer. Int Orthop. 2002;26:377–80.

12. Steinlechner CWB, Mkandawire NC. Non-vascularised 252 fibular transfer in the management of defects of long bones after sequestrectomy in children. J Bone Joint Surg Br. 2005;87(9):1259–63.
13. Beris AE, Lykissas MG, Korompilias AV, Vekris MD, Mitsionis GI, Malizos KN, Soucacos PN. Vascularized fibula transfer for lower limb reconstruction. Microsurgery. 2011;31(3):205–11.
14. De Boer HH, Wood MB, Hermans J. Reconstruction of large skeletal defects by vascularised fibular transfer. Factors that influenced the outcome of union in 62 cases. Int Orthop. 1990;14:121–8.
15. Paley D, Catagni MA, Argnani F, et al. Ilizarov treatment of tibial nonunions with bone loss. Clin Orthop. 1989;241:146–65.
16. Ilizarov GA. Clinical application of the tension-stress effect for limb lengthening. Clin Orthop. 1990;250:8–26.
17. Yazar S, Lin CH, Wei FC. One-stage reconstruction of composite bone and soft-tissue defects in traumatic lower extremities. Plast Reconstr Surg. 2004;114(6):1457–66.

Chapter 20
Our Experiences with Complications

20.1 Our Experiences with Complications

As already described in the book, we have used improved non-vascularized fibular grafts with enhanced quality and quantity in our cases. Hence, the complications have been minimal. However, there are some complications observed in the form of:

1. Superficial infection.
2. Deep infection without damaging the construct.
3. Exposed L-plate observed at the proximal end of the tibia (Figs. 20.1a, b, 20.2a–c, and 20.3a, b).
4. The proximal tibia is subcutaneous, and any necrosis of the skin exposes the grafts. As a standard procedure, the medial head of the gastrocnemius has been used to cover the graft (Figs. 20.4a–d and 20.5).
5. Non-union was observed at one end in this case of twin fibular graft (Fig. 20.6a, b).

S. S. Yadav, *Non-Vascularised Fibular Grafts in Orthopaedic Practice*,
https://doi.org/10.1007/978-981-95-1794-7_20

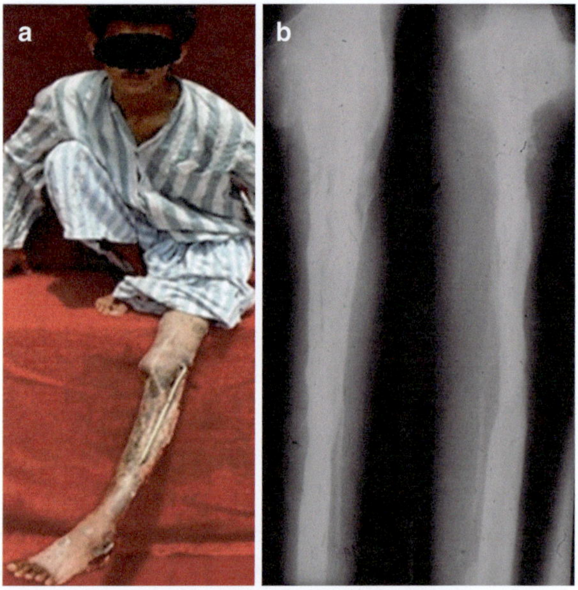

Fig. 20.1 (**a**) A case of GCT at the proximal end of the tibia with twin fibular grafts fixed with an L-plate. As the tibia is subcutaneous, the plate has been exposed. (**b**) However, the radiograph reveals healing of the construct with lateral union. The plate was removed and the wound healed

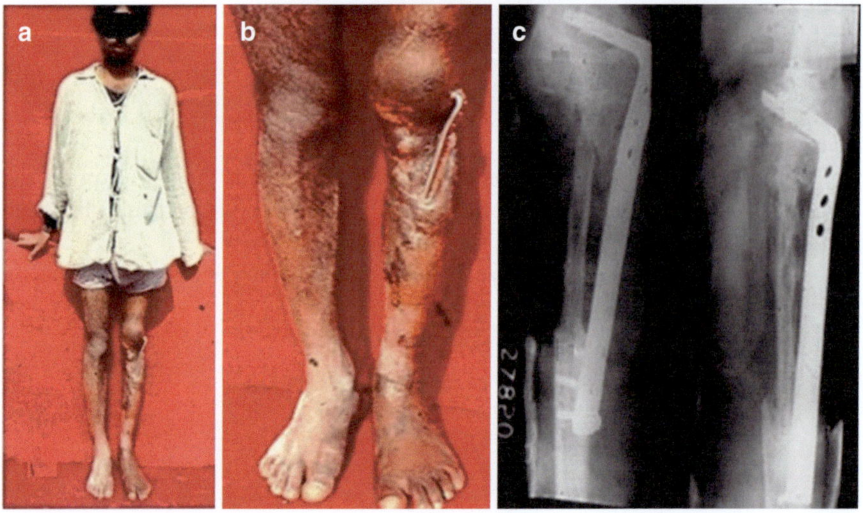

Fig. 20.2 (**a**, **b**) In another patient, although the plate is exposed, the construct had united. (**c**) Radiograph showing the L-plate (exposed) at the proximal end of the tibia. The plate was removed, and the wound healed

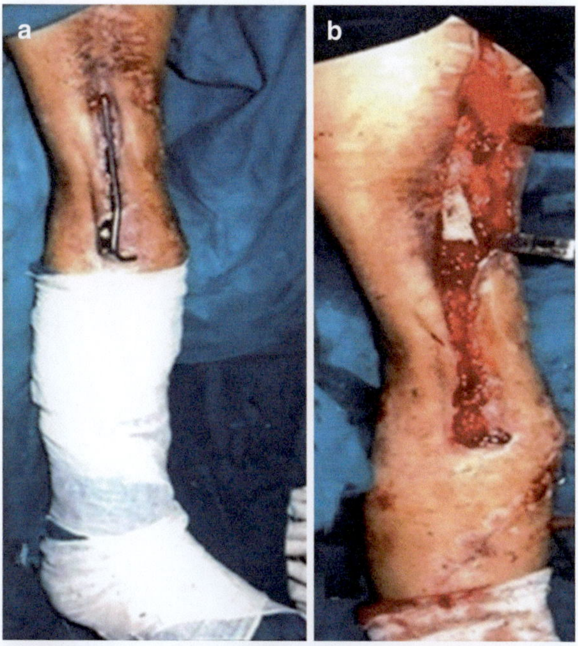

Fig. 20.3 (**a**) Clinical picture of the lower end of the femur showing the exposed plate. (**b**) The plate has been removed. However, the twin graft had healed

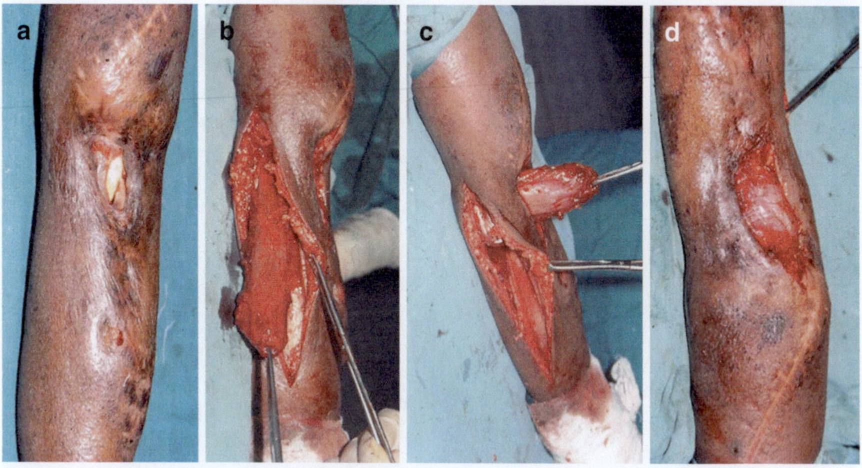

Fig. 20.4 (**a**) Clinical photograph of the proximal leg showing the exposed graft in a case of GCT of the proximal end of the tibia fixed with Kirschner wires. (**b**, **c**) Intraoperative photographs with the standard procedure of covering the graft with the medial head of the gastrocnemius. (**d**) The bone graft is fully covered with muscle. A split skin graft had been performed

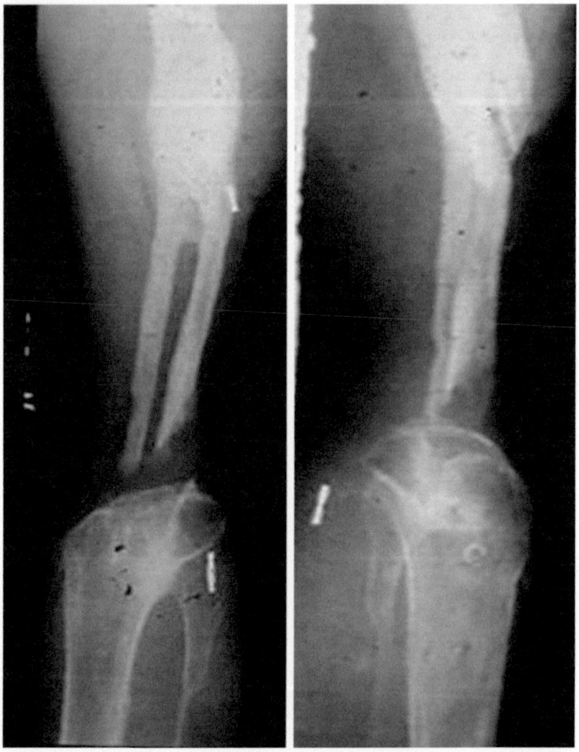

Fig. 20.5 Radiograph reveals non-union at the distal end of the twin grafts attempted in a case of GCT of the lower end of the femur. Since the grafts are separately placed in this case, lateral union had not taken place, resulting in non-union at the distal end of the twin grafts

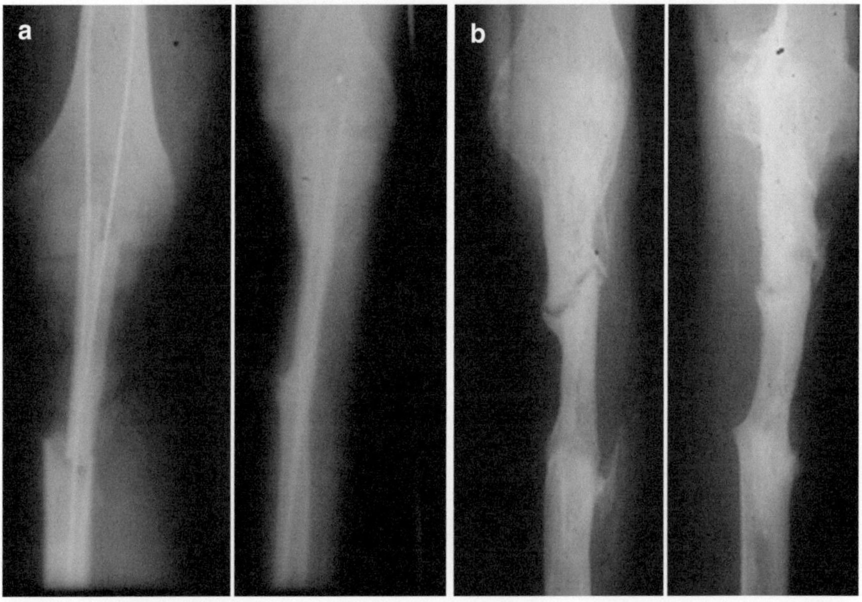

Fig. 20.6 (**a**) A case of GCT of the proximal tibia excised and reconstructed with twin fibular graft stabilized with Kirschner wires. (**b**) Although the graft had united at the ends, there has been a fracture in the centre which had healed in an above-knee plaster of Paris cast

Chapter 21
Observations Made by the Author on the Improved NVFG

21.1 Observations Made by the Author on the Improved NVFG

The literature review aims to analyse the characteristics of different bone grafts. The goal is to identify which option can give the optimal result for a patient being treated for a bone defect. During the period 1970–1980, I realized that there was a great bias against non-vascularized fibular grafts. However, I continued my presentations at various fora and published my work on improved NVFG in ACE Journals. The journey for an innovator is not easy.

The use of vascular fibular bone transfer is becoming more preferred due to benefits such as good osteogenic property, early healing and hypertrophy. However, such an aim has not been fully achieved as vascular grafts have their own drawbacks. Still, the advantages of the improved NVFG as compared to use of VSG consist of (1) an easier operative technique, (2) shorter operative time and (3) better remodelling capacity at the donor site.

The author has been using the improved NVFG in various clinical conditions for the last five decades. With the enhanced quality and quantity, the improved NVFG has many advantages as described earlier in the book. Out of these, there are two major innovative additions related to the improved NVFG that require consideration.

1. As a simple step, immediate transplantation and fixation of the graft at the host site retain its osteogenic cells and add to the quality of the graft. Through early transfer, these cells can draw their oxygenation and nutrition from the blood at the host site. In this way, the graft faces only transient ischemia. These vital surviving osteoblasts and osteocytes interact with mesenchymal cells of the host bone and result in simultaneous and early bone formation. In delayed fixation of the graft, these vital bone-forming cells die and the graft acts as a dead graft, resulting degenerative changes so commonly described earlier in the NVFG.

S. S. Yadav, *Non-Vascularised Fibular Grafts in Orthopaedic Practice*, https://doi.org/10.1007/978-981-95-1794-7_21

2. The other important observation made during this long period is that twin fibular grafts not only add to the quantity of the construct but, when the twin grafts are put together, they result in 'lateral union' throughout the length of these struts and finally form a sheet of bone. When remodelled, the construct simulates the diameter of the parent bone such as the femur, tibia and humerus. Such a construct is strong enough and does not result in a subsequent fracture, which is commonly observed in NVFG. These facts have been amply demonstrated in various clinical conditions in the book.

There is a general perception that a vascular graft should be used when large fibular bone grafts are needed, particularly those greater than 6 cm in length. The article cited by Taylor et al. describes the first human VBG, in which it is suggested that a vascularized graft might be indicated for long bone defects. However, in the literature, there is inconclusive evidence for the existence of a relationship between length and the need for vascularization. The author has been using a large (22 cm) twin NVFG for a long time and found no evidence to support the idea that grafts longer than 6 cm require vascularization. Moreover, it may not be necessary to expose the patient to a larger and riskier surgical procedure. The healing of the graft depends more on the quality and quantity of the graft, time duration and stability of its fixation to the host bone and other systemic evaluations of the patient.

Destiny prevails. It is possible that the creator has entrusted me to identify the additional advantages of this precious and priceless bone called 'fibula'. The recommended improved NVFG is biological and dependable. It is also true that for excellence of biological procedures, we do need simple and biological thinking which will enable more orthopaedic surgeons to practise this technique for the needy and poor patients in a cost-effective manner. Taking all the above in 1993, the Indian Orthopaedic Association had awarded the author with the title of 'Fibula man'.

It is expected that future studies will be carried out to further improve the status of these NVFGs, enabling them to be more acceptable to most surgeons. However, a further assessment of histopathological evaluation of such grafts is recommended. Such an attempt will serve the needs and requirements of most patients across the globe who are unable to afford the heavy cost of extensive procedures with frequent complications.

Research must be or has to be 'need-based', suited to the most needy patients. Our publications on the improved status of the NVFG have made the orthopaedic colleagues aware of these simple concepts while using the NVFG. Although the fibula has always been under our nose, we could not exploit this 'wonder bone' to this extent. The orthopaedic surgeons who have used the advocated technique believe in the usefulness of the proposed improved NVFG. 'It appears that the fibula is the future for most of the difficult ailments of the speciality—let us wait and see'.

I hear it and forget it
I think it and remember it
I do it and understand it
I practice it and recommend it

S S Yadav

MIX
Papier aus verantwortungsvollen Quellen
Paper from responsible sources
FSC® C105338

If you have any concerns about our products,
you can contact us on
ProductSafety@springernature.com

In case Publisher is established outside the EU,
the EU authorized representative is:
Springer Nature Customer Service Center GmbH
Europaplatz 3, 69115 Heidelberg, Germany

Printed by Libri Plureos GmbH
in Hamburg, Germany